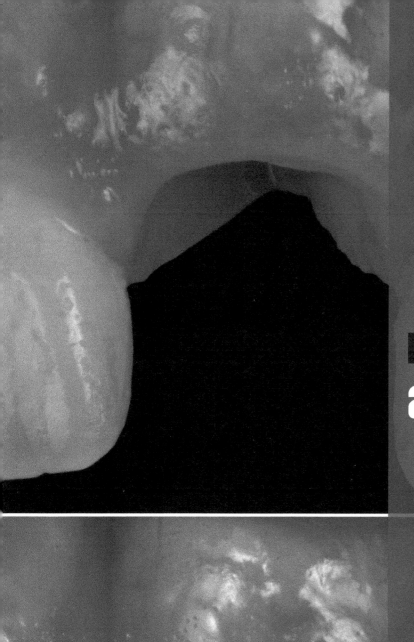

Implant Dentistry
at a Glance

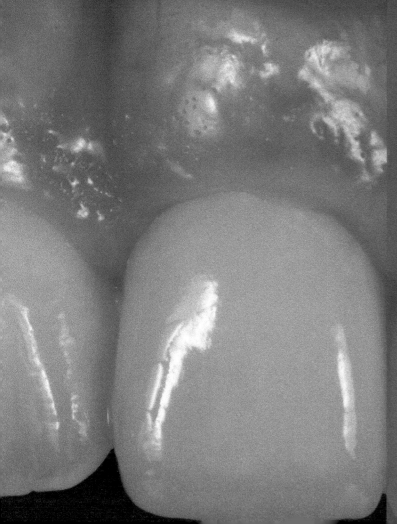

This title is also available as an e-book.
For more details, please see
www.wiley.com/go/malet/implant
or scan this QR code:

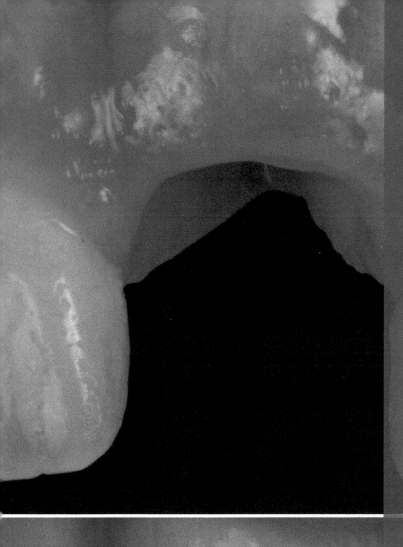

Implant
Dentistry
at a
Glance

Second Edition

Jacques Malet
France

Francis Mora
France

Philippe Bouchard
France

WILEY Blackwell

This edition first published 2018
© 2018 John Wiley & Sons Ltd.

Edition History
John Wiley & Sons (1e, 2012)

The right of Jacques Malet, Francis Mora and Philippe Bouchard to be identified as the authors of this work \has been asserted in accordance with law.

Registered Offices
John Wiley & Sons, Inc., 111 River Street, Hoboken, NJ 07030, USA
John Wiley & Sons Ltd, The Atrium, Southern Gate, Chichester, West Sussex, PO19 8SQ, UK

Editorial Office
9600 Garsington Road, Oxford, OX4 2DQ, UK

For details of our global editorial offices, customer services, and more information about Wiley products visit us at www.wiley.com.

Wiley also publishes its books in a variety of electronic formats and by print-on-demand. Some content that appears in standard print versions of this book may not be available in other formats.

Library of Congress Cataloging-in-Publication Data applied for
9781119292609

Cover Design: Wiley
Cover Images: Courtesy of Jacques Malet

Set in 9.5/11.5pt MinionPro by SPi Global, Chennai, India

Printed and bound by CPI Group (UK) Ltd, Croydon, CR0 4YY

C9781119292609_091024

Dedication

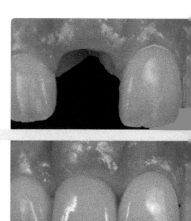

Dr Jacques Malet wishes to thank his children, Jeanne, Lou, Leo and Victor, and his wife Lisa, for their love and support; and would like to dedicate this second edition to those who inspire us every day to improve our knowledge and skills: our patients.

Dr Francis Mora wishes to thank his wife Anne-Sophie, his wonderful children, Paul-Louis, Victor and Josephine, for their ever-present love and devotion; he dedicates this book to his mother and to the memory of his father who has taught him the importance of the family.

Pr Philippe Bouchard dedicates this book to his wonderful grandchildren Charlie, Elio and Juliette, and to all the students and teachers who have contribute much to periodontology and implant dentistry.

The authors also wish to thank the teachers, post-graduate students, and staff of the Department of Periodontology, Rothschild hospital, AP-HP (Paris, France).

A special debt of gratitude to Pr Jean Pierre Ouhayoun and Dr Daniel Etienne, our mentors, without whom this book would not have been.

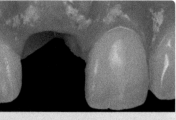
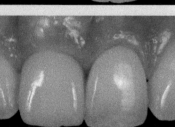

Contents

Preface

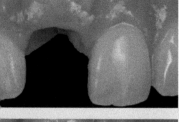
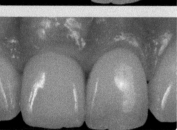

The first edition of this book was published in 2012. This means that the very preparation of the manuscript started in 2010. Jacques, Francis and I were nevertheless surprised when we were contacted about a year ago by the editor to prepare a second edition, even if seven years had passed since the first.

The first edition of this textbook was designed to help general practitioners and students in their approach to implant dentistry. It was written to streamline dental implant practice by using as much as possible available evidence-based procedures. We were pleased to learn that specialists were also interested in our book, as a tool for learning or as a memo in some fields with which they were not familiar. Nevertheless, the book was not dedicated to the most advanced specialists in dental implant surgery or prostheses, and we did not see the necessity for an updated version, precisely because as specialists robust clinical information was directly implemented in our daily practice. This information became invisible, and efforts had to be made to realise how important changes in implant dentistry research had impacted daily practice.

When we did this, it suddenly became obvious that many chapters had to be updated, and new chapters created. With our editor's agreement, the number of chapters jumped from 50 to 63. In-depth changes were implemented all through the book, not only in the text but also in the illustrations. In addition, because this textbook aims to be didactic and contemporary in terms of communication, some chapters are supplemented by multiple-choice questions (MCQs) and videos. We hope the reader enjoys this new format, which aims to improve the learning curve of students, and the accessibility of general practitioners to some complex surgical procedures.

The preface to the first edition stressed that dental implant therapy was a relatively young area of interest in dentistry. This is still true, and unanswered questions remain. However, since 2010 considerable efforts have been made in clinical and basic research. Two journals dealing with implant dentistry are today in the top ten of dental journals. Over the last 20 years, the profile of the candidate for implant dentistry has slowly evolved. Implant therapy is no longer reserved for the elderly, and at the same time the number of elderly in the world is increasing.

Aesthetic improvement and time reduction in procedures have been of utmost importance in research in the last ten years. Nowadays, digital implant dentistry has demonstrated clear progress. Oral health quality of life, cost–benefit and cost-effectiveness are invited in the field of dental implant research. These new areas of interest testify to the spread of implant dentistry to more and more people in need of teeth replacement.

It is often claimed that dental implant therapy is highly predictable. This is true, but predictability remains a challenge, not only because of the increasing number of dental implants placed, but also due to the increasing number of professional users. In the near future, there is little doubt that digital techniques will reduce the risk of error.

In the fifth edition of his landmark textbook (Lindhe J, Lang N.P, Karring T. Clinical Periodontology and Implant Dentistry, Fifth Ed, Blackwell Munksgaard Ed, 2008.), Jan Lindhe maintained: 'Implant dentistry has become a basic part of periodontology.' There is no doubt that periodontal thinking and practice form the best and the safest approach to implant dentistry to prevent and treat not only peri-implantitis but also to maintain aesthetics.

We hope the second edition of this book will give the reader the feeling that implant dentistry can be achieved by non-specialists, providing the clinical case is not complex; that is, dealing with aesthetics and/or soft and hard tissue reconstruction. The chapters go beyond the description of simple procedures, but we do hope the practitioner will be enticed by these advanced techniques, and consequently encouraged to undertake further training.

Philippe Bouchard

Acknowledgments

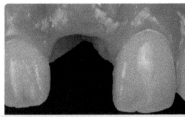

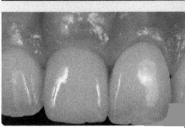

We would like to acknowledge the following colleagues for providing the figures listed:

- Dr Bernard Schweitz: Chapter 9, Figure 9.4.
- Dr Murielle Mola: Chapter 18, Figure 18.2.
- Dr Catherine Artaud: Chapter 18, Figure 18.3.
- Dr May Feghali: Chapter 24, Figure 24.3.
- Dr Alexandre Sueur: Chapter 29, Figure 29.3.
- Dr Eric Maujean: Chapter 52, Figure 52.2.

We are very grateful to Pr Pierre Carpentier (Chapters 4 & 5), Dr Olivier Fromentin (Chapter 24), and Dr Leonardo Matossian (Chapter 9) for their contribution to our book.

Special thanks to Dr Olivier Etienne for agreeing to write the CAD-CAM chapters 43 and 44.

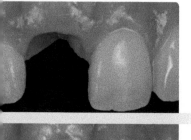

About the companion website

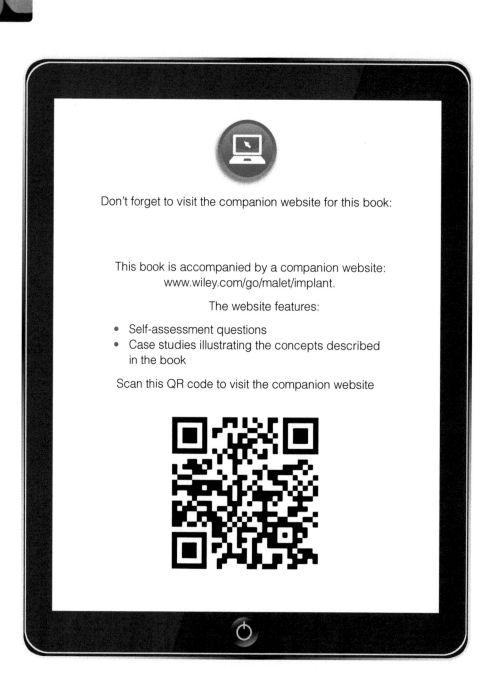

Don't forget to visit the companion website for this book:

This book is accompanied by a companion website:
www.wiley.com/go/malet/implant.

The website features:

- Self-assessment questions
- Case studies illustrating the concepts described in the book

Scan this QR code to visit the companion website

2

Chapter 1 Quality of life associated with implant-supported pr...

1 Quality of life associated with implant-supported prostheses: An introduction to implant dentistry

According to the World Health Organization, 'Health is a state of complete physical, mental, and social well-being and not merely the absence of disease, or infirmity' (WHO, 1946). Based on this definition, the WHO defines quality of life (QoL) 'as individuals' perception of their position in life in the context of the culture and value systems in which they live and in relation to their goals, expectations, standards and concerns' (WHO, 1997). In other words, 'QoL is a popular term that conveys an overall sense of well-being, including aspects of happiness and satisfaction with life as a whole' (CDC, 2000).

The concept of health-related quality of life (HRQoL) on an individual level 'includes physical and mental health perceptions (e.g., energy level, mood) and their correlates including health risks and conditions, functional status, social support, and socioeconomic status' (CDC, 2000). In short, the Centers for Disease Control and Prevention have defined HRQoL as 'an individual's or group's perceived physical and mental health over time'.

Oral health quality of life

Questionnaires have been developed to assess the impact of oral conditions on HRQoL. Oral health-related quality of life (OHRQoL) encompasses a collection of metrics such as Dental Impact on Daily Living (DIDL), Geriatric/General Oral Health Assessment Index (GOHAI), Oral Health Impact Profile (OHIP) and Oral Impacts on Daily Performances (OIDP). Among these metrics, the 14-item OHIP-14 is the most popular. The diversity of measures makes it difficult to adopt a global approach to assess the impact of missing teeth on OHRQoL.

Dental implants and oral health

Implant dentistry aims to replace missing teeth. This is a very challenging aspect of dentistry: Should dentists replace the teeth that have been lost? However, from the patient's perspective, it makes sense to ask the question: What are the benefits of dental implant placement? In other words, the following issues should be addressed:
- Should missing teeth be replaced?
- Does implant dentistry improve a patient's quality of life?
- Is implant dentistry a cost-effective option?

We hope that this chapter will help the practitioner, not to convince patients to have dental implants, but to provide them with sufficient information to assist in the decision-making process.

Should missing teeth be replaced?

It is beyond the scope of this book to explore the scientific rationale supporting the replacement of missing teeth. However, logic dictates that we need a minimum number of teeth and functional masticatory units (FMUs, defined as pairs of opposing teeth or

dental restoration allowing mastication, excluding incisors) to ensure an acceptable OHRQoL.

Number of teeth

A significant link has been established between the number of teeth and OHRQoL (Tan et al., 2016). Fewer than 17 teeth is associated with poor OHRQoL in the elderly (Jensen et al., 2008).

The concept of shortened dental arches (SDAs) has been proposed (Witter et al., 1999). This concept refers to dentition with intact anterior teeth and loss of posterior teeth; that is, molar teeth. It has been suggested that at least 20 teeth are required in order to maintain functional, aesthetic and natural dentition, and to meet oral health targets (Petersen and Yamamoto, 2005). Dentists advocate the practical applicability of SDAs. A recent multicentre survey showed that about 80% of participating professionals agreed with the SDA concept (Abuzar et al., 2015).

Moreover, there is no significant difference in terms of OHRQoL between subjects with SDAs and those with removable dentures (Antunes et al., 2016; Tan et al., 2015). This means that a worse OHRQoL is not SDA related and that the concept of directing treatment and resources to anterior and premolar teeth, without molar teeth replacement, is an acceptable option. In other words, there is a need to replace some but not all missing teeth.

Functional masticatory units

FMUs are needed to facilitate the chewing process. Masticatory function differs somewhat from masticatory capacity. Evaluation of masticatory function is based on complex laboratory methods. Qualitative assessment is based on video or electromyographic examination (Hennequin et al., 2005). Quantitative assessment focuses on measuring particle size values for masticated raw carrots collected just before swallowing (Woda et al., 2010). However, in clinical and epidemiological studies, the number of FMUs is a validated parameter for discriminating between functional and dysfunctional masticatory capacities (Godlewski et al., 2011). A threshold of five FMUs generally serves as the cut-off in epidemiological studies (Adolph et al., 2017; Darnaud et al., 2015).

A limited biting/chewing capacity is not conducive to a healthy diet and can lead to a high glycaemic index, increased fat consumption and reduced fibre consumption. In other words, 'good nutrition is a cornerstone of good health' (WHO, 2017) and masticatory capacity is one of the most important factors for ensuring a healthy diet. A systematic review of longitudinal studies reported that signs of impaired swallowing efficacy were deemed a risk factor for malnutrition in elderly people (odds ratio [OR] = 2.73; $p = 0.015$; Moreira et al., 2016). The number of FMUs has been positively linked (OR = 2.79, 95% confidence interval [CI]: 1.49–5.22) with

Implant Dentistry at a Glance, Second Edition. Jacques Malet, Francis Mora and Philippe Bouchard.
© 2018 John Wiley & Sons Ltd. Published 2018 by John Wiley & Sons Ltd.
Companion website: www.wiley.com/go/malet/implant

poor nutritional status in individuals over 65 years of age, according to the Mini-Nutritional Assessment (MNA; El Osta *et al.*, 2014). Malnutrition is associated with an increase in inflammatory biomarkers in post-menopausal women (Wood *et al.*, 2014). A higher morbidity/mortality risk was observed among haemodialysis patients with a high malnutrition-inflammation score (Pisetkul *et al.*, 2010). To conclude, a minimum of five FMUs is needed not only to ensure an adequate masticatory capacity, but also to guarantee a healthy diet.

Finally, it must be emphasised that the number of teeth and FMUs is not sufficient to portray the overall picture of edentulism. Teeth also contribute to an individual's appearance; that is, they have an aesthetic connotation. Dental aesthetics are known to be associated with OHRQoL (Broder and Wilson-Genderson, 2007; Klages *et al.*, 2004). Teeth are also important for phonation. Last but not least, missing teeth are associated with poor self-esteem and can thus have a psychological impact.

Does implant dentistry improve the patient's quality of life?

Most studies evaluate the advantages of implant-supported overdenture in the mandible. Limited research has focused on maxillary overdentures. Many different studies from various centres using a range of protocols suggest that patients positively rate their QoL after dental implant therapy. OHRQoL is generally better in patients with fixed prostheses than in those with a removable prosthesis (OHIP-14; Brennan *et al.*, 2010). Based on OHIP-21 metrics, assessment of post-implant therapy confirmed a significant improvement in terms of OHRQoL (Nickenig *et al.*, 2008). However, a recent systematic review indicates that the use of implant-supported overdentures to treat individuals with 100% dentures improves chewing efficiency, bite force and patient satisfaction. Nevertheless, no effect on nutritional status is apparent and QoL results remain inconclusive (Boven *et al.*, 2015).

Studies dealing with fixed implant-supported prostheses in the maxilla region are few and far between, and are mostly based on single-implant placement. A significant implant-related improvement in OHRQoL is evident from aesthetic and functional perspectives in patients with at least one implant in the anterior dental region (Pavel *et al.*, 2012). In addition, an extremely positive response in OIDP has been reported in all patients treated for single-tooth replacement with an anterior maxillary implant (Angkaew *et al.*, 2017). Finally, based on a seven-question customised, mailed questionnaire, elderly patients receiving dental implants had an excellent QoL score (Becker *et al.*, 2016).

Is implant dentistry a cost-effective option?

Of completely edentulous elderly individuals with implants, 70% were willing to pay three times the cost of conventional dentures for implant prostheses (Esfandiari *et al.*, 2009); the willingness to pay [WTP] is the maximum amount a person would be willing to pay for an implant in order to obtain effective treatment or avoid an undesirable event such as disease or discomfort. In the anterior area, 94% of edentulous patients chose implant-supported prostheses instead of conventional prostheses to replace missing teeth and, on average, a high number of patients are willing to pay for this type of treatment (Leung and McGrath, 2010). In other words, the question of cost-effectiveness in implant dentistry is important and cost is the first obstacle to growth in the dental implant market.

The average cost-effectiveness of the tooth-supported prosthesis strategy is higher than that of the implant strategy, even if greater initial costs are associated with implant-supported prostheses (Bouchard *et al.*, 2009). A systematic literature review including 14 studies revealed that, in the case of single-tooth replacement, one dental implant placement is a cost-effective treatment option compared to a three-unit fixed dental prosthesis (Vogel *et al.*, 2013). A two-implant overdenture is a cost-effective option for restoring complete edentulism in the lower jaw (Feine *et al.*, 2002; Thomason *et al.*, 2009). However, there is little evidence to show that implant-supported fixed prostheses perform better than implant-supported overdentures, especially from a cost-effectiveness perspective. No significant difference in muscular activity during clenching has been observed when comparing implant-supported overdentures and implant-supported fixed prostheses (von der Gracht *et al.*, 2016).

To conclude, implant dentistry as a first-line strategy appears to be the 'dominant' strategy compared to conventional tooth-supported prostheses, especially for single-tooth replacement and complete edentulism in the mandible using overdentures retained with two dental implants. However, further well-designed studies are essential in order to establish the extent of the improvement in OHRQoL with fixed and removable implant-supported prostheses, especially in the upper jaw.

Key points

- There is no need to replace all missing teeth.
- The concept of shortened dental arches – 20 teeth without molar teeth replacement – is an acceptable and cost-effective option.
- A minimum of five to six functional masticatory units is required to chew.
- Impaired chewing not only has impacts on general health but also on oral health-related quality of life.
- Implant dentistry improves the patient's quality of life.
- A two-implant overdenture is a cost-effective option for restoring complete edentulism in the lower jaw.

2 The basics: Osseointegration

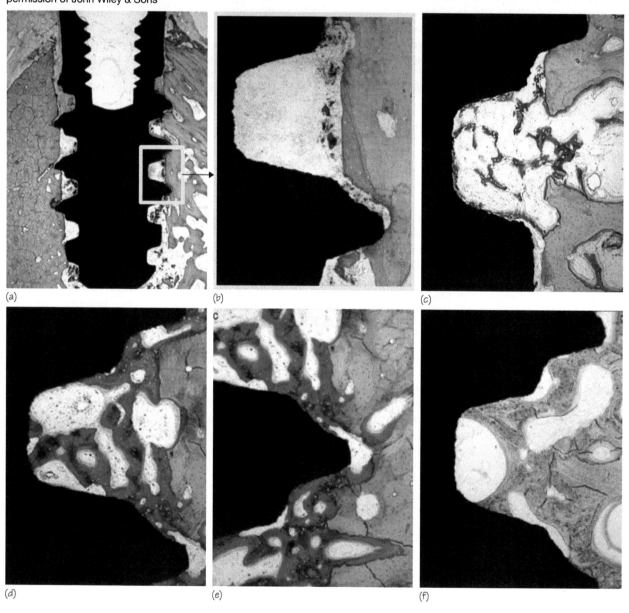

Figure 2.1 Healing phases of 'non-cutting' dental implants placed in Labrador dogs (Berglundh *et al.*, 2003). (a, b) *Four days of healing*. The fibrin clot has been replaced by granulation tissue. (c) *One week*. Woven bone formation. (d, e) *Four weeks*. The newly formed bone includes woven bone combined with lamellar bone. In the pitch regions, the bone remodelling appears to be intense (e). (f) *Twelve weeks*. Mature bone (lamellar bone and marrow) is in close contact with the implant and covers most of the surface. Reproduced with permission of John Wiley & Sons

(a) (b) (c) (d) (e) (f)

Implant Dentistry at a Glance, Second Edition. Jacques Malet, Francis Mora and Philippe Bouchard.
© 2018 John Wiley & Sons Ltd. Published 2018 by John Wiley & Sons Ltd.
Companion website: www.wiley.com/go/malet/implant

The aim of the surgical procedure for implant placement is to prepare, in an atraumatic manner, an intraosseous bed into which a dental implant is inserted. Following soft tissue elevation, a channel is drilled into the cortical and spongy bone and the dental implant (screw-type titanium device), slightly wider than the channel, is slowly inserted within the 'implant bed' (the channel) surgically created.

The compression of the bone surrounding the implant reduces the peripheral vasculature, and the lack of an adequate blood supply leads to non-vital tissue at the bone/implant interface. The inflammatory response to the surgical injury aims to remove the damaged tissues and to initiate the healing process leading to osseointegration; that is, the direct connection between newly formed bone and the metal device.

Implant neck

The initial stability of the interface between the implant and the mineralised bone is a critical factor to initiate the osseointegration process. The primary stability of the dental implant is often achieved at the cortical bone level. In the cortical compartment at the implant neck, the non-vital lamellar bone is first resorbed before new bone formation occurs onto the implant surface.

Implant body

At the implant body, in the cancellous compartment, the wound healing includes the following phases (Berglundh *et al.*, 2003; Abrahamsson *et al.*, 2004).

1 Clot formation

The blood fills the space between the threads of the implant. Erythrocytes, neutrophils and macrophages are trapped in a fibrin network. The fibrin clot is replaced by granulation tissue. Mesenchymal cells and blood vessels proliferate in the new granulation tissue, which is rich in collagen fibres (Figure 2.1a, b).

2 Bone modelling

A first line of osteoblasts, migrating from bone marrow, invades the granulation tissue. After one week an osteoid matrix is observed in the mesenchymal tissues surrounding the blood vessels. In the osteoid, deposition of hydroxyapatite leads to woven bone formation (immature bone). Woven bone formation (Figure 2.1c) is associated with increased local angiogenesis. The woven bone is characterised by randomly oriented collagen fibrils, numerous osteocytes and low mineral densities. It fills the space between the implant threads, constructing the first bony

bridges between the inner bony wall of the surgical channel and the external surface of the dental implant. This direct contact between the woven bone and the implant surface represents the first phase of osseointegration. Gradually, woven bone covers most of the implant surface.

3 Bone remodelling

During subsequent weeks, concentric layers of lamellar bone (osteon) are seen in the newly formed tissue (Figure 2.1d, e). Woven bone is progressively replaced by lamellar bone and marrow (mature bone; Figure 2.1f). The lamellar bone is the strongest type of newly formed bone and the most elaborate type of bone tissue; it is composed of collagen fibrils densely packed into parallel layers with alternating courses.

Implant loading

Micromovements along the bone/implant interface have a tolerance limit during the healing phase, and micromotion beyond this tolerance limit may result in connective tissue encapsulation of the implant body. On the other hand, it has been shown that immediate occlusal loading can present a high level of bone-to-implant contact (BIC) in humans. It must be understood that the degree of primary stability achieved depends on several factors, including bone density and quality, implant shape, design and surface characteristics, and surgical technique.

Even once the healing phase is completed – that is, after about three months – BIC is not 100%. It has been shown that functional loading of dental implants may enhance the BIC value (Berglundh *et al.*, 2005). This important finding indicates that the biological process of osseointegration is continuous, related to bone remodelling, and does not stop with the healing phase, and that a site-specific bone adaptation response to mechanical loading may result in increasing osseointegration over time. This emphasises the importance of controlling the occlusal load as well as the bacterial load during the maintenance phase.

Key points

- The surgical technique should be as atraumatic as possible.
- Good primary stability is a key factor in the osseointegration process.
- The degree of primary stability achieved depends on several factors.
- After the healing phase, functional loading of dental implants may enhance the bone-to-implant contact value.

3 The basics: The peri-implant mucosa

Figure 3.1 (a,b) Clinical appearance of the peri-implant mucosa. Red circles indicate the implant-supported prosthesis

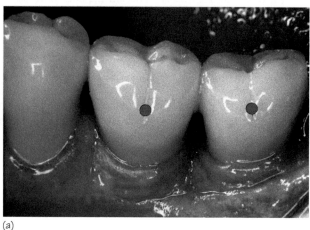

(a)

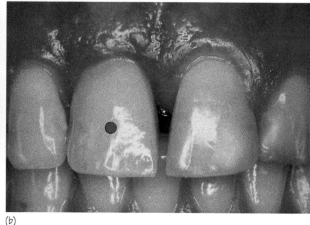

(b)

Figure 3.2 Histological differences between tooth and dental implant. AB, alveolar bone; BE, barrier epithelium; BII, bone/implant interface; C, cementum; CT, connective tissue; CTF, connective tissue fibres; GE, gingival epithelium; JE, junctional epithelium; P, periosteum; PIB, peri-implant bone; PIE, peri-implant epithelium; PL, periodontal ligament

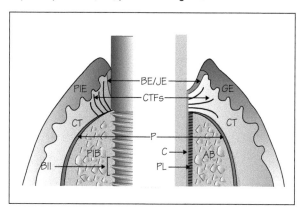

Figure 3.3 The biological width around dental implants

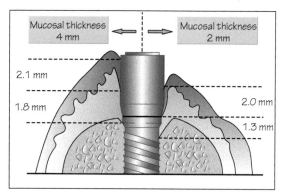

After implant placement, a delicate mucosal attachment is established. The peri-implant mucosa is sealed to the implant surface to protect the bone tissue, and to prevent the penetration of micro-organisms and their products. Limited data exist in humans. Most of the following information is extrapolated from animal studies. Thus, data on healing time might not always be directly transferable to the clinical situation.

The peri-implant mucosa results from the healing process of the soft tissues surrounding the implant, following the closure of the flap around the transgingival part of the implant.

From a clinical point of view, the outer surface of the peri-implant mucosa is covered by a keratinised oral epithelium. It has a pink colour and a firm consistency, and does not differ from the clinical appearance of the gingiva (Figure 3.1a, b). The

Implant Dentistry at a Glance, Second Edition. Jacques Malet, Francis Mora and Philippe Bouchard.
© 2018 John Wiley & Sons Ltd. Published 2018 by John Wiley & Sons Ltd.
Companion website: www.wiley.com/go/malet/implant

peri-implant mucosa clinical dimension tends to be thicker and lower in height than the gingiva surrounding teeth.

From a histological point of view, compared to the periodontal model, the dental implant model has the following main features (Figure 3.2):
- lack of cementum
- lack of periodontal ligament
- the attachment apparatus is different
- the collagen/fibroblast ratio is different.

Soft tissue interface dimensions

The epithelium barrier is about 2 mm long, and the connective tissue seal is 1–1.5 mm high.

These dimensions are maintained whatever the thickness of the mucosa. This means that when the mucosa is thin (i.e. ≤2 mm), bone resorption occurs to maintain these soft tissue dimensions. In short, as for teeth, a *biological width* must be respected around implants (Figure 3.3).

Soft tissue seal

The epithelium barrier is sealed to the implant surface via hemidesmosomes and must be considered identical to that of the epithelial seal around teeth.

The connective tissue compartment is in direct contact with the implant surface. The connective fibres are parallel to the implant surface without attachment to the metal body (adhesion). Consequently, the resistance to probing around implants is decreased compared to that around teeth. However, when probing in healthy tissues, the tip of the probe seems to reach similar levels at the implant and tooth sites. Marginal inflammation around implants is associated with a deeper probe penetration compared to that around teeth.

Soft tissue components

Compared to the gingiva, the peri-implant mucosa exhibits more collagen fibres, fewer fibroblasts and fewer vessels.

Soft tissue healing

Due to the lack of the vascular plexus of the periodontal ligament, the implant blood supply comes from two sources: the peri-implant mucosa and the supraperiosteal blood vessels.

A mature barrier epithelium is seen after eight to nine weeks of healing, and the collagen fibres are organised after four to six weeks of healing.

The potential for repair is limited due to the:
- lack of periodontal ligament
- reduction of the cellular components of the mucosa
- reduced vascularisation.

Key points

- The peri-implant mucosa is sealed and not attached to the implant.
- A biological width is maintained, whatever the thickness of the mucosa.
- Compared to the gingiva, the peri-implant mucosa is a scar-like tissue, rich in collagen fibres, poor in fibroblasts and with limited blood supply.
- The potential for repair is more limited than with gingival tissue.

4 The basics: Surgical anatomy of the mandible

Figure 4.1 Mandible: mental foramen. Two anatomical variations of the inferior alveolar nerve. (a) Anterior extension: incisive canal. (b) Anterior loop. 1. Inferior alveolar nerve; 2. mental nerve; 3. incisive canal; 4. anterior loop of the inferior alveolar nerve.

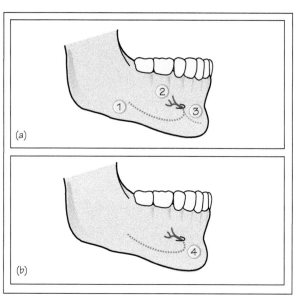

(a)

(b)

Figure 4.2 Mandible: horizontal section/occlusal view. 1. Mandibular foramen; 2. mandibular canal (inferior alveolar nerve); 3. mental foramen; 4. lingual nerve; 5. incisive canal.

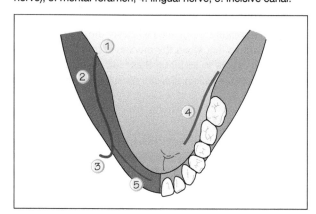

Figure 4.3 Mandible: posterior vertical section. 1. Lingual cortex concavity: submandibular fossa; 2. mandibular canal (inferior alveolar nerve); 3. lingual foramen; 4. mental spines: (a) genioglossus, (b) geniohyoid.

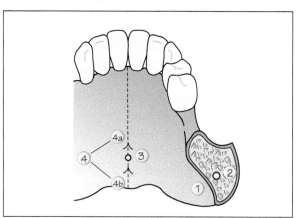

Figure 4.4 Mandible: lingual view. 1. Mandibular foramen; 2. lingual nerve.

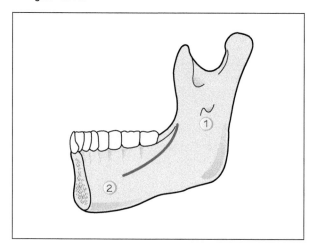

Implant Dentistry at a Glance, Second Edition. Jacques Malet, Francis Mora and Philippe Bouchard.
© 2018 John Wiley & Sons Ltd. Published 2018 by John Wiley & Sons Ltd.
Companion website: www.wiley.com/go/malet/implant

Placing dental implants requires access to bone tissue (usually by raising a flap) to achieve an osteotomy. The handling of soft tissues (gingiva and alveolar mucosa) and bone osteotomy must respect some anatomical structures to avoid injuries leading to damage which may be difficult to manage: reversible or irreversible nerve injury, haemorrhage and intrusion into unwanted anatomical areas. The risk level (high, moderate, low) and the approach to prevention will be described.

Anterior area

This region is usually considered at low risk for surgical damage. However, some anatomical structures have to be identified.

The *incisive canal* (Figures 4.1 and 4.2) is an anterior extension of the *mandibular canal* with neurovascular content. The lesion of this structure usually has no clinical consequences, except in the first premolar area and sometimes in the canine area.

The *lingual foramen* (Figure 4.3) can be observed on X-rays or computed tomography (CT) scan in more than 80% of subjects near the *mental spines*. A branch of the sublingual artery enters the foramen to supply the bone.

Neurovascular structures

- *Osseous*: incisive nerve in the incisive canal
- *Buccal*: mental artery, submental artery, mental nerve
- *Lingual*: sublingual artery.

> **Key points**
>
> - *Sublingual and submental artery* (moderate risk): in the lateral incisor or canine region, the risk of damage to the artery cannot be ignored when a basal mandibular perforation is performed during osteotomy, resulting in potential bleeding in the oral floor and the parapharyngeal space. Elevation of the periosteum of the lingual aspect during surgery and adequate compression or ligature will prevent problems.

Posterior area

The *inferior alveolar nerve* (see Figure 4.2) enters the mandibular ramus distally through the *mandibular foramen* and runs in the *mandibular canal*, from the lingual to the labial side. At the *mental foramen* (most often between the first and second premolars) it becomes the *mental nerve*, which divides into three branches for the skin and gingiva. The mean distance between alveolar crest and superior margin of the mental foramen is about 10 mm ± 5 mm, in non-edentulous areas. Occasionally, the *inferior alveolar nerve* describes an anterior loop (see Figure 4.1).

Rare variations (bifid mandibular canal, multiple foramina) have been described.

The posterior area of the mandibular body often shows lingual concavities (see Figure 4.3) facing the submandibular gland.

The *lingual nerve* (Figures 4.2 and 4.4) runs near the inner surface of the mandible in the region of the wisdom tooth, and then has an oblique course forward and inward, down to the tip of the tongue.

Neurovascular structures

- *Osseous*: inferior alveolar nerve, inferior alveolar artery
- *Buccal*: buccal nerve, facial artery branches, mental nerve
- *Lingual*: lingual nerve.

> **Key points**
>
> - *Inferior alveolar nerve* (high risk): laceration or compression of the nerve in the mandibular canal or section of the anterior loop during osteotomy will result in permanent paraesthesia. Precise 3D preoperative imaging (CT scan or cone beam computed tomography, CBCT) is thus essential in this region.
> - *Mental nerve* (moderate risk): section (during dissection) or compression (with instruments) of the mental nerve can occur. This is why good visualisation of the mental foramen is recommended during surgery.
> - *Lingual nerve* (moderate risk): injury or compression of the lingual nerve can occur when raising a full-thickness lingual flap, if the technique is not careful enough.

5 The basics: Surgical anatomy of the maxilla

Figure 5.1 Maxilla: palatal view. 1. Incisive foramen; 2. greater palatine foramen; 3. descending palatine artery; 4. greater palatine nerve; 5. nasopalatine nerves

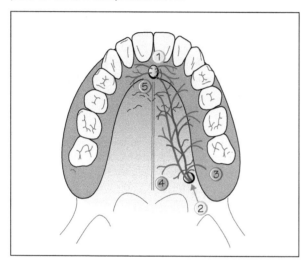

Figure 5.2 Maxilla: front view. *Right side: intra-bony structures*: 1. nasal cavity; 2. infraorbital artery and nerve; 2a. anterior superior alveolar arteries and nerves; 2b. middle superior alveolar arteries and nerves. *Left side: soft tissue structures*: 2c. infraorbital artery and nerve branches; 3. infraorbital foramen; 4. facial artery and superior labial artery; 5. facial nerve

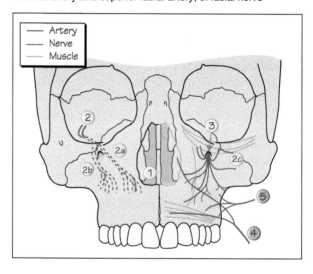

Figure 5.3 Maxilla: horizontal section. 1. Lateral pterygoid plate; 2. maxillary sinus; 3. inferior nasal meatus; 4. nasal septum

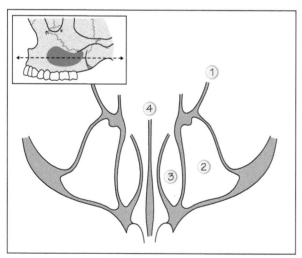

Figure 5.4 Maxilla: lateral view. 1. Maxillary sinus; 2. maxillary tuberosity; 3. lateral pterygoid plate; 4. palatine bone (pyramidal process); 5. anterior nasal spine; 6. alveolar antral artery; 7. posterior superior alveolar artery and nerve; 8. infraorbital artery branch

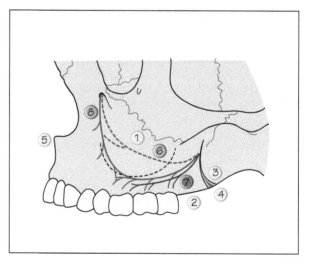

Implant Dentistry at a Glance, Second Edition. Jacques Malet, Francis Mora and Philippe Bouchard.
© 2018 John Wiley & Sons Ltd. Published 2018 by John Wiley & Sons Ltd.
Companion website: www.wiley.com/go/malet/implant

Anterior area

Located between the anterior walls of the maxillary sinus, this area is usually of good bone quality. The region is apically limited by the *nasal cavity* (Figure 5.1) that communicates with the *maxillary sinus* (through the middle meatus). Slight penetration or perforation of the *nasal floor* may be uneventful.

The canine region is a strategic area due to mechanical stress dispersion.

The *incisive foramen* (continuous with the *incisive canal*) is located between the two medial incisors, slightly palatal (see Figure 5.1). Its volume can prevent implant placement. Its content is not essential (accessory vascularisation and innervation) and can be replaced by a bone graft or substitute to improve the bone bed.

Neurovascular structures
Buccal (see Figure 5.2)
Intra-bony structures:
• infraorbital artery branches: anterior superior alveolar arteries
• infraorbital nerve terminal branches: anterior superior alveolar nerves.

Soft tissue structures (labial vestibule):
• infraorbital artery branches
• infraorbital nerve terminal branches
• facial artery (superior labial artery) and facial nerve branches.

Palatal (see Figure 5.1)
Incisive foramen and incisive canal: final branches of the greater palatine artery running to the nasal cavity, and nasopalatine nerves coming from the nasal cavity.

> **Key points**
> The risk is low, but we recommend avoiding penetration of the nasal floor and staying away from the incisive foramen (or removing its content if necessary).

Posterior area

This region is characterised by limited bone volume (due to the presence of the *maxillary sinus*) and poor bone quality.

The maxillary sinus is a large aerial cavity lined with a thin membrane. Slight penetration or perforation of the sinus floor in a healthy sinus can be uneventful.

Maxillary sinus and advanced surgeries

Sinus lift procedures are indicated to augment bone volume in this region. This surgery is frequently complicated by the presence of septa in the maxillary sinus. Septa occur in about 30% of sinuses, and they are most commonly located in the first and second molar area. The permeability of the *maxillary sinus ostium* must be checked before surgery.

Tuberosity and *pterygopalatine* region (Figures 5.3 and 5.4): in order to avoid the sinus region, the tuberosity can be used for implant placement. Occasionally, primary stabilisation could be necessary in the suture (*palatine bone–pterygoid process–maxillary tuberosity*).

Neurovascular structures
Buccal (see Figure 5.4)
• Maxillary artery branches: posterior superior alveolar artery, alveolar antral artery
• Maxillary nerve branches: posterior superior alveolar nerve, middle or anterior superior alveolar nerve
• Cheek: facial artery and facial nerve branches.

Palatal (see Figure 5.1)
Greater palatine artery branches, greater palatine nerve branches, greater palatine foramen: on the palatal side the *greater palatine foramen* (located in the hard palate near the second or third molar apex) contains a large vessel: the *greater palatine artery*. The artery runs along the alveolar process and hard palate corner in a more or less deep groove, to reach and penetrate the incisive canal after giving off a lot of small branches.

> **Key points**
> • Alveolar antral artery (moderate risk): haemorrhage during sinus lift procedures (see Chapter 51) can occur, by sectioning the artery during the osteotomy. It is recommended to locate the artery on CT scan and then in the sinus wall during osteotomy, and to avoid it if possible.
> • Greater palatine artery (moderate risk): haemorrhage during soft tissue graft harvesting. The risk is limited if the technique is performed carefully. Incisions must be distant from the greater palatine foramen. High risk: haemorrhage during posterior implant placement into the greater palatine canal will reach the soft palate and the parapharyngeal space. Precise knowledge of the greater palatine canal localisation and of the pathway of the neurovascular pedicle is recommended.

6 The basics: Bone shape and quality

Figure 6.1 Classification of the host bone. (A–E) Bone shape. (Group 1 to Group 4) Bone quality: 1. cortical bone; 2. dense cortico-cancellous bone; 3. sparse cortico-cancellous bone; 4. thin cortical and very sparse medullar bone

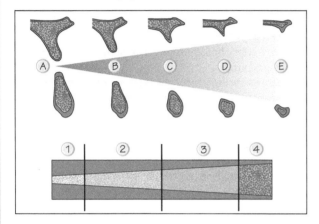

Figure 6.2 Bone volume resorption and interocclusal relationship. (a) The axis of the dental implant and the natural axis of the tooth are similar (blue arrow) when the postextractional bone resorption is moderate. (b) After advanced vertical and horizontal bone resorption, the axis of the implant (red arrow) does not allow an adequate interocclusal relationship

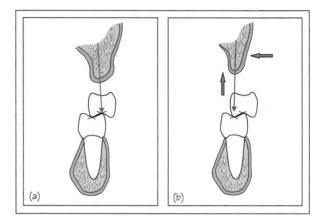

Figure 6.3 (a, b) Clinical examination shows a thin edentulous alveolar ridge with horizontal and vertical bone resorption. (c) The clinical conditions are confirmed by tomography

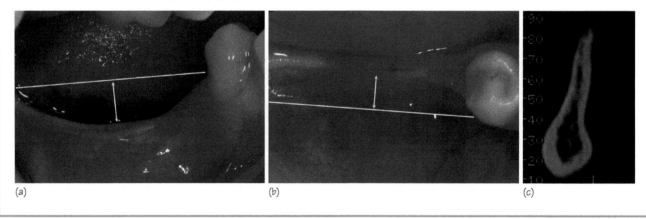

The volume, shape and quality of the bone are important parameters in establishing the treatment plan. They strongly influence the choice of surgical procedure and implant dimensions.

The bone volume determines the available bone; that is, the bone dimension that can be used for dental implant placement. The quality of the bone – that is, the density, strength and elasticity – may determine the ability of the bone to support the stress induced by the prosthetic restoration.

Bone shape

Bone volume atrophy depends on numerous factors such as tooth loss, trauma, infection, periodontitis and tooth extraction procedures. After tooth extraction, the alveolar bone resorption is more important at the facial aspect than at the palatal/lingual cortical plates, irrespective of the alveolar preservation techniques. The alveolar bone loss is almost ten times greater three months postoperatively than in the years following tooth

Implant Dentistry at a Glance, Second Edition. Jacques Malet, Francis Mora and Philippe Bouchard.
© 2018 John Wiley & Sons Ltd. Published 2018 by John Wiley & Sons Ltd.
Companion website: www.wiley.com/go/malet/implant

extraction. The resorption is higher at the posterior maxilla than in other areas of the jaws.

Several classifications have been proposed. The classification of Lekholm and Zarb (1985) is based on the residual jaw morphology and deals with the insertion of dental implants. They described five levels of jaw resorption in edentulous patients, ranging from minimal to severe osseous atrophy (Figure 6.1).

Bone quality

The quality or density of the internal structure of bone exhibits a number of biomechanical properties. Poor bone quality may be associated with implant failure. According to Wolff's laws (1892), the shape and function of bone depend on biomechanical concepts based on mathematical models. Consequently, the mandible is designed as a force absorption unit with a dense outer cortical bone and a coarse or dense trabecular bone. The maxilla is a force distribution unit: the zygomatic arch and palate dissipate mechanical stress to protect the brain and orbit. The maxilla has thin cortical and trabecular bone when teeth are present. Bone modelling and remodelling processes are considered as adaptive phenomena associated with alteration of the mechanical stress and strain environment in the bone.

Lekholm and Zarb (1985) classified bone density using a four-point ordinal scale (see Figure 6.1). The G1 density is localised in the anterior area of the mandible. G2 is the most common bone density observed in the mandible. G3 is very common in the anterior maxilla. G4, the poorest bone quality, is found in the posterior maxilla.

Several studies using finite element analysis models with various implant designs and bone quality have evaluated the stress/strain distribution. The titanium/cortical bone interface shows less microstrain than the titanium/sparse medullar bone interface.

According to the type of bone density, the surface and design of dental implant can be selected. It is also important to evaluate the bone quality to determine the optimal drilling sequence, the healing time and the implant loading protocol.

Clinical examination

The horizontal discrepancies between the upper and lower arches must be assessed to prevent biomechanical complications (Figure 6.2). The difference between vertical bone level at the adjacent teeth bordering the edentulous area and the bone level at the dental implant site must also be evaluated (Figure 6.3a). The interocclusal distance is measured as the height between the antagonist teeth and bone crest.

The available bone volume may be evaluated by clinical palpation to assess the shape of the alveolar crest and the depth of the vestibule (Figure 6.3b). A CT scan confirms the clinical examination (Figure 6.3c).

Osseous bone density may be assessed by probing through the mucosa, under local anaesthesia and/or during the implant surgical site preparation. Strong correlations have been found between tactile perception and osseous density during bone drilling.

Key points

- The shape and quality of the bone strongly influence treatment planning in dental implant therapy.
- Bone shape can be evaluated before radiographic analysis, during the clinical examination.
- Bone quality cannot be evaluated during the clinical examination.

7 Implant macrostructure: Shapes and dimensions

Figure 7.1 Implant dimensions. L, length; D, diameter; P, platform

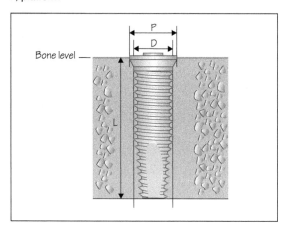

Figure 7.2 Selection of implant diameter depending on the location (tooth dimension)

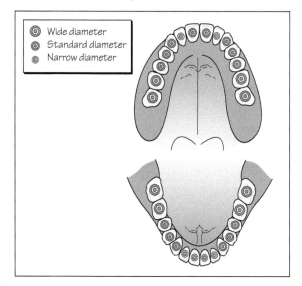

Wide diameter
Standard diameter
Narrow diameter

Figure 7.3 Wide implants (teeth 36 and 37, diameter 5 mm, length 8.5 mm)

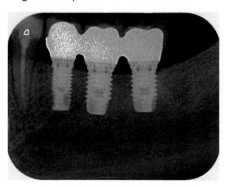

Figure 7.4 Narrow implant (length 13 mm, diameter 3.3 mm)

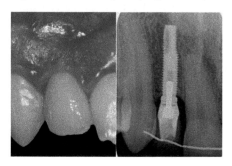

Figure 7.5 Currently available implant thread patterns. (a) V threads; (b) square threads; (c) buttress threads; (d) reverse buttress threads; (e) spiral threads. Adapted from Abuhussein et al., 2010. Reproduced with permission of John Wiley & Sons

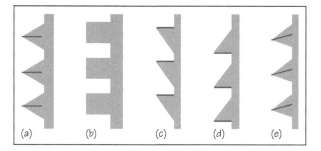

(a)　(b)　(c)　(d)　(e)

Table 7.1 Commercially available dental implants

	Length (in mm)	Diameter (in mm)
Minimum	5	2
Standard implant	10	3.75–4.1
Maximum	20	6.9

Implant Dentistry at a Glance, Second Edition. Jacques Malet, Francis Mora and Philippe Bouchard.
© 2018 John Wiley & Sons Ltd. Published 2018 by John Wiley & Sons Ltd.
Companion website: www.wiley.com/go/malet/implant

Most screw-type implant systems are available in different shapes and dimensions. This allows clinicians to select the most appropriate implants according to the clinical situation (see Chapter 28).

Treatment planning in implant dentistry aims to maximise the implant surface in contact with the bone bed, to provide a good *bone-to-implant contact* (BIC). This surface increases with the length, diameter and design of the implant, but also with the surface characteristics (see Chapter 10). Most of the time, an optimal contact can be obtained with a standard implant.

Another major goal of implant surgery is to achieve a good *primary stability*. In this view, numerous dental implant dimensions and designs are commercially available (Table 7.1).

Standard implants are well documented in the literature, and show excellent success rates in normal conditions; that is, sufficient amount and good quality of bone. In case of limited bone volume (height or width), an alternative to bone augmentation is to adapt the implant at the existing anatomy, through the use of narrow, short or wide implants.

Limited evidence is available regarding the impact of dental implant dimensions on the survival/success rate. Therefore, except for the standard dimensions, clinical guidelines are based on biomechanical theories confirmed (or not) by clinical trials.

Implant length

The length of an implant can be defined as the distance from the most coronal part of the implant inserted into the bone to the more apical part of the implant (Figure 7.1). Most implant systems provide implant lengths from 4 mm to 20 mm or greater.

Long implants (more than 10 mm) are indicated in particular situations where primary stability requires an apical anchorage: immediate implant, bone defect, tilted implants, poor bone quality. Otherwise, they are not recommended, particularly at the lower jaw, because of the risk of apical overheating.

Short implants can be a good alternative to bone augmentation procedures (see Chapter 28).

Implant diameter

Implant diameter (Figure 7.2) represents the distance between the external parts of the threads engaged into the bone. It can be different from the diameter of the prosthetic platform (see Figure 7.1).

Most implant systems provide implant diameters ranging from 3 mm to 6 mm (Figures 7.3 and 7.4). The optimal diameter selection should allow:

- engagement of a sufficient amount of bone (cortical plates)
- respect for adjacent roots (distance >1.5 mm)
- adequate emergence profile for aesthetic and oral hygiene.

The use of *wide-diameter implants* (5 mm or greater) has benefits and risks (Table 7.2).

Scientific data are limited for wide implants. A higher failure rate in the literature is described with implants placed in compromised sites, poor bone density or during an operator learning curve.

An adapted surgical protocol is recommended to assure primary stability (soft bone) and avoid overheating (dense bone). A one-stage procedure is recommended for wide implants.

The use of *narrow-diameter implants* (3–3.3 mm) is a good alternative to horizontal bone reconstruction (bone width <5 mm). Narrow implants are particularly adapted to the replacement of mandibular incisors and maxillary lateral incisors, and when mesiodistal prosthetic or bone space is limited.

The reduced mechanical resistance of these implants implies a good control of occlusal loading.

Implant shape

As implant shape can modify *surgical outcomes* (primary stability, bone compression) as well as *biomechanical parameters* (force distribution during occlusal function), different designs of commercially available screw-type implants have been developed.

Thread design of implants

The shape of the implant thread is designed to optimise force distribution at the bone/implant interface on the one hand, and to increase BIC on the other hand (primary stability and quantity of osseointegration).

Different thread patterns are commercially available (Figure 7.5).

It seems that a square thread design enhances the quality of osseointegration (BIC and reverse torque; Steigenga *et al.*, 2004) and transmits better shear forces compared to other designs.

Greater thread depth enhances the implant surface in contact with bone and therefore is indicated in cases of poor bone quality and high occlusal loading conditions, while a shallow thread depth allows easier insertion in dense bone.

Table 7.2 Implant length and diameter: indications compared to standard implants

	Advantages	Disadvantages	Indications
Long implants (>10)	Primary stability	Apical overheating risk	Immediate implant
			Bone defect
			Tilted implants
			Poor bone quality
Short implants (<9)	Alternative to bone grafts	Primary stability difficult to obtain	Limited bone height
Wide implants (>4)	Primary stability	Lateral overheating risk	Limited bone height
	Cortical anchorage		Poor bone quality
	Crestal bone contact		Molar
	Stress distribution		Bruxism
	Resistant components		Wide sites (failure)
Narrow implants (<3.7)	Alternative to bone grafts	Low mechanical resistance	Small-diameter teeth
			Limited space

Data on implant design should be interpreted with caution, since most of them come from finite element analysis studies (theoretical models).

Cylindrical versus tapered dental implants

Tapered implants are supposed to lead to a reduced need for bone augmentation and an improved primary stability in immediate implant placement, as the shape is more similar to the extraction socket. However, such differences could not be detected (Lang *et al.*, 2007).

There is no evidence that a particular implant has a better success rate or a clinical advantage than another (Esposito *et al.*, 2007). The surgeon's individual perception is the major selection criterion for a specific implant design.

Key points

- Standard implants are the best documented.
- Wide implant use requires an adapted surgical protocol.
- Narrow implants are not recommended with excessive occlusal load.
- There is no evidence that implant shape is a factor that may influence the survival rate of dental implants.

8

Implant macrostructure: Short implants

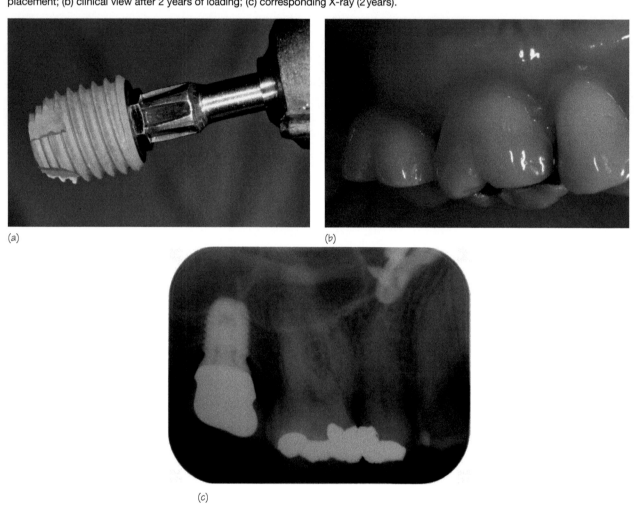

Figure 8.1 Single tooth (#17) restoration supported by a short implant (7 mm length, 6 mm diameter). (a) Dental implant before placement; (b) clinical view after 2 years of loading; (c) corresponding X-ray (2 years).

(a)

(b)

(c)

Short and extra-short dental implants seem attractive options as an alternative to vertical bone augmentation. They eliminate further surgical procedures in addition to dental implant placement. Short and extra-short dental implants appear cost-effective and more comfortable than classical pre-implant surgeries aiming to increase bone dimension. Thus, it is of clinical interest to explore the short implant option, and to compare with the use of conventional surgical approaches. Recent data encourage the use of short dental implants in atrophic ridges. However, even if small dental implants (including short and narrow-diameter bodies) are intuitively attractive, cost–benefit and cost-effective-ness analyses are needed to evaluate the long-term efficacy of these options.

Definition

Dental implants with a body ≤ 8 mm length are short (Figure 8.1), while dental implants with a body ≤ 5 mm length are extra-short (Nisand and Renouard, 2014). Given the current lack of consensus, this opinion-based definition seems convenient. In any case, regardless of definition, it does not change the prognosis associated with the implant length.

Implant Dentistry at a Glance, Second Edition. Jacques Malet, Francis Mora and Philippe Bouchard.
© 2018 John Wiley & Sons Ltd. Published 2018 by John Wiley & Sons Ltd.
Companion website: www.wiley.com/go/malet/implant

Figure 8.2 Fixed partial denture supported by two short implants (7 mm length, 4 mm diameter) in positions 35 and 36 and one wide implant (8.5 mm length, 5 mm diameter) in position 37. (a) clinical view; (b) radiographic control.

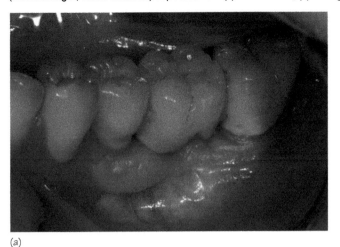

(a)

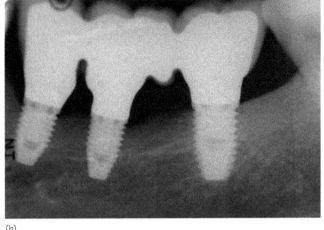

(b)

Figure 8.3 Patient at risk for sinus lift procedure. Fixed partial denture supported by three dental implants. Standard implants are used for 25 and 27 replacement. One short implant (7 mm length, 4 mm diameter) in position 26 avoids bone augmentation procedure. Radiographic control after 5 years of loading.

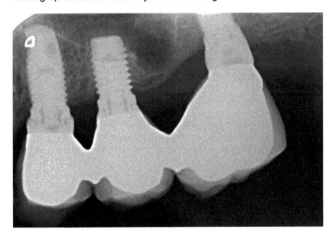

Survival and success rates
Short implants compared to standard implants in native bone

Implant length per se has no impact on marginal bone loss (Monje *et al.*, 2014). Survival and success rates are affected by the primary stability of short implants, which is sometimes hard to achieve in low-density bone (Javed *et al.*, 2013). Thus, in the posterior maxilla, the survival and success of short implants appear to be lower than in the mandible, where bone density is normally higher than in the maxilla (Telleman *et al.*, 2011). Overall, prospective studies now indicate similar survival and success rates for short and standard dental implants (Thoma *et al.*, 2015). The use of rough surfaces as well as adapted surgical techniques may explain the improvement in outcomes.

Short implants compared to standard implants following sinus grafting

Despite a limited number of comparative clinical trials, systematic reviews indicate fewer complications and similar survival rates

Figure 8.4 Short implant use in aesthetic areas. (a) Buccal bone concavity (arrow) does not allow the use of standard implant; (b) standard implant simulation showing the protrusion of the apex out of the cortical plate; (c) optimal 3D short implant position; (d) one-year follow-up.

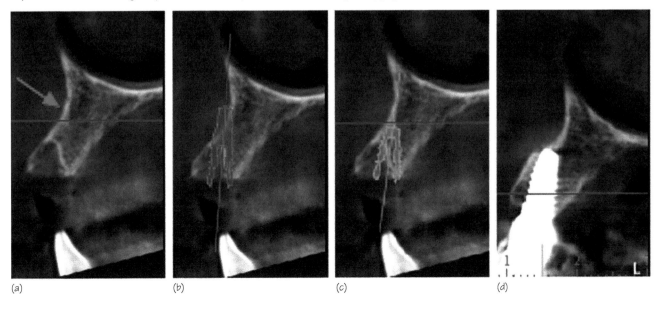

(a) (b) (c) (d)

with short implants compared to standard implants placed in regenerated bone following sinus lift procedures (Fan *et al.*, 2017; Thoma *et al.*, 2015). In addition, patient-reported outcomes and costs favour the short implant approach because sinus lift implies further surgical procedures and morbidity (Thoma *et al.*, 2015).

Extra-short implants

A few case reports highlight some success with extra-short dental implants in the posterior mandible. Nowadays, there is no strong evidence to support the recommendation of extra-short dental implants instead of pre-implant bone graft in the atrophic posterior mandible.

Limitations

Short dental implants can be recommended regardless of prosthetic design or type of edentulism (Figures 8.1 and 8.2). However, consideration of short dental implants normally corresponds to significant bone resorption. This resorption not only leads to a reduction in residual bone dimensions, but also increases the restorative dimension. Consequently, an increased crown/implant ratio is often observed because of the reduction in implant length and augmentation in crown-height space. A recent systematic review indicates that the crown/implant ratio affects peri-implant marginal bone levels (Garaicoa-Pazmino *et al.*, 2014). Within the range of 0.6/1 to 2.36/1, the higher the crown/implant ratio, the lower the peri-implant marginal bone loss. Thus, an excessive interarch distance should not preclude the use of short dental implants. Unfortunately, there are no evidence-based guidelines to indicate a security threshold for an adequate crown/implant ratio, and published crown/implant ratio information is both limited and conflicting. Nowadays, the decision is still based on the practitioner's experience.

The decision-making process is impacted by several parameters. Firstly, the decision to use short implants instead of standard implants in regenerated bone must be balanced against morbidity and surgery-related risks (Figure 8.3). Secondly, the operator's technical skills must be taken into account. Primary stability is sometimes difficult to achieve. There is no stability-related tolerance with short dental implants. They must be completely stable at the end of the surgical procedure. Thirdly, bone density is an important clinical parameter. It has been suggested that, for an acceptable density – that is, no more than type 2 – short or extra-short dental implants may be used even in 5–6 mm of residual bone height. Fourthly, in aesthetic zones, short implants may be indicated when bone dimension makes optimal 3D implant positioning either hazardous or impossible (buccal bone concavities, unfavourable axis, etc.; Figure 8.4). Finally, short implants are not generally recommended for patients at risk of marginal bone loss, such as periodontally compromised patients and heavy smokers.

Clinical recommendations

The following recommendations are adapted to the use of short dental implants:
- Allow a sufficient time laps after extraction (1) to avoid residual bone remodelling, and (2) to achieve coronal cortical anchorage that improves primary stability.
- Underdrilling is recommended in soft bone to promote primary stability.
- Moderately rough implant or bioactive surfaces must be used.
- Avoid heat accumulation, such as excessive bone compression in very dense bone, through strict sequential bone drilling.
- Immediate implant or immediate loading is not recommended.

Key points

- Short dental implants are an option when complex bone augmentation procedures are considered.
- There is no sufficient evidence to recommend extra-short dental implants.
- Bone quality and primary stability are the cornerstones of surgical success.
- Short dental implant placement is technically demanding and requires skilled operators.

Implant macrostructure: Special implants

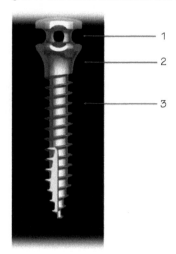

Figure 9.1 A classical orthodontic mini-implant (OMI) design. 1: Head; 2: gingival portion; 3: body. Note the hole of the head's groove that allows orthodontic wire insertion

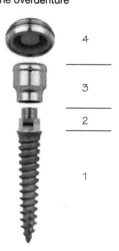

Figure 9.2 A classical mini dental implant (MDI) design (denture stabilisation). 1: Body; 2: implant-abutment connection; 3: abutment; 4: prosthetic component. Note the abutment design matching with the prosthetic component (attachment) included in the overdenture

Figure 9.3 Orthodontic mini-implant (OMI) used as distal anchorage to increase the interdental distance. (a) Preoperative view – note the tilting of the second molar; (b) clinical view at six months; (c) detail of the orthodontic appliance

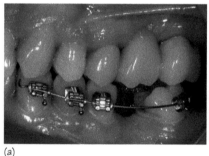
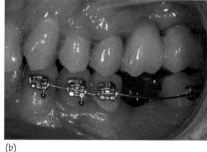
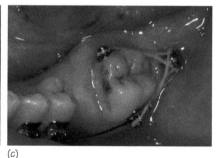

(a)   (b)   (c)

A special implant is a dental implant with a diameter of less than 3 mm, which is not intended to support permanent fixed prostheses. Special implants are mostly used for a limited period of time. They should not be confused with long-term narrow implants, which can be used with any type of prosthetic design. Two types of special implants can be identified according to use: (1) orthodontic mini-implants (OMIs), used as a temporary anchorage device in orthodontic patients (Figure 9.1); and (2) mini dental implants (MDIs), which can be used to support either a temporary prosthesis or a removable overdenture (Figure 9.2).

Orthodontic mini-implants

Orthodontists consider these implants an effective anchorage tool (Antoszewska-Smith *et al.*, 2017; Reynders *et al.*, 2009). Therefore,

the terms 'mini-implant', 'mini-screw' and 'orthodontic implant' are sometimes used interchangeably for this purpose. Orthodontic mini-implants are indicated to shorten the treatment time or as an alternative to extra-oral anchorage (Figure 9.3), which is an issue for most patients.

As the osseointegration process is not a prerequisite for their use, mini-implants can be loaded at different times ranging from 1 day to 4 weeks. An immediate loading protocol (within 48 hours) seems to enhance the mini-implant success rate (Melsen and Costa, 2000).

Orthodontic mini-implant failure is defined by OMI loss or mobility. Failures are more frequent with OMIs than with conventional dental implants. More OMI failures are observed in teenagers than in adults, primarily affecting mini-implants

Implant Dentistry at a Glance, Second Edition. Jacques Malet, Francis Mora and Philippe Bouchard.
© 2018 John Wiley & Sons Ltd. Published 2018 by John Wiley & Sons Ltd.
Companion website: www.wiley.com/go/malet/implant

Figure 9.4 Mini dental implants (MDIs) used to support a provisional fixed restoration. (a) Preoperative view – treatment plan includes extraction of teeth 43, 33 and 34; (b) preoperative X-ray; (c) immediate provisional bridge (34–43) supported by three MDIs after teeth extractions; (d) immediate X-ray control; (e) clinical view at six weeks – note the location of MDIs between the future implant sites (black circles)

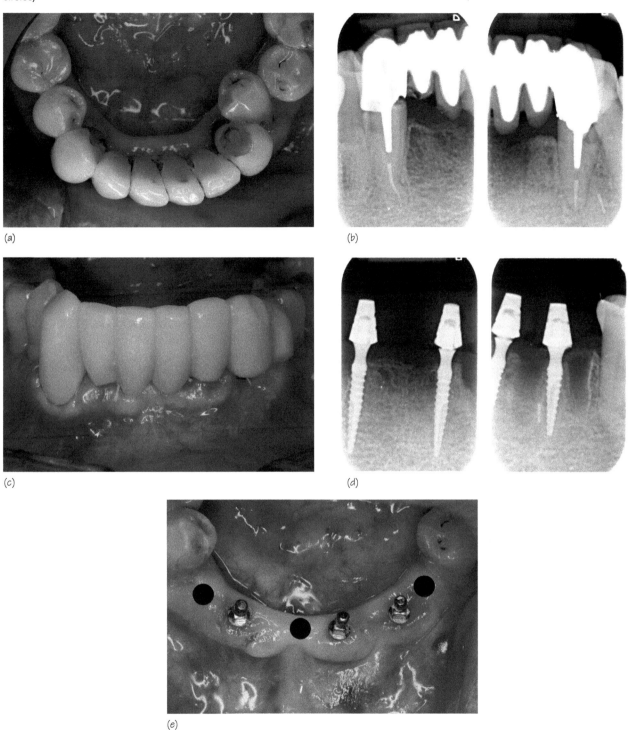

(a)

(b)

(c)

(d)

(e)

placed in the mandibular arch as opposed to the maxilla (Chen *et al.*, 2007; Watanabe *et al.*, 2013).

Pre-implant diagnostic protocol

Soft and hard tissues must be carefully examined before mini-implant placement. The OMI must be placed as closely as possible in the keratinised tissues. A combination of plaster cast and X-ray identifies the precise area of implantation. A thorough periodontal examination indicates the gingival biotype, the location of the mucogingival line and frenal attachments. The

orthodontist indicates the appropriate location of the OMIs on the plaster cast.

A periapical X-ray of the implant placement area is mandatory. The X-ray is used to evaluate bone density and to determine a safe area for implantation; that is, one free from anatomical and dental structures that could be damaged.

Surgical technique

Basically, mini-implant transmucosal placement appears to be a straightforward surgical procedure because it is a flapless approach. However, OMI placement is technically demanding.

Local anaesthesia is performed in the implantation area. Most OMIs are self-tapered. Consequently, no drilling is required, except in the case of thick cortical plates. The OMI should preferably be placed using a manual screwdriver provided that there is adequate surgical accessibility.

Otherwise, the OMI is connected to a contra angle and placed at low speed. Following cortical perforation with a firm grip, manual pressure is decreased to allow soft OMI progression within the alveolar bone between the dental roots. Increased resistance at manual pressure may indicate root contact. Primary stability of the OMI is mandatory. Once stability is achieved, the OMI is loaded within 48 hours. If the OMI is not immediately stable, another location should be considered, as delayed stability cannot be achieved with this type of implant.

Complications such as mucositis, root trauma, nerve and/or microvascular injury, implant fracture and sinus perforation have been described. Care must be taken during patient follow-up, because complications can develop over time. These complications may be of late onset, sometimes occurring 12 months after OMI placement. In the case of late failure, another OMI can be positioned in the same location 3 months later.

Mini dental implants

Mini dental implants are mainly used during the provisional phase of dental implant therapy. Because of the minimally invasive surgical approach and the low cost of MDIs, this indication has been now extended to overdenture. In addition, the small diameter of MDIs allows implant placement in narrow ridges, without bone augmentation procedures.

Many MDIs are now commercially available. Their diameters and lengths range from 1.8 to 2.9 mm and from 6 to 15 mm, respectively. The MDI design depends on the prosthetic indication: denture stabilisation (Figure 9.2) or provisional fixed restoration (Figure 9.4).

Scientific background

Limited data indicate that after 1 to 3 years' follow-up, implant survival rate (ISR) and marginal bone-level changes in MDI-supported overdentures are similar to those in standard implants (Zygogiannis et al., 2016). A systematic review shows that the ISR is higher in the mandible than in the maxilla and an improvement in variables is related to patient satisfaction and quality of life (Lemos et al., 2017). The lack of long-term data precludes the recommendation for MDIs to be used as a straightforward alternative to dental implants (Bidra and Almas, 2013). However, the short-term survival of MDI appears encouraging when used with overdenture. Nowadays, MDIs can be recommended only when validated, conventional surgical approaches cannot be achieved.

Indications

Temporary prosthodontic treatment:
• Stabilisation of dentures or provisional fixed restorations (Figure 9.4) to avoid implant compression during the healing phase
• Treatment of tooth agenesis before the end of growth (Lambert et al., 2017).

Permanent prosthodontic treatment:
• Mandibular overdenture supported by four mini-implants
• Maxillary overdenture supported by six mini-implants.

Clinical procedure

Mini dental implants are usually placed with a flapless procedure in class I and class II native bone. Where possible, cortical bone is recommended in order to achieve optimum MDI stability. After occlusal cortical perforation, the implant is carefully screwed between the cortical plates, with a self-tapping placement, to avoid bone perforation. When used for overdenture stabilisation, MDIs should be placed as parallel as possible. When MDIs are placed for provisional restoration, they must be distal from dental implant sites (Figure 9.4). Insertion torque must be compatible with implant strength (15 to 35 Ncm). Both immediate and delayed loadings are feasible, depending on primary stability, but immediate loading is recommended.

Key points

• Special implants require thorough clinical and X-ray examinations.
• Orthodontic mini-implants are effective orthodontic anchorage devices.
• Short-term data encourage the use of mini dental implants (MDIs) to support overdentures at the mandible.
• MDIs can be recommended only when validated conventional surgical approaches cannot be achieved.
• There is no evidence for the long-term survival of MDIs.

Implant macrostructure: Implant/abutment connection

10

Figure 10.1 Three types of implant/abutment connection. Coronal part of the implant

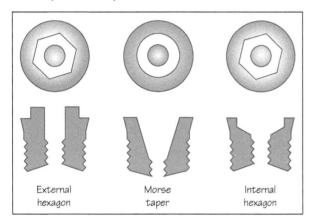

External hexagon   Morse taper   Internal hexagon

Figure 10.2 Three types of implant/abutment connection. Schematic abutment connected

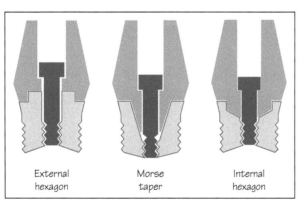

External hexagon   Morse taper   Internal hexagon

Figure 10.3 Interface location (arrows) for submerge-designed implants (1, subcrestal; 2, crestal) and transmucosal-designed implants (A, sulcular; B, supragingival)

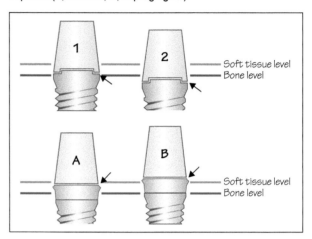

Soft tissue level
Bone level

Soft tissue level
Bone level

Figure 10.4 The standard implant/abutment interface

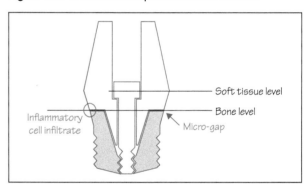

Soft tissue level
Bone level
Inflammatory cell infiltrate
Micro-gap

Figure 10.5 The platform switching concept

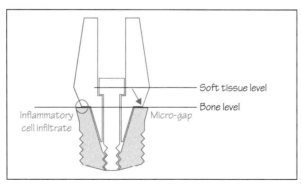

Soft tissue level
Bone level
Inflammatory cell infiltrate
Micro-gap

Implant Dentistry at a Glance, Second Edition. Jacques Malet, Francis Mora and Philippe Bouchard.
© 2018 John Wiley & Sons Ltd. Published 2018 by John Wiley & Sons Ltd.
Companion website: www.wiley.com/go/malet/implant

Abutment connection

This is defined as the interface between the fixture and the prosthetic abutment. The interface may have different designs (Figure 10.1), and is always secured by an abutment screw (Figure 10.2). The implant/abutment connection must be precise and stable. It includes an antirotation device for single-tooth restorations.

Over time, the connection should allow mechanical stability and adequate occlusal load distribution at the implant/abutment interface. From a clinical point of view, the connection enables the clinical recording of the three-dimensional implant position during prosthetic impression (indexing).

The relevant question is: does the connection design influence implant survival rate, marginal bone loss and implant complications?

External connection

Historically, the first implants were designed with a flat butt-joint interface and an *external hexagon* to allow for the recording of the implant location, and to avoid rotation for single-unit restorations. This very well-documented connection allows some micromotion of the interface, and less rigidity during occlusal load transmission.

Internal connection

Different designs of internal connections are available: internal hexagon, Morse taper and cylinder (Table 10.1).

Several implant systems include a Morse taper connection; that is, an internal connection with a conical design (5–10° of conicity) frequently supplemented by a geometric recording device (triangle, hexagon, octagon, dodecagon and so forth). The Morse taper design offers an intimate contact between implant and abutment. It is intended to prevent the rotation of the abutment and to eliminate the microgap.

Table 10.1 Some commercially available implant connection designs

	Connection type	Index device
External		
Nobel Biocare (Branemark)	Hexagon	Hexagon
Internal		
Straumann (massive abutment)	Morse taper	No
Straumann (Synocta)	Morse taper	Octagon
Astra	Morse taper	Dodecagon
Biomet 3i (Certain)	Hexagon + dodecagon	Hexagon + dodecagon
Nobel Biocare (Replace)	Cylinder	Three channels
Zimmer (Screw vent)	Hexagon friction-fit	Hexagon
Ankylos	Morse taper	Six channels

Load transmission

Finite element analysis indicates that occlusal forces (horizontal and axial) are essentially transmitted at the coronal part of the marginal bone. This could explain marginal bone resorption. With a Morse taper connection located at the bone level, it seems that axial loads are transmitted deeper in the bone (Hansson, 2003). The separation between horizontal and vertical stresses could be beneficial to bone stability.

Abutment screw loosening

This is the most common mechanical complication in single-tooth restorations. Screw loosening is the result of stress distribution at the interface (connection design), but it may be influenced by the screw design and material. Machined titanium screws tend to loosen.

Suprisingly, internal connections, whatever the design, and external connections have a similar resistance to screw loosening (Piermatti *et al.*, 2006). In fact, it seems that abutment screw material (gold alloy, coated titanium) and the abutment design prevent screw loosening more than the type of connection.

Interface location

Depending on the system or the surgical procedure, the implant/abutment connection can be located at the bone level (crestal or subcrestal) or at the soft tissue level (above or below the soft tissue interface; Figure 10.3).

For implants initially designed to be used in a submerged protocol (two-stage surgery), the implant/abutment interface is positioned crestally or subcrestally. These implants can also be inserted with a non-submerged protocol (one-stage surgery). In any case, there is a microgap close to the bone level between the abutment and the implant.

On the other hand, transmucosal implants are designed to be placed with a one-stage procedure. For these implants, the fixture/abutment interface is located above the bone level; that is, below or up to the soft tissue margin. Consequently, transmucosal implants eliminate the microgap at the bone level.

Bacterial colonisation

When the prosthetic abutment is connected to the fixture, there is a bacterial colonisation of the microgap between the dental implant and the abutment. On paper, implant connection design may influence this colonisation. Depending on the location of the microgap and the level of micromotion, a potential risk of inflammatory reaction leading to bone resorption occurs.

However, the clinical relevance of this phenomenon is unclear, since marginal bone loss occurs during the first year of function, even for non-submerged implants, and it stabilises over time for most implant systems.

Platform switching

As explained previously, the implant/abutment connection is associated with an inflammatory cell infiltrate localised at the microgap, close to the bone crest (Figure 10.4). This crestal inflammation could explain some peri-implant bone loss located around the dental implant neck. To prevent the crestal bone loss, a reduction of the abutment diameter (*platform switching*) has been proposed to displace the inflammatory infiltrate closer to the abutment; i.e. distant to the crestal contact between the dental implant and the bone. (Figure 10.5). Furthermore, the platform-switching design could modify the biomechanical characteristics of implant/abutment connection by partially moving stress distribution from the compact bone to the cancellous bone.

It should be noted that evidence supporting this concept is weak. Only one comparative study indicates that implants placed in fresh sockets showed no difference in bone-level changes between conventional and platform switching configurations (Crespi *et al.*, 2009).

Key points

- There is no evidence that internal connections have better biomechanical properties than external connections.
- There is no evidence that the type of implant/abutment connection has an impact on the survival rate of dental implants.
- The connection design seems to influence stress distribution.
- The location of the microgap influences peri-implant bone morphology.
- Screw loosening is more influenced by the material and design of the screw than by the type of implant/abutment connection.

Implant microstructure: Implant surfaces

11

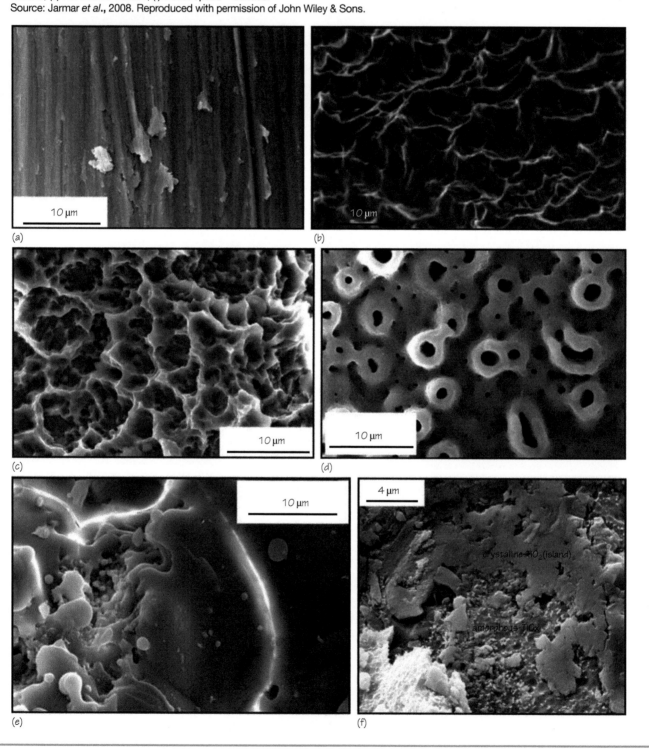

Figure 11.1 Scanning electron microscopy images showing the surface morphology of some commercially available implants. (a) Machined surface; (b) Osseotite™ surface (data from www.biomet3i.com.br/implantenanotite_pg04.asp); (c) SLA™ surface; (d) TiUnite™ surface; (e) HA-coated surface; (f) OsseoSpeed™ surface.
Source: Jarmar *et al.*, 2008. Reproduced with permission of John Wiley & Sons.

Implant Dentistry at a Glance, Second Edition. Jacques Malet, Francis Mora and Philippe Bouchard.
© 2018 John Wiley & Sons Ltd. Published 2018 by John Wiley & Sons Ltd.
Companion website: www.wiley.com/go/malet/implant

Titanium is commonly used for dental implants. There is ongoing development to obtain better anchorage and surface properties. The first generation of dental implants had smooth machined (turned) surfaces (Figure 11.1a). The extensive use of dental implants has led to more and more challenging clinical situations; that is, implant placement in fresh extraction sockets, grafted bone, low bone density and immediate loading. The attachment of transitory structural proteins, such as fibrin, to the machined surfaces was quite poor, and increased failure rates were reported in challenging clinical situations.

The employment of microtextured-surface implants has been shown to improve the retention of these proteins at the implant surface, and to facilitate contact osteogenesis. It has also been demonstrated that microtopographically complex surfaces could increase the bone-to-implant contact (BIC) compared to smooth (machined) surfaces.

Consequently, rough surface implants have been proposed because they integrate more rapidly and have a better BIC than machined implants.

Surface topography

Surface roughness is characterised in terms of amplitude, spacing and hybridity. Spatial parameters describe the texture of the surface. Hybrid parameters describe a combination of spatial and amplitude characteristics. The use of three-dimensional scanning electron microscopy (3D-SEM) provides a set of parameters for detailed description of all kinds of engineering surfaces.

The amplitude is considered to be the most important property of surface topography, and the average height parameter (S_a) is the parameter most frequently used for describing dental implant surfaces. Minimally roughened surfaces ($S_a < 1.0\,\mu m$), such as those of machined implants ($S_a = 0.71\,\mu m$), have been abandoned in favour of moderately roughened surfaces ($S_a = 1–2\,\mu m$).

A surface can be characterised according to microtopography, nanotopography and surface chemistry. However, it is not easy to document in vivo if the biological response to a surface modification is specifically due to one of the characteristics mentioned above.

Surface configurations of some commercially available implants

Some machining procedures aim to create surfaces with bumps (convex surfaces) in contrast to other techniques that create pores (concave surfaces; Wennerberg and Albrektsson, 2010).

Therefore, the machining process is subtractive or additive. In addition, a previously roughened implant surface can be chemically modified.

Blasting
Topography is created by blasting by particles of titanium dioxide (TiOblast™).

Acid etching
The surface is etched in a two-step procedure (Osseotite™; see Figure 11.1b).

Blasting + acid etching
The surface is modified by sand-blasting followed by acid etching (SLA™; $S_a = 1.98 \pm 0.08\,\mu m$; see Figure 11.1c).

Anodic oxidation
The surface is oxidized progressively by increasing the thickness of the oxidized layer in the "apical" direction (TiUnite™; $S_a = 1.55 \pm 0.01\,\mu m$; see Figure 11.1d).

Hydroxyapatite-coated surface
The surface of the dental implant is coated with a deposit of more or less fine particles of hydroxyapatite by a chemical process (Nobel Biocare Steri-Oss® HA-coated; $S_a = 3.29 \pm 1.15\,\mu m$; see Figure 11.1e).

Surface chemistry

Different surfaces are commercially available, including NanoTite™ (nano-scaled calcium phosphate crystals incorporated to the surface of the implant), OsseoSpeed™ (fluoride modification of titanium-blasted surface; see Figure 11.1f), SLActive™ (hydrophilic modification of the SLA™ surface) and Inicell™.

Key points

- Surface modifications have shortened the healing time.
- Rough surfaces may improve the short-term prognosis of the immediate loading protocol.

12 Choice of implant system: General considerations

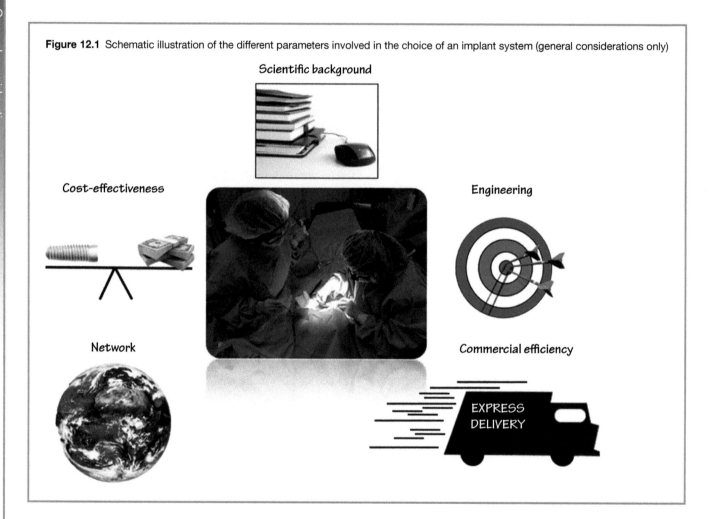

Figure 12.1 Schematic illustration of the different parameters involved in the choice of an implant system (general considerations only)

Scientific background

Cost-effectiveness

Engineering

Network

Commercial efficiency

EXPRESS DELIVERY

The choice of an implant system is a key clinical decision. The decision-making process is based not only on scientific evidence and the ergonomic efficiency of the system, but also on commercial supply (Fig. 12.1). One implant system cannot cover all clinical situations, even if each system tends to advocate a universal approach. The range of implants currently available is rather large and complex within any one system.

Extensive product catalogues are now available. Given the diversity of the implant designs, it is impossible to remember all of the commercial options. In addition, from a practical perspective, it is pointless building up a collection of different implant systems. Instead, practitioners should familiarise themselves with a selective, albeit limited, number of systems.

Scientific background

Scientific background should be of paramount importance when choosing a dental implant system. The choice should normally be limited to implants that have featured in long-term studies published in high-quality scientific publications.

However, most dental implant companies support new concepts in implant dentistry to meet the demands of patients and clinicians alike. These concepts aim (1) to simplify and/or shorten procedures to ensure the timely delivery of prostheses; (2) to improve patients' comfort and quality of life; and (3) to improve immediate or long-term implant stability. New concepts in implant dentistry are mostly based on the rapid commercial availability of new implant designs. It should be noted that, in essence, new concepts are not adequately documented. Many new concepts promoted in the last 20 years have since been taken off the market because of poor short-term outcomes. This applies to some ceramic implants (Cionca *et al.*, 2017) and one-piece implants (Sennerby *et al.*, 2008), for instance.

Nevertheless, it is obviously difficult to wait a decade before marketing an innovation – the fruit of straightforward research and development (R&D) projects. In other words, the dental implant company should be able to provide a sound scientific dossier and professionals should be able to assess the quality of that dossier. If the advantages of the new concept largely outweigh

Implant Dentistry at a Glance, Second Edition. Jacques Malet, Francis Mora and Philippe Bouchard.
© 2018 John Wiley & Sons Ltd. Published 2018 by John Wiley & Sons Ltd.
Companion website: www.wiley.com/go/malet/implant

the limitations associated with a short clinical follow-up, the clinician can carefully consider using the new device.

Dental implant engineering

A biocompatible implant system should provide ergonomic efficiency and prosthetic versatility.

Ergonomic efficiency

The system must be:

• *Easy to use.* A dental implant must be profiled for strength, stability and ease of insertion. Each implant system is delivered with a specific set of instruments for drilling and implant placement. It is important to simplify the drilling protocol to prevent any distortion between the drill hole and the implant. Consequently, a reduced range of drills with well-defined sequences is recommended.

• *Precise and flexible.* The drill set must allow accurate bone preparation in accordance with the pre-planned implant position. Guided drills are recommended to maintain the initally planned dental implant direction, but should allow for any per-operative change in dental implant direction, when necessary. Visible depth marks on dental implant drills, and possibly depth stops, improve drilling pecision. The implant driver should be sufficiently retentive, but easy to remove from the implant with minimal pressure in the event of low primary stability.

• *Easy to clean.* The reprocessing of instruments depends on the design of the surgical cassette, which must comply with current sterilisation techniques. Ideally, disposable drills should allow efficient bone preparation, thereby limiting the bone-heating risk and avoiding cleaning problems.

Prosthetic versatility and precision

• The implant system(s) should cover a wide range of prosthetic options. Such systems should facilitate screw-retained and cemented restorations. Although both options are effective, there are specific indications for each solution (see Chapter 32). The implant system should also be compatible with current prosthetic computer-aided design and manufacture (CAD/CAM) technologies (see Chapters 43 and 44).

• In addition, the precision of the implant/abutment connection is crucial, because a stable connection prevents micromotion and reduces the risk of unscrewing or microgap opening during occlusal loading.

Cost-effectiveness

Professional choice must be guided by the most efficient and least expensive implant system that provides optimal teeth replacement in the long term. The cost of dental implant systems has a substantial impact on the patient's fees and the clinician's profits! Thus, the cost-effectiveness of each dental implant system must be carefully weighed, bearing in mind not only the immediate costs but also costs over time.

Commercial efficiency

Swift turnaround times in terms of implant delivery, after-sales service and warranties must be considered when choosing an implant system. Most companies offer next-day deliveries and issue warranties of 5–10 years. A warranty covers replacement of the dental implant and prosthetic components. A detailed questionnaire generally accompanies the warranty in support of the post-marketing monitoring programme.

The dental implant 'network'

Local professional networking systems are important. Some companies work closely with practitioners in the same geographical area. This may be useful when advice is required. It is also important to identify the system used in nearby hospitals. These hospitals often organise continuing training courses and seminars which will benefit private practitioners. Some companies also have training and professional development departments that offer training at various levels of experience.

Key points

• Scientific background is pivotal when selecting an implant system.
• Surgical and prosthetic precision are key factors.
• Cost-effectiveness and commercial efficiency must also be considered.

13 Choice of implant system: Clinical considerations

Figure 13.1 Choice of implant collar according to aesthetic requirements. (a) This implant collar is designed to be placed at the bone level; (b) this implant collar is smooth and is not indicated in aesthetic zones

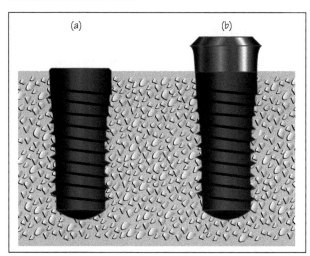

Figure 13.2 Choice of implant design according to primary stability requirements. (a) This implant body is cylindrical and is advisable in standard situations when the bone is completely healed; (b) this implant body is tapered and is advisable to improve primary stability in low-density bone and/or non-completely healed bone

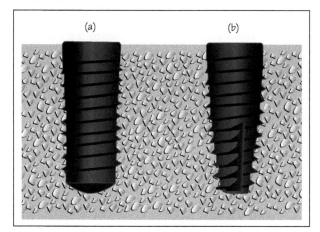

Table 13.1 Main characteristics of five well-documented implant systems

	Material	Surface		Body design	Collar design	Implant-abutment connection
BIOMET 3i Certain®	Cp-Ti Ti6Al4V	Osseotite® *MR*		Parralel *PW* NT® *T*	Smooth or rough	Internal double hex
DENTSPLY Astratech®	Cp-Ti	Osseospeed® *MR*		Straight *PW* Conical *T*	Rough + microgrooves	Internal cone
NOBELBIOCARE Branemark®	Cp-Ti	Ti Unite® *MR*		MKIII® *PW* MKIV® *T*	Smooth Rough	External hex
STRAUMANN®	Cp-Ti Roxolid®	SLA® *MR*	SLA Active *MR/H*	Tissue level® *PW* Bone level® *PW* Bone level tapered® *T*	Smooth/two heights Rough Rough	Synocta® Crossfit®
THOMMEN®	Cp-Ti	SPI® *MR*	SPI Inicell® *MR/H*	Element® *PW* Contact® *T*	Smooth/four heights	Internal hex + stabilisation ring

Cp-Ti, commercially pure titanium; Crossfit®, internal cone + grooves; H, hydrophilic surface; MR, moderately rough surface; mR, minimally rough surface; PW, parallel walls; Synocta®, morse taper + octagon; T, tapered.

Implant Dentistry at a Glance, Second Edition. Jacques Malet, Francis Mora and Philippe Bouchard.
© 2018 John Wiley & Sons Ltd. Published 2018 by John Wiley & Sons Ltd.
Companion website: www.wiley.com/go/malet/implant

Many clinical cases require standard protocols (see Chapter 40). Therefore, in 'classical' situations in non-aesthetic areas without excessive ridge deficiency, implant selection is straightforward, and standard implants are mostly indicated (see Chapter 28). Nowadays, regardless of anatomical constraints, patients are increasingly demanding in terms of aesthetics and functional stability. Various implant designs are commercially available to satisfy patient demands and numerous dental implant systems are adapted to most clinical situations.

Table 13.1 provides an overview of the main characteristics of five documented dental implant systems. This table highlights the key dental implant parameters taken into account in the decision-making process when an implant choice arises. These parameters include the material and surface of the dental implant, the design of the body and collar, and the abutment connection. Aesthetics, surgical timing, bone dimension and density, as well as periodontal history, are clinical features that affect the choice of dental implant. Most of these parameters are discussed in detail in other chapters.

Aesthetics

Two major requirements must be considered in aesthetic zones to achieve dental implant success over time.

Firstly, the dental implant must guarantee soft tissue stability. The dental implant collar must be located subgingivally at bone level (Figure 13.1). It has been suggested that dental implants without a collar or with a minimally smooth collar are preferable to rough collar implants, especially when the soft tissue phenotype is thin. However, a recent meta-analysis indicates less marginal bone loss with rough-surface implants and rough-surface microthreaded neck than with machined-neck implants (Koodaryan and Hafezeqoran, 2016). As the implant neck is often located at depth, the stability of the *implant–abutment connection* is a major determinant of long-term implant success. Micromotion at the implant–abutment level has been identified. No perfect implant collar geometry or perfect manufacturing technique that would result in undetectable micromotion has been identified to date (Karl and Taylor, 2016).

Secondly, guided bone regeneration (GBR) procedures are often required in aesthetic zones. Thus, dental implants are often placed into grafted bone. When a GBR procedure is planned, dental implants with rough surfaces should be chosen (see below).

Finally, zirconia ceramics have been proposed to replace titanium, first for the abutment, then for the implant body, in order to improve aesthetics. Zirconia implants are commercially available. They display high biocompatibility and aesthetic integration, but cannot yet be recommended because of a high incidence of early failures (Cionca et al., 2017).

Timing of implant placement

A dental implant can be inserted before the extraction socket bone has completely healed, even at the time of tooth extraction (Chapter 41). The primary stability of the dental implant as well as the speed of the osseointegration are key factors in immediate, immediate-delayed and delayed implantation approaches. Because of their self-tapping property, tapered implants appear to be particularly suitable for achieving good primary stability in a fresh extraction socket (De Bruyn et al., 2014; Figure 13.2). Various types of surface roughness have been proposed in order to accelerate osseointegration and improve bone-to-implant contact (BIC). The cutting design of the implant threads in the body, especially at the apex, also appears to be an important parameter for primary stability.

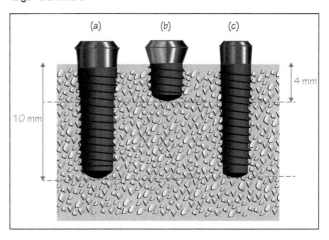

Figure 13.3 Type of dental implant adapted to bone dimensions. (a) Standard implant; (b) very short implant; (c) narrow implant. Standard and very short dental implants are also available with larger diameters

Bone dimension

The dimensions of the edentulous area may be insufficiently large for the surgical placement of standard dental implants. 'Small' implants, including narrow-diameter and very short implants (Figure 13.3), may be used when bone augmentation procedures cannot be performed or when the patient refuses any surgery in addition to the implant placement (Figure 13.4). Implant survival rates (ISR) and success rates of narrow-diameter dental implants range from 93.8% to 100% and 91.4% to 97.6%, respectively (Klein et al., 2014). No significant differences have been shown between narrow-diameter implants and standard implants in terms of ISR and success rates.

The major drawback to the use of narrow-diameter dental implants is the risk of body fracture. Most commercially available dental implants are manufactured from titanium, because of its high biocompatibility and strength. Commercially pure titanium (cp-Ti) and titanium alloys (Ti6Al4V and TiZr) display excellent corrosion resistance and biocompatibility. Commercially pure titanium is classified into four categories according to oxygen content, ranging from grade 1 (lowest oxygen content) to grade 4 (highest oxygen content), which is the strongest.

Titanium alloys have been developed to improve the mechanical properties of titanium for specific indications such as very short or small-diameter implants. Most documented titanium alloys are titanium–aluminium–valadium (Ti6Al4V) and titanium–zirconium (TiZr1317). It has been suggested that the addition of different components to cp-Ti may decrease biocompatibility. Recent experimental data indicate that cp-Ti, TiZr and Ti6Al4V fail to demonstrate differences in osseointegration and biomechanical anchorage (Saulacic et al., 2012; Shah et al., 2016). However, TiZr and cp-Ti implants display faster osseointegration than Ti6Al4V implants. Furthermore, there is no comparative clinical trial showing a significant long-term clinical difference between the types of material.

Bone density
Native bone

Low bone densities (types 3 and 4) are sometimes found, especially in the posterior maxilla area. Provided that dental implant stability is sufficient and the healing time extended, osseointegration is predictably achievable in this type of bone. The posterior maxilla exhibits similar ISR to other locations when rough-surface dental implants are used (Stach and Kohles, 2003).

Figure 13.4 (a) Narrow-diameter implant used to avoid bone augmentation procedure at a mandible narrow ridge, allowing placement of a 3.3 mm diameter implant (right) instead of a standard implant with a bone dehiscence (left/red arrow). (b) Clinical view (five-year follow-up) of the four-units fixed partial dentures, including standard dental implants (4.0 mm diameter) to replace teeth #34 and 37, and a narrow dental implant to replace tooth #36. (c) radiographic control 5 years after dental implant placement.

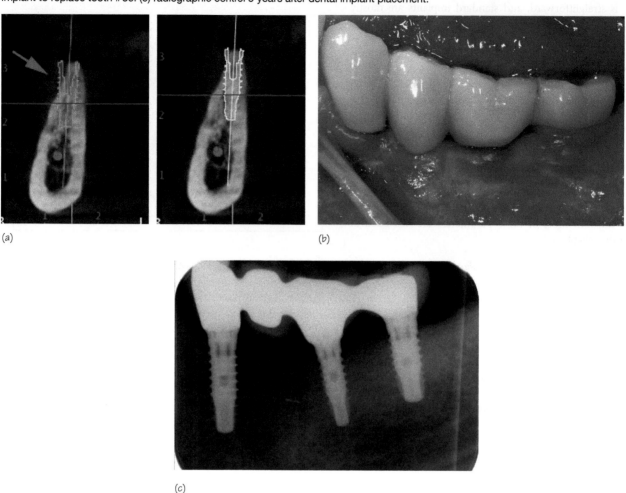

(a) (b)

(c)

In addition, as shown above, tapered dental implants are suitable for soft bone (Figure 13.2).

Regenerated bone

Regardless of the graft material, the initial BIC in the regenerated bone is lower than the BIC in native bone. Thus, the healing time for osseointegration is longer into grafted bone than into native bone. Compared to turned or minimally rough surfaces, rougher surfaces may enhance bone response to improve the initial BIC and reduce healing periods (Bornstein *et al.*, 2005; Sullivan *et al.*, 2005). Bioactive surface coatings (mostly hydrophilic) seem to promote osseointegration during the early stages of healing, and may improve the healing time (Lang *et al.*, 2011; Smeets *et al.*, 2016).

Periodontally compromised patients

Patients with a history of treated periodontitis are more susceptible to peri-implantitis than non-periodontal patients (see Chapter 21). The reduction in initial peri-implant marginal bone remodelling after abutment connection and the prevention of peri-implantitis are clinical considerations in terms of implant choice. The stability of the implant–abutment connection and the location of the microgap are two major factors in preventing or reducing marginal bone remodelling.

Ideally, the microgap should be placed distant from the bone crest to prevent crestal bone remodelling and implant surface exposure. Fig 13.1 (b) shows an implant design that fullfil this recommendation. The machined collar is only in contact with the soft tissue and the microgap is distant from the bone crest. The smooth surface of the dental implant neck may also reduce the risk of peri-implantitis because it may prevent peri-implant plaque formation.

Key points

- Rough bone-level dental implants without a neck are recommended in aesthetic zones.
- Tapered implants with a rough surface should be used in fresh extraction sockets.
- Ti6Al4V and titanium–zirconium alloys are adequate materials for small implants.
- Tapered implants with a rough surface are indicated in areas of low bone density.
- Rough implants with bioactive surface modification are indicated in regenerated bone areas.
- Dental implants with a smooth collar design at the soft tissue level are recommended in periodontally compromised patients.

14 Success, failure, complications and survival

Figure 14.1 Factors that may influence implant longevity

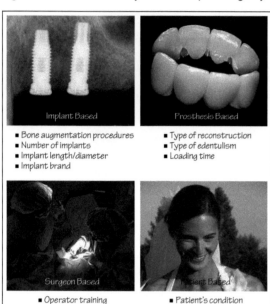

Figure 14.2 Estimated implant loss after five years of function according to the type of prosthesis. FPDs, fixed partial dentures
Data sources: 1. Lang *et al.*, 2004; 2. Berglundh *et al.*, 2002. Reproduced with permission of John Wiley & Sons

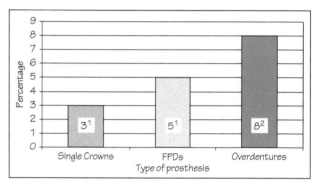

Figure 14.3 Ten-year survival estimate of tooth-supported fixed partial dentures (FPDs), implant-supported FPDs, tooth-implant FPDs and implant-supported single crowns (SCs)
Data source: Pjetursson, 2008. Reproduced with permission of John Wiley & Sons

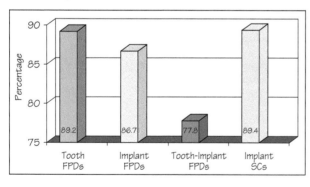

Figure 14.5 Implant-supported single crowns: cumulative five-year biological complications
Data source: Pjetursson, 2008. Reproduced with permission of John Wiley & Sons

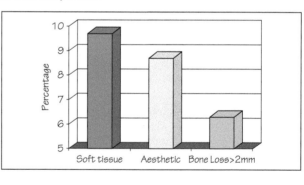

Different factors may influence implant longevity (Figure 14.1). Therefore, from a statistical point of view, it is difficult to draw a definitive conclusion on the percentage of 'success' of a dental implant. In 2008, the School of Bern produced estimates to give a comparative overview of prevalence values in implant dentistry (see Figures 14.3–14.5), and they are still valid. Figure 14.2 gives some data that provide a picture of the longevity of dental implants according to the type of reconstruction. A more recent systematic review, including 23 studies with a mean follow-up time of 13.4 years, indicates survival rates and mean marginal bone resorption values of 94.6% and 1.3 mm, respectively (Moraschini *et al.*, 2015). The first attempts to evaluate dental implant 'success' were the measurement of the overall survival of implants using life table analyses. The statistical unit was the dental implant. Nowadays, the evaluation of dental implant success takes into account the lack of complications.

Implant Dentistry at a Glance, Second Edition. Jacques Malet, Francis Mora and Philippe Bouchard.
© 2018 John Wiley & Sons Ltd. Published 2018 by John Wiley & Sons Ltd.
Companion website: www.wiley.com/go/malet/implant

Figure 14.4 Cumulative five-year biological and mechanical complications
Data source: Pjetursson, 2008. Reproduced with permission of John Wiley & Sons

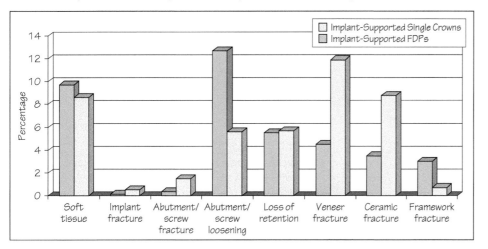

Dental implants: The best treatment option?

Regarding the single tooth replacement, there is no doubt that an implant single crown is the dominant strategy (less costly, more efficient and more cost-effective) when compared with tooth-supported fixed partial dentures (FPDs; Bouchard *et al.*, 2009; Popelut *et al.*, 2010a). In other cases, the literature indicates that the success rate of dental implant therapies is predictable (Figure 14.3).

What is a success?

Taking into account that dental implant therapy is an elective procedure, a patient-centred approach may be the best choice in terms of evaluation. Thus, it seems that the modern definition of 'success' can be simply stated as follows: *A dental implant therapy is successful when there are no complications over time and when the patient is satisfied.*

Nowadays, the following definitions, related to implant stability after surgical placement, are commonly used.

Success

Definition: the dental implant and the prosthetic reconstruction are present in the mouth of the patient without any complications.

Many attempts have been made to establish success criteria in implant dentistry. Success should ideally evaluate the long-term primary outcome of an implant–prosthetic complex as a whole (Papaspyridakos *et al.*, 2012). The most frequently reported criteria are listed in Box 14.1.

Failure

Failures can be divided into two types, depending on whether they relate to the dental implant or to the prosthetic reconstruction.

Implant failure (synonym: implant loss)

Definition: the dental implant and the prosthetic reconstruction, if any, cannot be used or are no longer present in the mouth of the patient.

Traditionally, two types of implant failures can be observed:
• Primary failure (synonym: early failure): failure to establish osseointegration.
• Secondary failure (synonym: late failure): failure to maintain the achieved osseointegration.

Box 14.1 Most frequently reported criteria for success in implant dentistry according to different levels.
Source: adapted from Papaspyridakos *et al.*, 2012

Implant
• Lack of mobility
• Lack of pain
• Lack of radiolucency
• Lack of peri-implant bone loss (>1.5 mm)

Peri-implant soft tissue
• Lack of suppuration
• Lack of bleeding

Prosthesis
• Lack of technical complications/prosthetic maintenance
• Adequate function
• Aesthetics

Patient
• Lack of discomfort
• Lack of paraesthesia
• Satisfaction with appearance
• Ability to chew/taste

The terms 'early' and 'late' failure relate to the implant loss before or after loading. The immediate loading procedure has changed this approach. Thus, the terms 'primary' and 'secondary' failure are nowadays more appropriate.

Prosthetic failure

Definition: the reconstruction cannot be used or is no longer present in the mouth of the patient.

Trends indicate that implant single crowns perform better than FPDs and overdentures (see Figure 14.2). A systematic review dealing with the loading times – that is, including immediately, early and conventionally loaded implants – indicates that, after one year of function, 2.6% of placed dental implants failed (48/1,852) and 4.7% of placed restorations failed (36/767; Esposito *et al.*, 2009). The authors indicate that the risk of failure depends on patient selection and operator training. More failures occur among the early than the immediately loaded implants, which appear to be at higher risk of failure than conventionally loaded implants.

A recent pooled analysis of systematic studies indicates a mean annual implant failure rate of about 1% (Popelut *et al.*, 2010b). The annual failure rate was 2.73% when the studies were not sponsored by the industry and 0.88% when the studies were supported by the industry.

Survival

Theoretically, survival rates should be divided into two types, depending on whether they relate to the dental implant or to the prosthetic reconstruction.

Implant survival

Definition: the dental implant is present at the follow-up examination.

Prosthetic survival

Definition: the prosthetic reconstruction is present at the follow-up examination.

Complication

Definition: the dental implant and/or the reconstruction show problem(s) that compromise their prognosis or their normal use by the patient.

Data indicate that complications occur in about 50% of patients after five years of function (Lang *et al.*, 2004).

Complications can be divided into two types, depending on whether they are related to the surrounding tissues (biological complications) or to the prosthetic restoration (technical complications; Figures 14.4 and 14.5).

Biological complications

• *Mucositis*: reversible peri-implant inflammation limited to the soft tissues. Meta-analysis estimated a weighted mean prevalence for peri-implant mucositis of 43% (confidence interval [CI]: 32–54%; Derks and Tomasi, 2015).
• *Peri-implantitis*: non-reversible peri-implant inflammation extended to the bone and characterised by bone loss around the dental implant. The same meta-analysis estimated the prevalence for peri-implantitis at 22% (CI: 14–30%).
• *Peri-implant abscess*: acute peri-implant infection with localized collection of pus.

Technical complications (synonym: mechanical complications)

• *Fractures*: implant, screw, abutment, veneer, metal framework
• *Loosening*: screw, abutment
• *Loss of retention* (fracture of the luting cement).

Data indicate that implant-supported reconstructions may have up to a threefold higher incidence of technical complications than tooth-supported reconstructions (Lang and Salvi, 2008).

The crown-to-implant ratio does not seem to influence peri-implant crestal bone loss (Blanes, 2009).

Key points

• The risk of failure in dental implants can be substantially minimised by proper patient selection and well-trained operators.
• Complications are frequent (50% after five years).
• More failures occur among the early than the immediately loaded implants.

The implant team

Figure 15.1 The basic team

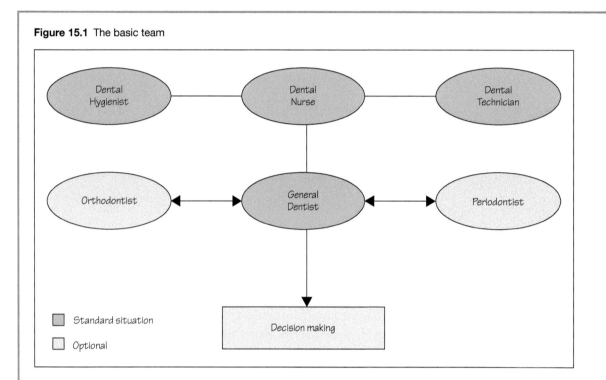

Figure 15.2 The extended team

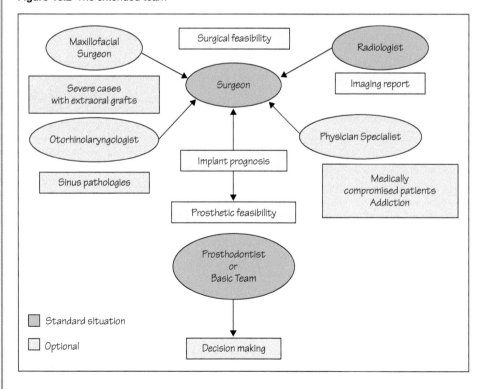

Implant Dentistry at a Glance, Second Edition. Jacques Malet, Francis Mora and Philippe Bouchard.
© 2018 John Wiley & Sons Ltd. Published 2018 by John Wiley & Sons Ltd.
Companion website: www.wiley.com/go/malet/implant

Basically, dental implant therapy combines (i) surgical treatment aiming to place the implant in the jaws, and (ii) restorative treatment aiming to replace the teeth supported by the implants. In addition, prior to the treatment, a radiographic examination is mandatory.

Over time, the sophistication of surgical and prosthetic techniques has led to unlimited possibilities for the placement of dental implants in the oral cavity. Therefore, apart from some drastic medical contraindications, from a technical point of view *it is always possible to place implants*, even when there is a lack of supporting bone. Consequently, patient demands are now higher in terms of success. The term 'success' not only includes a functional demand, but also an aesthetic result and minimum complications.

In the dental implant team, a well-trained general dentist may assume the full treatment of simple cases; that is, when a sufficient amount of bone is present in non-aesthetic areas and when the periodontal status of the patient does not require a specialist. In other cases, which are increasingly frequent, a more extended team approach must be considered.

The basic dental implant team should include at least the following (Figure 15.1):
• a general dentist competent in basic dental implant diagnosis and therapy, basic periodontal diagnosis and therapy, basic dental implant surgery and prostheses
• a dental nurse competent in surgical assistance and perioperative care
• a dental hygienist competent in dental implant maintenance
• a dental technician competent in dental implant prostheses.

In addition, some cases may necessitate the collaboration of dental specialist consultants such as:
• a periodontist
• an orthodontist
• an endodontist
• a specialist in paediatric dentistry.

The extended team should include at least the following (Figure 15.2):
• a radiologist competent in dental digital imaging
• a surgeon competent in the surgical management of advanced periodontal diseases and conditions, and dental implant placement and ancillary intraoral grafting procedures
• a prosthodontist or a general dentist competent in dental occlusion and aesthetics.

In addition, some advanced cases may require the collaboration of the following:
• a maxillofacial surgeon competent in autogenous bone grafting from extraoral sources
• an otorhinolaryngologist competent in maxillary sinus pathologies
• physician specialist(s) competent in the patient's condition and in the management of addiction such as tobacco smoking, alcohol consumption and drug abuse.

Who is the head of the team?

In all cases, *the general dentist/prosthodontist should be the team captain*; that is, the person who collects the information and ensures treatment follow-up in accordance with the patient's need. They are the cornerstone of the decision-making process because they are the project manager.

Before surgical decision making, the surgeon must answer the following questions:
• What is the periodontal status of the patient?
  • Does the patient need periodontal treatment before the implant placement?
  • What is the risk of loss of the teeth bordering the implants?
• What are the surgical constraints of the prosthetic treatment plan?
  • What are the surgical risks for the patient?
  • What percentage of success can be expected following the surgical procedure(s)?
  • What is the full length of the surgical procedure(s)?
  • What are the total fees for the surgical part of the treatment?
• What are the alternative surgical options if the patient does not accept the initial treatment plan?

Key points

• A simple case is one where a sufficient amount of bone is present in non-aesthetic areas.
• There is no need for an extended team in simple cases.
• For complex cases, patient demand and conditions determine the team composition.
• In all cases, the general dentist/prosthodontist is the head of the team.
• A periodontal examination is mandatory before implant placement.

16 Patient evaluation: Medical evaluation form and laboratory tests

Figure 16.1 A basic physical examination that can be performed in the dental practice. (a) Body Mass Index: scales and a measuring rod should be used to calculate the patient's BMI. (b) High blood pressure: the blood pressure should be measured with a sphygmomanometer and stethoscope. The patient must be in a sitting position and at rest. (c) Diabetic patients: the surgeon may use a blood glucose meter to measure the glucose level before a surgical procedure.

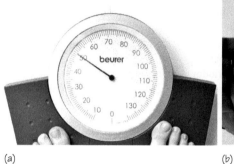

(a)

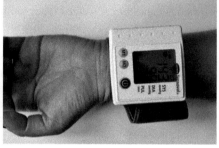

(b)

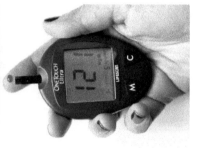

(c)

Table 16.1 International normalised ratios (INR) for specific conditions

Patient condition	INR value
Normal	1.0
Prevention of myocardial infarction	2.0–3.0
Treatment of pulmonary embolism	2.0–3.0
Treatment of atrial fibrillation	2.0–3.0
Pulmonary embolism	2.0–3.0
Prosthetic heart valves	2.5–3.5
Prevention of venous thrombosis	2.5–3.5

Box 16.1 Routine laboratory screening and vital signs that may be useful before dental implant surgery

Laboratory tests
- Complete blood count
- Prothrombin time (INR test)
- Glycaemic control: glycated haemoglobin measurement (normality: 4–6%)

Vital signs
- Blood pressure (normality: 140/90 mmHg)
- Pulse rate (normality: 60–80 bpm)
- Oral temperature (normality: 36.8 ± 0.7 °C or 98.2 ± 1.3 °F)
- Respiration rate (normality: 12–20 breaths per minute)

bpm, beats per minute; INR, international normalised ratio.

Box 16.2 American Society of Anesthesiologists physical status classification system

P1 A normal healthy patient
P2 A patient with mild systemic disease
P3 A patient with severe systemic disease
P4 A patient with severe systemic disease that is a constant threat to life
P5 A moribund patient who is not expected to survive without the operation
P6 A declared brain-dead patient whose organs are being removed for donor purposes

Implant Dentistry at a Glance, Second Edition. Jacques Malet, Francis Mora and Philippe Bouchard.
© 2018 John Wiley & Sons Ltd. Published 2018 by John Wiley & Sons Ltd.
Companion website: www.wiley.com/go/malet/implant

The information on medical history in Chapters 16 and 17 is not to be construed as a standard of care or guidelines, which may legally vary based on locale. In view of the relatively low prevalence rate of postoperative complications in the general population, limited evidence is available to guide clinicians in regard to the possible increased risks of dental implant procedures associated with non-healthy patients.

The major difference between dental implant surgery and most of the other oral surgeries is that it does not treat an ongoing disease or a current infection, but treats an oral condition (edentulism). The implant failure may induce an unexpected infection that may have serious consequences in patients with poor health. Therefore, the famous precept of Hippocrates, *primum non nocere* (first, do no harm), is particularly relevant to this type of elective surgery. Consequently, it is mandatory to take the medical history of candidates for implant therapy and to include it in the medical records.

The medical history informs the surgeon on:
• the surgical risk (Chapter 17)
• the implant failure risk (Chapter 18).

Completion of a medical history form is requested to obtain a written record for every individual patient (Appendix D). The past medical history and medication usage within the preceding six months are of particular importance. This form is not a sufficient medical evaluation, and must be supported by a medical interview. The implant surgeon reviews it with the patient. Any health conditions/problems must be documented in the patient's records (Chapter 26).

Dental implant surgery is not specific in terms of contraindications as compared to other intraoral surgeries. There are very few absolute contraindications. However, there are many situations of risk that must be carefully evaluated.

As a rule of thumb, dental implant placement should be postponed in patients who have a disease that can be treated, until the patient is cured or stabilised. This is also true for oral conditions such as dental caries or periodontal diseases, which must be treated *before* dental implant placement.

The clinical risk assessment for perioperative complications must be individually based on the medical history of the individual patient. In light of the interview and the medical examination (Figure 16.1), if necessary the surgeon may record vital signs and prescribe common laboratory tests (Box 16.1, Table 16.1). The American Society of Anesthesiologists (ASA) classification system (Box 16.2) may also be used, but this classification merely provides a general idea of patient risks during surgery. In addition, only P1 patients are safe candidates for dental implant placement.

It must be understood that the lists on the medical history form are not all-inclusive and represent the more commonly occurring diseases and conditions. In addition, physician approval is required for treatment of all medically compromised patients.

Key points
• Dental implant placement should be postponed in patients with a treatable disease until the patient is cured or stabilised.
• Physician approval is required for treatment of all medically compromised patients.

17 Patient evaluation: Surgery and the patient at risk

Figure 17.1 The patient at risk during the surgical procedure: the risk of bleeding. (a) Extraction socket in an anticoagulated patient. (b) A collagen sponge is inserted in the socket. (c) Clinical view of the collagen sponge in situ. (d) The soft tissues are tightly sutured over the resorbable material. Note the immediate cessation of bleeding

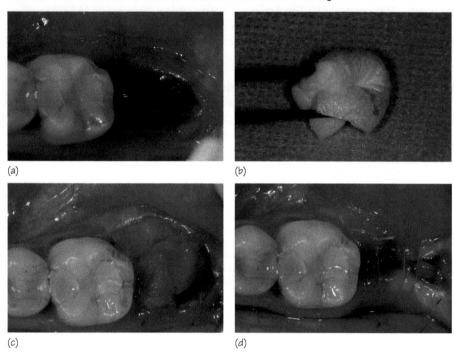

(a)

(b)

(c)

(d)

Box 17.1 How to prevent the risk of bleeding in anticoagulated patients

Before the surgery
- Good plaque control is important before performing the surgical procedures
- The surgery should ideally be scheduled at the beginning of the day and early in the week

During the surgery
- A local anaesthetic containing a vasoconstrictor should be administered
- Regional nerve blocks should be avoided
- Efforts should be made to make the procedure atraumatic
- Absorbable haemostatic dressings (Surgicel®, Haemocollagen®, Spongostan® or others) should be used
- Resorbable sutures are preferable as they attract less plaque
- Following closure, the patient bites down on a wet gauze pad for 20 minutes; the gauze may be soaked with tranexamic acid (Exacyl®)

After the surgery
- Patients should be given clear written instructions on management of the clot
- The following medications should be avoided because they may interact with the anticoagulants: metronidazole, aspirin and non-steroidal anti-inflammatory drugs (NSAIDs)

Box 17.2 How to prevent stress

Before the surgery
- Premedication on the night before the appointment (anxiolytic)
- Setting an early morning appointment
- Minimising waiting room time

During the surgery
- Duration of the surgery not exceeding the patient's limits
- Profound anaesthesia

After the surgery
- Excellent postoperative pain control

Implant Dentistry at a Glance, Second Edition. Jacques Malet, Francis Mora and Philippe Bouchard.
© 2018 John Wiley & Sons Ltd. Published 2018 by John Wiley & Sons Ltd.
Companion website: www.wiley.com/go/malet/implant

Absolute contraindications

An absolute contraindication is a condition that makes a particular treatment or procedure, such as dental surgery, absolutely inadvisable.

ASA P5 and P6 patients

See Box 16.2.

Chemotherapies in malignancies

The potential side-effects, including immunosuppression and myelosuppression, prevent any dental implant surgery during the active phase of chemotherapy.

Radiotherapy

The risk of osteoradionecrosis exists, even six months after radiotherapy treatment (Brasseur et al., 2006). Hyperbaric oxygen therapy does not seem to offer an evident clinical benefit (Esposito et al., 2008).

Cardiac conditions

The most critical risk is infective endocarditis, which is a life-threatening infection. The following cardiac conditions associated with the highest risk of adverse outcomes from endocarditis prohibit any dental implant surgery:
• Prosthetic cardiac valve or prosthetic material used for cardiac valve repair
• Previous infective endocarditis
• Congenital heart disease (CHD):
  • Unrepaired cyanotic CHD, including palliative shunts and conduits
  • Completely repaired congenital heart defect with prosthetic material or device, whether placed by surgery or by catheter intervention, during the first six months after the procedure
  • Repaired CHD with residual defects at the site or adjacent to the site of a prosthetic patch or prosthetic device (which inhibits its endothelialisation)
• Cardiac transplantation recipients who develop cardiac valvulopathy.

Transplantation

After a transplant, patients are given immunosuppressive medications to prevent the body from rejecting the new organ. Therefore, they may have an increased risk of infection, especially during the first months when dosages are higher because of the increased risk of rejection. The dental implant surgery must be postponed, and the dental implant indication discussed at a later time with the specialists.

Dialysis catheters

Catheter-related infection is one of the major causes of morbidity in dialysis patients, such as those treated for end-stage renal disease (ESRD). Thus, any non-vital surgery that may potentially induce bacteraemia must be postponed.

Intravenous bisphosphonates

These are administered to patients with breast cancer, multiple myeloma, hypercalcaemia of malignancy, and bone metastasis in breast, prostate, lung and other cancers. Nowadays, dental implant surgeries are contraindicated for patients who take intravenous bisphosphonates because these have been associated with the onset of bisphosphonate-related osteonecrosis of the jaws (BRONJ). The prevalence of BRONJ in patients receiving intravenous bisphosphonates is 5–12% (Sanz and Naert, 2009). When bisphosphonate treatment has started before dental implant placement, it has been shown that clinical signs of BRONJ may appear more than one year after dental implant surgery (Lazarovici et al., 2010).

Relative contraindications

Relative contraindications are conditions that make a particular treatment or procedure somewhat inadvisable but do not rule it out, unless it is absolutely necessary. Dental implant therapy is never absolutely necessary. Thus, relative contraindications may not exist per se in this area. However, for the reader's ease of understanding, a gradation can clarify the medical risk in implant therapies.

ASA P3 and P4 patients

See Box 16.2. The indication for dental implant surgery must be discussed with the physician according to the level of the surgical treatment (number of dental implants, pre-implant surgery) and the severity of the systemic disease.

Cardiac conditions

Cardiovascular diseases that are not an absolute contraindication (see above) may constitute relative contraindications that must be discussed with the cardiologists.

Oral bisphosphonates

These are used in the treatment of diseases such as osteoporosis (post-menopausal and steroid induced) and Paget's disease of bone. The prevalence of BRONJ in patients receiving oral bisphosphonates is 0.01–0.04% (Sanz and Naert, 2009). The placement of an implant may be considered in patients taking oral bisphosphonates (Madrid and Sanz, 2010). However, there are no diagnostic techniques to identify those at increased risk of developing BRONJ.

Diabetes

Severe type 1 diabetes or uncontrolled type II diabetes is a significant relative contraindication, as healing is delayed due to poor peripheral blood circulation.

Chronic kidney disease

The healing process is deeply modified by chronic kidney disease and the specialist must be consulted.

AIDS/HIV

Limited published scientific evidence is available to guide clinicians with regard to the possible increased risks of dental implant procedures associated with the HIV status of the patient. However, patients who are immunocompromised due to viral infection (HIV) or medication have a clearly reduced wound-healing capacity and an inappropriately responding immune system.

Patients at risk for poor wound healing

Gastroesophageal reflux disease creates an acid reflux, which may modify the oral pH and thus compromise the healing process.

Lichen planus, erythema multiforme and lupus erythematosus may compromise soft tissue healing. A fixed prosthesis will be preferred to a removable prosthesis to avoid any soft tissue compression.

Long-term, high doses of glucocorticoids inhibit the immune system, which may lead to severe infections following dental implant surgery.

Patients at risk during the surgical procedure

Regarding blood coagulation disorders and medications that may modify the coagulation process (anticoagulants and antiplatelet agents), the international normalised ratio (INR) should be checked within the 24 hours before surgery. For patients who have a stable INR, an INR measured within 72 hours before the procedure is acceptable (RPSGB/BMA, 2006; National Patient Safety Agency, 2007). There is no need to withdraw continuous oral anticoagulant therapy for ordinary surgical implant procedures with an INR <3.5 (Sanz and Naert, 2009). However, special attention must be given to anticoagulated patients (Figure 17.1, Box 17.1).

Hypertensive and epileptic patients need a stress reduction protocol (Box 17.2). Some respiratory diseases can make the surgical procedure impossible.

Key points

• Decision making for surgery in medically compromised patients should be the result of a consensus among the treating professionals; that is, dentists and physician specialists.
• It is the surgeon, not the physician, who makes the final decision.

Patient evaluation: The patient at risk for dental implant failure

Figure 18.1 Patient at risk for implant failure: combination of smoking and periodontitis. (a) Clinical view of a periodontitis patient four years after implant placement. The patient is a heavy smoker and has not received a periodontal treatment. (b) The panoramic radiograph indicates bone loss around teeth and implants (yellow arrows)

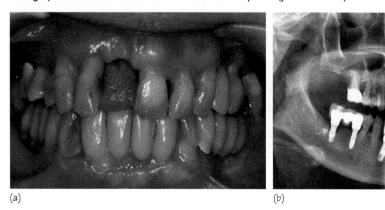

(a)

(b)

Figure 18.2 Complete edentulism in a 9-year-old boy with ectodermal dysplasia. (a) Clinical view of the maxilla. (b) Clinical view of the mandible. (c) Three-dimensional reconstruction of the mandible. Note the thin edge of the alveolar ridge that may preclude the placement of temporary dental implants. (d) Panoramic radiography. Courtesy of Dr Muriel Mola, Centre of Rare Oral Diseases (ORARES), Rothschild Hospital AP-HP, Paris, France. Reproduced with permission of Muriel Mola

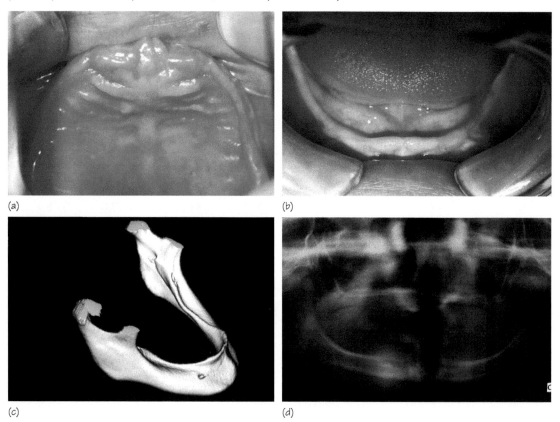

(a)

(b)

(c)

(d)

Implant Dentistry at a Glance, Second Edition. Jacques Malet, Francis Mora and Philippe Bouchard.
© 2018 John Wiley & Sons Ltd. Published 2018 by John Wiley & Sons Ltd.
Companion website: www.wiley.com/go/malet/implant

e have not identified in the literature an individual risk factor that might be a contraindication for implant survival. Most studies indicate that dental implants can be successfully placed and maintained in patients exhibiting a variety of systemic diseases and congenital defects. However, the level of evidence indicating a risk of dental implant failure or complication associated with the health state of patients is low; that is, restricted to case reports and case series. Thus, dental implant indications must be thoroughly and *individually* evaluated, according to the patient's profile. The decision-making process must include the severity of the risk factors and/or, maybe most importantly, their combination in the same individual (Figure 18.1). In any case, patients need to be informed of the possibility of implant complications.

The following sections indicate potential risk factors that have been adequately documented and the overall conclusions that can be drawn.

Age

There is no upper limit in terms of age, and old age alone should not be a limiting factor for dental implant therapy. At 10 years, the implant survival of elderly patients (≥65 years) is 91.2% (Srinivasan *et al.*, 2017). As a general rule, the lower limit for implant placement is 18–19 years, when an adolescent's jaw growth and development can be considered to be complete. However, this rule can be broken with children suffering from hypodontia or anodontia, such as in ectodermal dysplasia, because the benefit/risk analysis is in favour of implant placement.

Smoking

Smoking has been identified as an independent risk indicator for peri-implant mucositis (Renvert and Polyzois, 2015). Smoking increases the failure rates and the risk of postoperative infections, as well as the marginal bone loss (Keenan and Veitz-Keenan, 2016). There is strong evidence that smokers are at greater risk for peri-implantitis (odds ratio [OR] 3.6–4.6) and radiographic marginal bone loss (OR 1.95–10) than non-smokers (Heitz-Mayfield and Huynh-Ba, 2009). However, the majority of studies report implant survival rates of 80–96% in smokers (Cochran *et al.*, 2009). There is some evidence for a dose effect of cigarette smoking. There is no strong evidence of an increased risk of implant failure when sinus augmentation procedures are used (Chambrone *et al.*, 2014).

Figure 18.3 Complete edentulism of the mandible in a 3-year-old boy with ectodermal dysplasia. This young boy, born in 2000, was implanted in 2003. The clinical view was taken in 2007. The lower denture has been stabilised by two implants placed between the mental foramina. Courtesy of Dr Catherine Artaud, Rothschild Hospital AP-HP, Paris, France. Reproduced with permission of Catherine Artaud

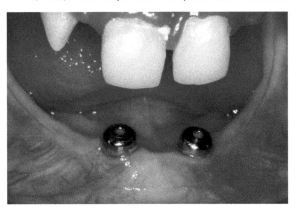

History of treated periodontitis

There is evidence that the history of treated periodontitis increases the risk for peri-implantitis (Chrcanovic *et al.*, 2014a; Sousa *et al.*, 2016). The risk ratio for failure in patients with aggressive periodontitis is significantly higher when compared with healthy patients (4.0) and those with chronic periodontitis (3.97; Monje *et al.*, 2014). Implant survival rates ranged from 59% to 100% in patients who have regular periodontal maintenance (Heitz-Mayfield and Huynh-Ba, 2009). However, the majority of studies report high implant survival rates (>90%; Cochran *et al.*, 2009). Consequently, implant placement in patients with a history of treated periodontitis is a viable option to restore oral function. This special patient category must be informed of an increased risk of failure, and the need for regular peri-implant and periodontal maintenance. Residual pockets and non-attendance at a periodontal maintenance programme have been shown to be negative factors for a good long-term implant outcome (Zangrando *et al.*, 2015).

Number of teeth

The number of remaining teeth (≥20) and the opposing unit being a removable partial denture or nothing have been shown to be risk indicators for implant failure (Noda *et al.*, 2015).

Ectodermal dysplasia

Studies indicate significantly lower survival and success rates in the maxilla than in the mandible (Bornstein *et al.*, 2009). Implant survival rates vary between 88.5% and 97.6%. Implants placed in patients younger than 18 years have a higher risk of failure (Yap and Klineberg, 2009). See Figures 18.2 and 18.3.

AIDS/HIV

Several case reports have shown successful dental implant therapies in HIV-positive, immunologically stable patients receiving highly active antiretroviral therapy. However, there are limited published data available to guide clinicians on possible increased risks of dental implant failure associated with the HIV status of the patient.

Diabetes/hyperglycaemia

There is evidence that diabetes increases the risk for peri-implantitis (Ferreira *et al.*, 2006), but not for peri-implant mucositis (Monje *et al.*, 2017). A significant small difference between diabetic and non-diabetic patients concerning marginal bone loss has been shown, favouring non-diabetic patients (Chrcanovic et al., 2014b), However, the difference between patients (diabetic vs non-diabetic) does not significantly affect implant failure rates. Other researchers have found that more diabetic patients experienced dental implant failures than non-diabetics, but the overall percentage of failing implants is within a normal range (Bornstein *et al.*, 2009). Thus, it may be assumed that the failure risk in diabetes is patient dependent. It may depend on the severity of the disease and the glycaemic status. When diabetes is well controlled, implant procedures are safe and predictable, with a complication rate similar to that of healthy patients (Shi et al., 2016).

Bone diseases

Severe bone diseases such as Paget's disease of bone, rheumatoid arthritis, osteomalacia or osteogenesis imperfecta must be considered as high-risk factors.

There is no evidence for higher failure rates and complications in osteoporotic patients. The major problem is associated with the use of bisphosphonate in these patients. Nevertheless, the intake of oral bisphosphonates does not influence short-term (one to four years) implant survival rates (Madrid and Sanz, 2009).

Radiotherapy

A similar failure rate has been shown for implants placed after radiation and those placed before radiation (3.2% and 5.4%, respectively). The implant failure was lower at the mandible (4.4%) than at the maxilla (17.5%). However, the sample size was small and the heterogeneity of the included studies was high.

Miscellaneous

The following non-exhaustive list indicates factors that have been suggested as being detrimental for dental implant survival, and where no conclusion can be drawn due to the paucity of evidence: alcohol consumption, asthma, autism, cardiac disease, Crohn's disease, Down's syndrome, drug abuse, genetic predisposition, Huntington's disease, hypertension, inadequate calcium intake, menopause, Parkinson's disease, schizophrenia, Sjögren's syndrome, xerostomia.

Key points

- Patients who are candidates for dental implants must be informed of the increased risk of dental implant failure and potential complications associated with their individual health profile.
- Smoking and diabetes can be considered as risk factors for dental implant complications.
- A history of treated periodontitis and severe bone diseases may be considered as risk indicators for dental implant complications.
- Further studies are required to define the true effect of medical parameters and smoking on dental implant survival rate and biological complications.

19 Patient evaluation: Local risk factors

Figure 19.1 (a) Loss of papilla (arrow) due to insufficient distance between the implant shoulder (22) and the proximal tooth (21). Note the inflammatory process of the soft tissues. (b) Note the proximity between tooth 21 and the dental implant on the X-ray corresponding with the clinical view

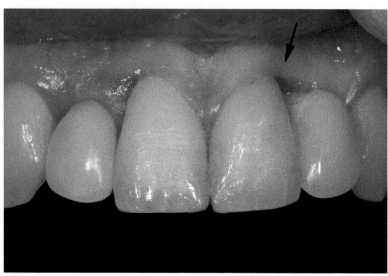

(a)

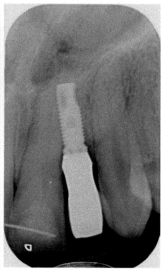

(b)

Figure 19.2 Apical peri-implantitis. (a) The dental implant has been inserted in a completely healed site. The tooth had been extracted for endodontic reasons. Note the presence of a fistulous tract two months after implantation. (b) A flap is raised. Note the apical localisation of the bone defect

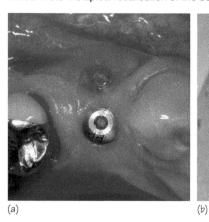

(a)

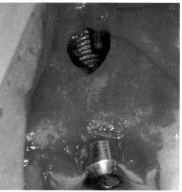

(b)

Figure 19.3 Mucosal recession due to a thin tissue biotype

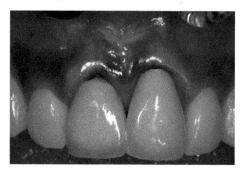

Any situation that poses a risk to successful osseointegration and restoration of a dental implant at the level of the implant site and surrounding teeth must be considered.

Implant stability

The primary stability of the implant is a critical factor for implant survival. Several methods and devices are used to measure implant stability, including subjective evaluation, resonance frequency analysis (RFA) and insertion torque. However, they are insufficient to assess the primary stability, or to provide any predictive value of implant outcome. From a clinical point of view, insertion torque value is routinely used. The surgeon should strive to achieve high insertion torque values whenever possible (35 Ncm).

Implant Dentistry at a Glance, Second Edition. Jacques Malet, Francis Mora and Philippe Bouchard.
© 2018 John Wiley & Sons Ltd. Published 2018 by John Wiley & Sons Ltd.
Companion website: www.wiley.com/go/malet/implant

Bone density

Poor bone quality must be considered as a local risk factor. In the scientific literature, bone quality is often referred to as bone density. It is defined in terms of metabolism, cell turnover, mineralisation, maturation and vascularity; each of these factors plays a role in the osseointegration success of dental implants. Bone density is measured according to histological and morphometric analyses (Molly, 2006). The clinical evaluation of bone quality is questionable, since no commercial instrument is currently available to measure bone density. Bone quality can only be evaluated by radiographic examination and confirmed during preparation of the surgical site.

Interproximal space

The three-dimensional position of the dental implant shoulder is defined as the relationship to the bone crest level of the teeth adjacent to the implant. This critical factor influences the position of the interdental papillae surrounding the implants.

Tooth–implant

The risk of proximal bone resorption increases when the distance between the implant shoulder and the adjacent tooth is less than 1.5 mm. In aesthetic areas, this lack of bone support may compromise papilla preservation (Figure 19.1). In narrow spaces, this risk can be prevented with the use of narrow implants. A decreased implant survival rate has been reported when the implant is placed too close to the tooth.

Implant–implant

Similarly, a 3 mm horizontal distance between two dental implant shoulders is the minimum required to prevent soft and hard tissue loss.

Infected sites

The evidence regarding implant placement into infected sites is poor. Dental implants should be placed in non-infected sites. However, the reasons for tooth loss are multiple, including endodontic infections, periodontal infections and fractures or trauma. Consequently, the implant site(s) cannot be considered as sterile. Micro-organisms might persist in the trabecular bone. Therefore, sites of neighbouring teeth with endodontic pathology, or extraction sites of infected teeth, constitute a risk for successful osseointegration (Figure 19.2). This risk can be prevented by a thorough examination of radiographs prior to implant insertion. The vitality of neighbouring teeth should also be evaluated.

The lack of infection at extraction sites is of particular importance for immediate extraction-implantation procedures in fresh extraction sockets. Thus, the procedure is deemed questionable in clinical situations with infected teeth. Nevertheless, there is no detectable difference between the percentages of bone-to-implant contact (BIC) for immediate implant placement in infected versus non-infected fresh extraction sockets (92–100% survival rate at 12 months; Martin *et al.*, 2009).

Soft tissue thickness

Periodontal biotype must be considered a potential risk factor. A thin tissue biotype increases the risk of recession (Figure 19.3). Peri-implant recessions are dependent on bone thickness surrounding the implant body as well as the three-dimensional position of the dental implant. In the aesthetic zone, the reinforcement of soft tissue with connective tissue graft contributes to an aesthetic result for the implant-supported prosthesis. However, the presence of keratinised attached peri-implant mucosa poses a challenging question in the health maintenance of peri-implant soft tissue. It seems that increasing the soft

Figure 19.4 The minimally invasive flapless procedure. (a) The alveolar mucosa is punched out over the implant site. (b) The tissue punch is removed to expose the alveolar ridge. (c) After drilling, a direction indicator is placed in the implant bed. (d) The dental implant is inserted. (e) Clinical view of the implant platform. (f) A prosthetic abutment is placed at the end of the surgery (one-stage procedure)

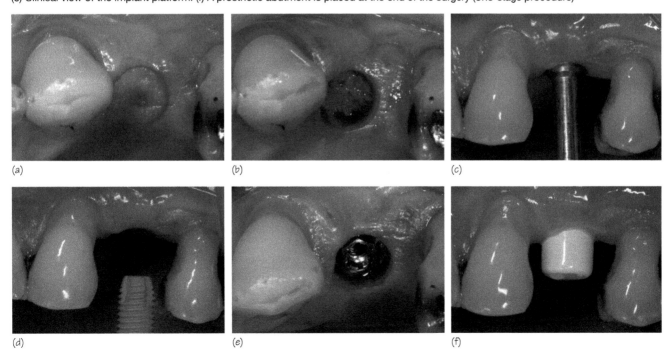

(a)   (b)   (c)

(d)   (e)   (f)

peri-implant tissue is advisable in order to limit marginal inflammation (Bengazi *et al.*, 1996). Nevertheless, there is no evidence to support soft tissue thickness as a risk factor in implant survival (Cochran *et al.*, 2009).

Keratinised soft tissue

It is often recommended that dental implants be surrounded by keratinised tissue to improve their long-term survival. There is no evidence that increasing the width of keratinised tissue improves the long-term prognosis of the dental implant. However, inflammation and plaque accumulation are greater when the keratinised mucosa width is less than 2 mm. No correlation has been found between the peri-implant mucosa width and marginal bone loss. Surgical augmentation of keratinised mucosa should be limited to situations where it can be beneficial for individual plaque control.

Surgical procedure

Following conventional flap surgery, a slight buccal alveolar resorption may occur due to bone exposure. The flapless approach has been proposed to reduce postoperative bone resorption and to preserve soft tissue contours (Figure 19.4). Furthermore, this procedure may reduce patient discomfort and surgical time. Favourable short-term implant survival rates have been reported (Esposito *et al.*, 2012). Because this is a blind approach, the technique is limited to experienced surgeons.

Key points

- Primary stability is a key factor for implant survival.
- Poor bone quality and inadequate interproximal space are true risk factors.
- Limited evidence indicates that site infection is a risk factor.
- There is no evidence that soft tissue condition is a risk factor for implant survival.
- Flapless procedures are limited to experienced surgeons.

20 Patient evaluation: Dental history

Figure 20.1 Extraction of the left cuspid after successive endodontic surgeries. (a) Successive surgeries have failed to treat the endodontic lesion. (b) Clinical view of multiple bone defects when extracting the canine. (c) The canine has been extracted and endodontic surgery has been performed on the lateral. Note the complete destruction of the buccal cortical plate at the canine site

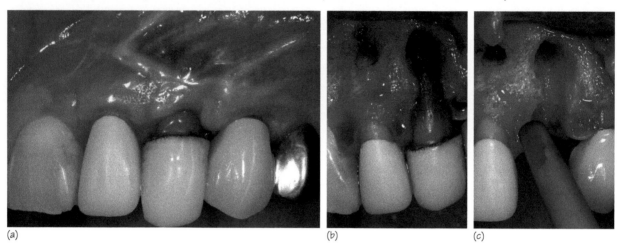

(a)   (b)   (c)

Figure 20.2 Traumatic injury of the anterior teeth. (a) The maxillary incisors have been knocked out following a trauma. Clinical view of the alveolar ridge one year after the trauma. The horizontal bone resorption beneath the soft tissue is clinically visible. (b) The thin alveolar ridge is confirmed during surgery

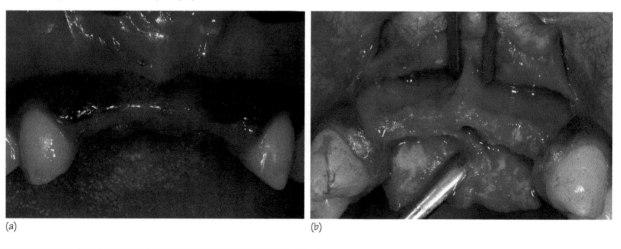

(a)   (b)

Not all patients are good candidates for dental implants, even if the clinical situation seems to be a good indication. Evaluation of dental history allows the clinician to establish a comprehensive treatment plan and to prevent the risk of failure or complication. Information is provided by the patient during initial interviews.

Compliance

Before surgery, during wound healing and after prosthesis delivery, a minimum of patient cooperation is essential to prevent complications. Some patients refuse to participate actively in their treatment, and their excessive 'passivity' may be a barrier to the development of an implant treatment plan. Early detection of

Implant Dentistry at a Glance, Second Edition. Jacques Malet, Francis Mora and Philippe Bouchard.
© 2018 John Wiley & Sons Ltd. Published 2018 by John Wiley & Sons Ltd.
Companion website: www.wiley.com/go/malet/implant

Figure 20.3 Bone and soft tissue collapse following extraction of teeth 21 and 22 for periodontal reasons (severe periodontitis)

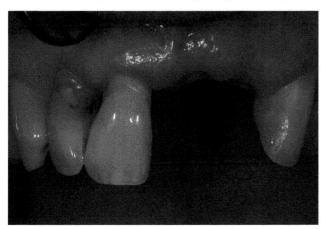

Figure 20.4 Posterior vertical bone resorption due to a removable denture worn for 20 years

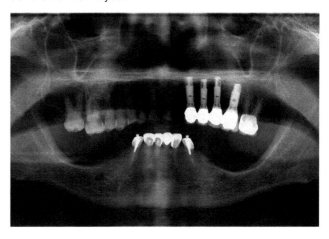

these unmotivated patients avoids unnecessary inconvenience for the clinician and the patient.

Oral hygiene

Effective dental plaque control is a prerequisite for successful implant therapy. A detailed description of the patient's brushing techniques and the type of professional support therapy must be reviewed, to be corrected if necessary. This point is particularly important for edentulous patients who no longer maintain effective plaque control habits.

Inadequate plaque control has a significant impact on:
• early implant failure in partially edentulous patients (bacterial contamination during surgery; Van Steenberghe *et al.*, 1990)
• excessive bone loss around osseointegrated implants, even in edentulous patients
• peri-implantitis (see Chapters 61 and 62).

Bruxism

Although this is a controversial issue, the trend is that excessive occlusal loading increases the risk of mechanical complications (prefabricated component), technical complications (laboratory fabricated) and failures (Salvi and Bragger, 2009). Despite this, bruxism (except in extreme cases) is not a contraindication for dental implants, but precautions are recommended for the selection of implants and elaboration of the restoration design.

History of tooth loss

The origin of the tooth loss must be stated, as it can compromise implant success or complicate dental implant placement.

In *endodontic infection/endodontic surgery failure*, in cases of incomplete debridement of the lesion, a latent inflammatory/infectious process may remain in the bone even after several years. This lesion is not always observable on radiographs, if not previously suspected, and can interfere with the osseointegration process. Moreover, successive endodontic surgeries are often associated with large postextraction bone defects (Figure 20.1).

Root fracture may be related to excessive occlusal forces (bruxism) or occlusal disorders. Substantial alveolar bone loss occurs after extraction of a root with a vertical fracture.

Traumatic tooth loss and traumatic surgery will result in large alveolar ridge defects and gingival scars. Bone and soft tissue reconstruction should be considered (Figure 20.2).

In *terminal periodontitis*, after tooth extraction periodontal bone loss and soft tissue migration limit the amount of available bone and jeopardise the aesthetic outcome (Figure 20.3).

For patients with *extensive caries*, caries risk does not directly influence implant success rates.

Age of edentulism negatively influences residual *bone volume*. For edentulous patients, removable dentures accelerate bone resorption (Figure 20.4).

Multidirectional *tooth migrations* must be anticipated for partially edentulous patients with old, non-compensated tooth loss. Orthodontic space management could be required.

Dental inflammatory or infectious processes

Implant site (immediate implant)

Although implant placement in an infected site (if correctly debrided) does not affect osseointegration outcome, delayed implantation is recommended to the extent possible.

Adjacent teeth

Infections/inflammatory processes within the jawbone in the vicinity of an integrating implant (apical lesions, root remnants, endodontic material) can interfere with osseointegration. They must be treated separately, before implant placement.

Periodontal history

Untreated periodontitis is a contraindication to implant therapy (see Chapter 21). Periodontal infection must be controlled before implant placement.

A history of treated periodontitis increases the risk of implant failure and peri-implant bone loss (Heitz-Mayfield and Huynh-Ba, 2009). Individual periodontal supportive therapy is essential.

> **Key points**
> • Taking a dental history is mandatory before implant placement.
> • The aim of taking a dental history is to identify potential risk factors/indicators for implant failure.
> • Knowledge of the history of tooth loss provides information on bone loss and infection risk.

Patient evaluation: Dental implants in periodontally compromised patients

21

Figure 21.1 Dental implant therapy in a well-maintained periodontitis patient. (a) Panoramic radiography, seven years after implant placement. (b) Clinical view at the time of the radiography

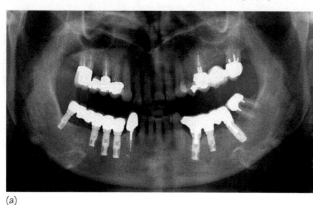

(a)

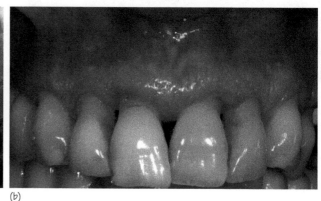

(b)

Figure 21.2 Full arch fixed restoration in a periodontitis patient. Note that without bone augmentation procedures, the aesthetic outcome is compromised by the restoration, which cannot compensate for bone resorption. In addition, plaque control may be difficult due to the reduction of the vestibule (see tooth 21)

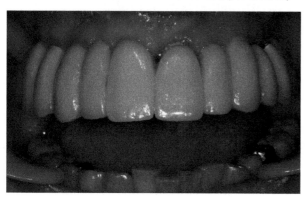

Figure 21.3 Treatment plan for dental implant therapy according to the periodontal status of the patient

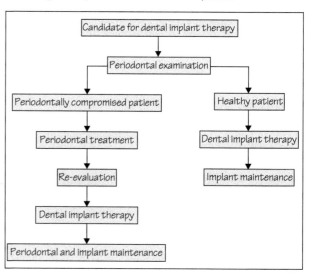

Treated periodontitis subjects
Implant outcomes

Patients with a history of periodontitis demonstrate a greater risk for peri-implantitis (odds ratio [OR] 3.1–4.7) and a lower implant survival rate (ISR) than non-periodontal patients (Ong *et al.*, 2008; Cochran *et al.*, 2009). Nevertheless, over a period of 3–16 years, the ISR remains high – that is, greater than 90% – when patients are periodontally well maintained (Heitz-Mayfield and Huynh-Ba, 2009). Meta-analysis shows that a history of periodontitis is not significant in short-term dental implant survival (Wen *et al.*, 2014). However, after long-term follow-up, periodontitis, especially aggressive or severe periodontitis, significantly but modestly affects implant survival within a period of 8–16 years (relative risk [RR] = 1.03, 95% confidence interval [CI]: 1.02–1.04).

Thus, a history of treated periodontitis does not contraindicate implant therapy (Figure 21.1). However, the patient must be

Implant Dentistry at a Glance, Second Edition. Jacques Malet, Francis Mora and Philippe Bouchard.
© 2018 John Wiley & Sons Ltd. Published 2018 by John Wiley & Sons Ltd.
Companion website: www.wiley.com/go/malet/implant

informed of an increasing risk of implant failure and peri-implantitis (see Appendix E). The completed prosthesis and its supporting components (teeth and implants) must be carefully monitored with a maintenance programme that includes systematic and continuous monitoring of the periodontal and peri-implant tissue conditions.

Risk factors

Smoking is a risk factor for periodontitis and peri-implantitis. Patients who combine cigarette smoking and a history of periodontitis should be considered at risk for implant failure, even if further research is required to properly assess the combination of these factors. Implant placement procedures do not affect the ISR (one-stage versus two-stage). The ISR does not change when immediate implant insertion and immediate loading procedures are applied. The characteristics of the implant surface seem to influence the ISR. Lower ISRs are observed for very rough surfaces.

Dental implant therapy

In cases of severe periodontitis, subsequent alveolar bone resorption poses a significant challenge to achieving aesthetic and functional restorations. Implant placement in periodontitis patients often results in long, unaesthetic teeth (Figure 21.2).

Care must be taken in bone and soft tissue preservation during periodontal therapy. The ridge resorption that results from removal of the teeth involved should be anticipated (see Chapter 39). During periodontal surgical treatment, attention should also be paid to regeneration of the periodontal tissues.

Vertical and/or horizontal bone augmentations are often required in order to reduce the crown/implant ratio, and to allow adequate three-dimensional implant positioning.

The soft tissue biotype significantly affects the aesthetic outcome. The thin-scalloped type (long and triangular teeth) often results in recession of the peri-implant soft tissues, exposing the gingival crown margins. Therefore, in aesthetic areas, soft tissue augmentation is also often required. Consequently, dental implant therapy in periodontitis patients is frequently more complex than in patients with no history of treated periodontitis, and necessitates an extended team (see Chapter 15).

Untreated periodontitis subjects

In light of the data on treated periodontitis subjects, one can understand that the placement of dental implants in the context of untreated periodontitis is questionable in terms of long-term success, and may dramatically jeopardise ISR. The possible translocation of micro-organisms, the recurrence of disease, poor oral hygiene and systemic disorders may contribute to colonisation of the peri-implant sulcus, and lead to peri-implantitis.

Any patient who is a candidate for dental implant therapy must have a periodontal examination.

Decision making for teeth extraction

In dental implant therapy, the main difference between periodontally compromised patients and healthy patients is the prognosis of the remaining teeth after periodontal treatment. Dental implant prognosis should be viewed on a long-term basis. Consequently, the long-term prognosis of the periodontally compromised teeth must be carefully evaluated.

Aggressive or chronic periodontitis can be successfully treated. This is well documented in the literature. The decision to extract or maintain a periodontally questionable tooth may be critical in the context of dental implant therapy, and often requires a specialist approach (Popelut et al., 2010). As a general rule, the projected survival rate of the residual teeth after periodontal treatment should not be less than 10 years, when implant-supported fixed partial dentures (FPDs) are planned for dental rehabilitation in partially dentate patients.

Treatment plan

The treatment may vary according to the periodontal condition of the individual patient. The following workflow may be used in periodontitis patients (Figure 21.3):
• Comprehensive clinical and radiographic examination to adequately diagnose the periodontal disease
• Initial therapy to reduce the bacterial load (including extraction of hopeless teeth and the conservative control of dental caries)
• Orthodontic treatment to improve tooth position
• Periodontal surgical treatments to improve the results of the initial therapy (including surgical regenerative procedures)
• Bone augmentation procedures to allow or improve implant placement
• Fabrication of a surgical template to guide implant placement
• Implant placement
• Interim maintenance to facilitate healing
• Re-evaluation to evaluate the stability of the remaining periodontally compromised teeth
• Prosthetic treatment.

Key points

• Dental implant therapy is a viable option in periodontally compromised patients.
• Periodontal examination is a prerequisite to dental implant therapy.
• Systematic and continuous monitoring of periodontal and peri-implant tissue conditions is critical for the survival of dental implants in patients with a history of periodontitis.

22 Patient evaluation: Aesthetic parameters

Figure 22.1 Patient with a high lip line ('gummy' smile)

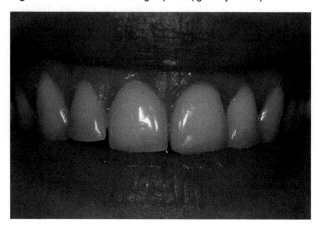

Figure 22.2 The determinants of aesthetics. 1. Symmetry; 2. gingival line; 3. crown shape and proportions; 4. interproximal papilla

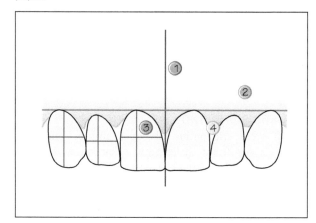

Figure 22.3 Thin scalloped biotype: high aesthetic risk

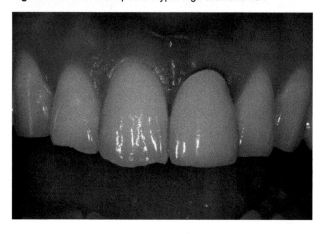

Figure 22.4 Three-dimensional ideal positioning of implant in the aesthetic zone

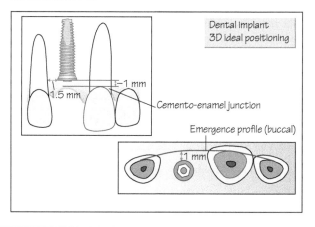

Dental implant 3D ideal positioning

1 mm
1.5 mm
Cemento-enamel junction
Emergence profile (buccal)
1 mm

The increasing demand for dental implants in the aesthetic zone (anterior maxilla) is a challenge for the clinician who is seeking not only implant success but also aesthetic predictability. With this in mind, the appearance and stability of the soft tissues are important factors to consider.

Acceptable aesthetic results in the anterior area necessitate more complex treatments than in non-aesthetic standard situations. However, the patient's request should be carefully evaluated to avoid overtreatment. Aesthetic evaluation comprises both an objective and a subjective aspect. A full photographic documentation is essential.

Compliance and the patient's demand

Patient compliance is a key factor. The patient must be informed of the complexity and limitations of the treatment (see Chapter 27). If the aesthetic demand of the patient is beyond the technical possibilities that can be offered by implant therapy, non-implant strategies should be considered.

Smile line

The smile line defines the lip position and its relationship to teeth during a 'natural' smile. Most patients show part of the interproximal papilla, but not the gingival margins.

Implant Dentistry at a Glance, Second Edition. Jacques Malet, Francis Mora and Philippe Bouchard.
© 2018 John Wiley & Sons Ltd. Published 2018 by John Wiley & Sons Ltd.
Companion website: www.wiley.com/go/malet/implant

Figure 22.5 Parameters to be considered to obtain a papilla filling after implant placement. PDL, periodontal ligament

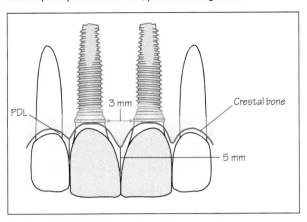

Figure 22.6 Adjacent implants 21–22. Red circles indicate the implant-supported prosthesis

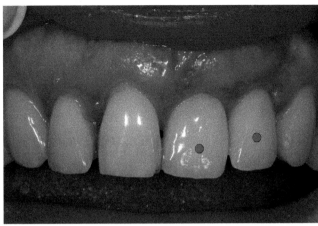

Patients with a high lip line ('gummy' smile) are challenging, as they will show all the tissues surrounding the future implant restoration (Figure 22.1).

A full dental and periodontal examination will highlight the following elements: teeth positions, teeth dimensions, gingival contour and midline position (Figure 22.2).

Biotype and soft tissue thickness

Biotype describes the periodontal morphology and it can be of two main types (Olsson and Lindhe, 1991): a thin-scalloped type (with long, triangular teeth) and a thick-flat type (with short, square teeth).

Patients with a thin-scalloped biotype are considered at 'high aesthetic risk' (Figure 22.3). Bone modifications after tooth extraction will be more pronounced for these patients and, in cases of impaired healing, the aesthetic consequences will be more evident than for patients with a thick-flat biotype.

Soft tissue integration of the prosthetic restoration is easier and more stable with thick tissues. As a result, soft tissue augmentation is often recommended for situations of high aesthetic risk.

Tissue modification after tooth extraction

Extraction of a tooth leads to a succession of healing events in the socket, resulting in a loss of alveolar bone on the labial side. This bone loss is variable (2–3 mm vertically) and is the consequence of bone remodelling (bundle bone; Araújo and Lindhe, 2005).

For a single tooth extraction, proximal periodontium (bone and soft tissue) is supported by adjacent teeth. However, extraction of two or more adjacent teeth will result in proximal bone resorption and papilla collapse (tissue flattening).

Buccal and proximal tissue modifications must be prevented or corrected for an optimal aesthetic result. Socket preservation, soft tissue augmentation, and bone augmentation procedures should always be considered in the aesthetic area.

Immediate implant

Although implant placement into a fresh socket is supposed to preserve bone and soft tissue, it is a very controversial subject.

The timing of the implant placement has less influence on the long-term aesthetic outcome than other parameters.

Three-dimensional positioning of implant

Clinical recommendations are proposed to achieve a good and stable aesthetic result (Figure 22.4). The crucial point is the precise three-dimensional (3D) positioning of the implant, which must respect some minimal distances (implant–tooth, implant–implant; Buser et al., 2004) and prosthetic guidelines (emergence point and general axis). As a general rule, palatal positioning has fewer negative consequences than buccal positioning.

Bone height and soft tissue position

If one agrees with the postulate that soft tissue position depends on supporting bone – that is, on the height of proximal and buccal bone surrounding implants – it is obvious that the stability of this bone is essential for long-term aesthetic success.

Proximal bone

For an implant adjacent to a natural tooth, the crestal bone height depends only on the natural tooth. For adjacent implants, the stability of the proximal bone depends on the interimplant distance (Tarnow et al., 2000): a distance of 3 mm or more helps maintain a stable bone position (Figure 22.5).

After prosthetic restoration, the amount of filling of interproximal papilla depends on the vertical distance between the top of the crestal bone and the prosthetic contact area (Choquet et al., 2001). A distance of 5 mm or less is required for a full filling.

Buccal bone

There is no evidence that a minimum bone width is required to ensure buccal bone stability, but 2 mm is usually recommended.

Aesthetic limitations in implant therapy

Because of proximal bone loss, the aesthetic result is unpredictable for multiple edentulous ridges. Reducing the number of implants can sometimes facilitate aesthetic predictability. The restoration of two *adjacent teeth* in a reduced prosthetic space is the most difficult situation (Figure 22.6).

Vertical bone augmentation is a very challenging procedure. A limited aesthetic outcome must be anticipated.

In cases of *advanced periodontitis*, the amount of bone and soft tissue loss is significant. This could result in longer clinical crowns and interdental black holes (incomplete papilla filling) after implant treatment. Preventive and reconstructive surgical procedures should be undertaken for these patients, if the aesthetic demand is high. Compensations with prosthetic devices may also be considered.

Key points

- Dental implant therapy in aesthetic areas is complex.
- Patient demand is central and must be thoroughly evaluated.
- Patients with a thin-scalloped biotype must be considered at high aesthetic risk.
- Bone remodelling after tooth extraction is predictable.
- A minimum of 3 mm is required between two implants.
- In aesthetic areas, adjacent implants should be avoided.

(23) Patient evaluation: Surgical parameters

Figure 23.1 A minimum of 40–45 mm of mouth opening is required for surgical and prosthetic accessibility

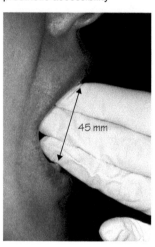

Figure 23.2 A drill extension may be necessary to avoid contact between the handpiece and the adjacent teeth, without altering the drilling direction

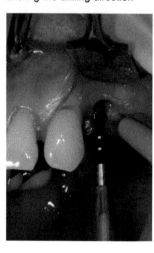

Figure 23.3 Buccal bone concavity. (a) A meticulous palpation of the alveolar process identifies a buccal bone concavity (white arrow). (b) The CT scan corroborates the clinical examination. In order to respect the prosthetic axis (red arrow), a short implant (8.5 mm) is selected. (c) The apical fenestration will require a guided bone regeneration (GBR) procedure

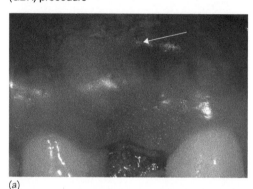

(a)

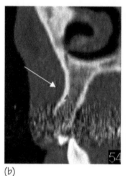

(b)

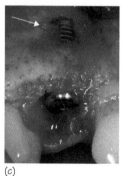

(c)

Figure 23.5 Prosthetic management of a reduced interdental space due to a mesial migration of 27. The implant is not placed in the middle of the original interdental space (red arrow), but slightly more mesial, in the middle of the residual interdental space (green arrow). The size of the crown is reduced (premolar design)

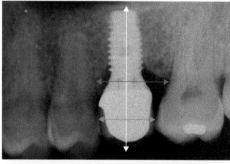

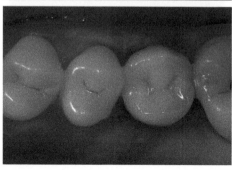

Figure 23.4 Management of the keratinised mucosa. The keratinised mucosa is located between the mucogingival junctions (white lines). The incision (black line) preserves sufficient keratinised tissue around the implant to allow a favourable environment after healing

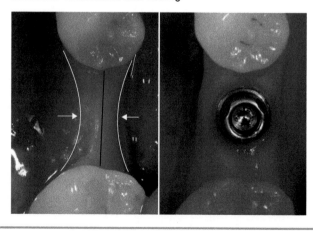

Implant Dentistry at a Glance, Second Edition. Jacques Malet, Francis Mora and Philippe Bouchard.
© 2018 John Wiley & Sons Ltd. Published 2018 by John Wiley & Sons Ltd.
Companion website: www.wiley.com/go/malet/implant

Before surgery, a clinical examination must be carefully conducted and cannot be replaced solely by a radiographic examination. A comprehensive patient examination is mandatory to anticipate surgical complications.

Surgical accessibility

A minimum of 40–45 mm (about three fingers' width) *mouth opening* is required to allow access to the posterior area of the mouth for drills and implants, while respecting prosthetic guidelines (Figure 23.1). A limited mouth opening will compel the surgeon and prosthodontist to use short instruments, short implants or tilted implants. In extreme situations, implant therapy can be contraindicated.

Teeth adjacent to the implant site can interfere with correct positioning of drills (bumping of the handpiece). The use of a drill extension may be required, but is not always possible in the posterior area (Figure 23.2).

Surgical access should be tested before confirming the surgery appointment.

Aesthetic complexity

Soft tissue manipulation during implant surgery of the anterior area can have detrimental consequences for patients with a thin biotype or multiple planned surgeries (see Chapter 22). Evaluation of aesthetic surgical complexity is essential. Complex situations require the most predictable therapeutic options (Table 23.1).

Alveolar mucosa

The presence of keratinised tissue on the surgical site is evaluated. The incision will be located, if possible, within keratinised mucosa to facilitate tissue manipulation and to allow for a more favourable environment after healing (Figure 23.4).

Probing of keratinised tissue thickness under local anaesthesia provides a good evaluation of the transmucosal part of the future restoration for prosthetic anticipation and bone volume evaluation.

Hypertrophic mucosa on an edentulous ridge, particularly if it is mobile, can require a surgical reduction.

Alveolar process dimensions

A first estimate of bone width and height is performed with meticulous palpation of the alveolar ridge. This allows the clinician to

identify some anatomical limits and to anticipate specific surgical troubles (Table 23.2). Tomographic examination will confirm this initial evaluation.

Diagnostic casts are sometimes needed to estimate the bone dimensions, after subtracting the thickness of the mucosa measured at several points.

Bone dimensions are compared to the prosthetic project to confirm the treatment decision.

Dimensions of the edentulous area

A minimum of 7 mm horizontal interdental distance is required to place a standard implant, 14 mm for two implants, 21 mm for three implants and so on. In cases of tooth migration, a reduction of the tooth gap is observed. Even if bone dimension is not altered, reduced interdental distance can prevent correct orientation of the drills or implant insertion. The position, orientation and even number of implants must be modified (Figure 23.5). Orthodontic space management is an alternative.

Adjacent teeth

Surgical access for implant placement can have detrimental effects on the adjacent periodontal tissues, in cases of thin biotype or reduced *periodontal support*. In order to prevent periodontal recessions, modified flap design or preventive soft tissue augmentation could be indicated.

It is crucial to estimate the direction of the roots of adjacent teeth, since they can converge with the implant axis and cause surgical interference. Modification of the implant direction (if compatible with the prosthetic project) or reduction of the implant length can avoid this drawback.

Table 23.1 Surgical options according to the risk factors

Complexity parameter	Associated risk	Therapeutic option
Thin biotype	Recession	Soft tissue thickening
Proximal bone collapse	Papilla lost	Papilla preservation
Prominent natural roots	Large bone dehiscences	Guided bone regeneration (GBR)
Incisors palatal version	Oblique bone orientation	Shorter implant in an adequate orientation
Buccal bone concavity (Figure 23.3)	Bone fenestration	Shorter implant, tapered implant, GBR

Table 23.2 Surgical complexity associated with anatomical deformities

Anatomical deformities	Surgical complexity
Bone concavities	Overdrilling risk
Horizontal resorption, narrow crest	Narrow implant or guided bone regeneration (GBR) indication
Vertical resorption	Anatomical risk
	Short implant indication
Shallow vestibule	Tension during healing
	Plaque control difficulty

Key points

• Before surgery, a clinical examination must be carefully conducted and cannot be replaced by a radiographic examination alone.
• A minimum of three fingers' width mouth opening is needed for surgical access.
• Soft tissue manipulation is evaluated before surgery.
• The amount of keratinised mucosa must be evaluated for the design of the incisions and for preservation.

24 Patient evaluation: Surgical template

Figure 24.1 Radiographic template: titanium guide sleeves allow visualisation of implant direction and indicate surgical placement

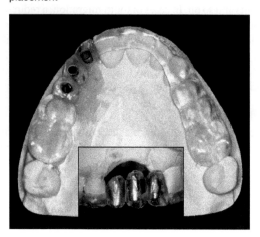

Figure 24.2 Surgical template with a denture design. Note the exact positioning of the implants

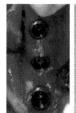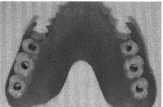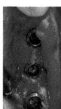

Figure 24.3 Radiographic/surgical template. (a) Artificial teeth are covered with barium sulfate. The drilling holes are filled with a radiopaque cement for radiographic examination. The cement is removed before the surgical procedure (white arrows). (b) CT scan (cross-sectional images): visualisation of tooth shape (green arrow) and identification of future implant position and direction (red arrow). (c) Drilling with a surgical guide

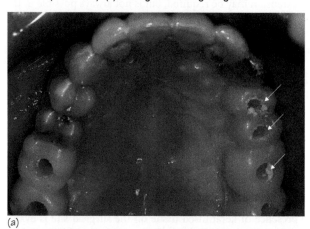

(a)

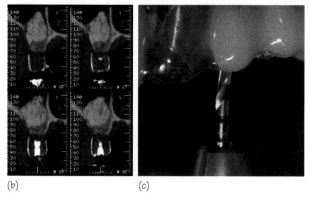

(b)   (c)

The surgical template is a device that prefigures the prosthetic project both (i) to enable its visualisation on X-rays (radiographic template) and (ii) to optimize the implant positioning during surgery (surgical guide). Placement of several contiguous implants often requires a surgical template.

Characteristics

Precision is essential, particularly in the aesthetic area, where even limited inaccuracy can have detrimental consequences. As a result, technical procedures are similar to those for temporary removable dentures.

Stability avoids any displacement of the template during radiographic examination and surgery. Stability is provided by non-mobile teeth if possible (teeth-borne template; Figure 24.1) or by the edentulous ridge (soft tissue–borne template; Figure 24.2).

The template must be *easy to use*, essentially because patients will wear it during radiographic examination. During surgery, positioning of and retrieving the device must be simple and reproducible, without alterations.

Radiopacity offers the possibility to visualise tooth shape and ideal implant direction on the radiographs. Radiographic markers should not cause any radiographic diffraction. Barium sulfate can be incorporated in the whole template body during fabrication (Figure 24.3). Radiopaque materials include:
- cavit
- gutta percha

Implant Dentistry at a Glance, Second Edition. Jacques Malet, Francis Mora and Philippe Bouchard.
© 2018 John Wiley & Sons Ltd. Published 2018 by John Wiley & Sons Ltd.
Companion website: www.wiley.com/go/malet/implant

Figure 24.4 Dental-borne surgical guide. (a) Surgical template stabilised on the proximal incisal edges. (b) A wide hole allows modification of drilling only in the palatal direction

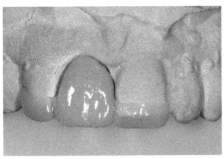

(a)

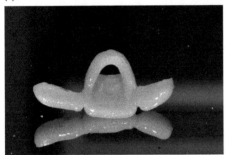

(b)

- titanium
- steel
- barium sulfate.

Resistance to heat is critical for decontamination and sterilisation of the template in order to use it during surgery.

The main information incorporated in the surgical template includes teeth shape (Figure 24.4), emergence crestal point and implant direction.

For aesthetic areas, the surgical template can include the soft tissue profile to adapt the implant position to the future gingival margin after flap elevation, and if necessary to perform a soft tissue augmentation procedure.

Technical procedures

The surgical template is made from a simulation of the future restoration. Special radiopaque devices are included in the template, in the optimal position and axis of the future implants; that is, compatible with the prosthetic project.

When residual teeth are present, they are used to stabilise the template. The existing partial or complete denture can also be modified (drill perforations in the implant positions) to be used as a template.

For partially edentulous patients, common manufacturing steps are the following:

- diagnostic casts
- wax-up or set-up
- duplicate casts
- vacuum-formed template
- ideal implant(s) location (position and axis)
- insertion of radiographic markers
- radiographic examination
- modification (opening) for irrigation and drills
- decontamination
- surgery.

Limitations

The fabrication of surgical templates requires additional chair time, for their fabrication, compared to surgical procedures that do not use them. Conventional templates are fabricated on dental casts, and thus their stability during surgery is lower than computer-generated surgical templates.

Furthermore, as they are made with the ideal prosthetic-driven implant position, conventional surgical templates do not allow intentional deviations to achieve a precise 3D implant placement considering the actual bone volume and anatomical structures.

Computer-generated surgical templates (optical scans, planning software, 3D printing) could overcome these limitations, by reducing chair time and improving accuracy (Vercruyssen *et al.*, 2015; see Chapter 42). The cost–benefit ratio should be evaluated to select the best option.

Key points

- In all cases, a surgical template is mandatory to allow optimal implant placement, except for single tooth placement in non-aesthetic areas.
- The surgical template mimics the future restoration.
- The surgical template must be stable, especially when it is supported by the mucosa.
- The placement and removal of the surgical template during surgery should be easy.

25 Patient evaluation: Imaging techniques

Figure 25.1 Conventional tomography image

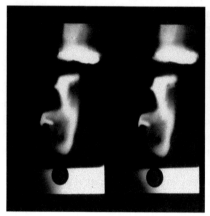

Figure 25.2 Computed tomography (CT) scan image

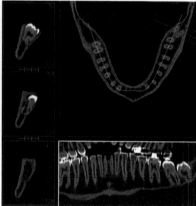

Figure 25.3 Cone beam computed tomography (CBCT) image

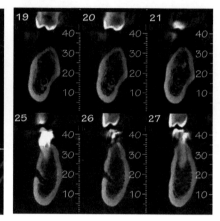

Figure 25.4 The periapical parallel technique: the detector (film, X-ray sensor) is positioned parallel to the long axes of the implants, and the central X-ray is directed perpendicular to both the film and the implant

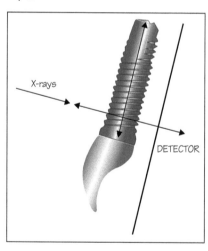

Figure 25.5 Proper parallel technique: good position of the film and correct orientation of the X-ray. Note the accurate appearance of the threads of the implant

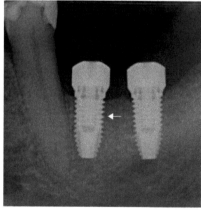

Figure 25.6 Incorrect technique: wrong position of the film and/or non-perpendicular orientation of the X-ray

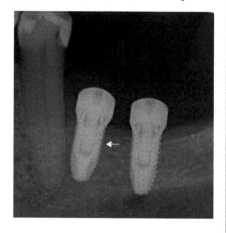

With the development of implant therapy, many imaging devices have been suggested. The objective of the clinician is to select the most appropriate technique to obtain optimal information with the minimal radiation dose and the best financial cost.

This follows the *ALARA principle*, meaning as low as reasonably achievable. The risk–benefit ratio must be evaluated to minimise the radiation dose, while obtaining the most reliable information.

Imaging techniques

See Table 25.1 for an overview.

Radiography

Intraoral (periapical) radiography, performed with the parallel technique, provides a good deal of information with a minimum radiation dose. It is the examination of choice for dental/

Implant Dentistry at a Glance, Second Edition. Jacques Malet, Francis Mora and Philippe Bouchard.
© 2018 John Wiley & Sons Ltd. Published 2018 by John Wiley & Sons Ltd.
Companion website: www.wiley.com/go/malet/implant

periodontal preoperative evaluation and for implant monitoring. If intraoral positioning of the detector is not possible, panoramic radiography can be an alternative.

Panoramic radiography is a good, quite systematic screening examination in implant therapy. It allows global visualisation of many anatomical structures. Its drawbacks include major distortion and variable magnification, making it inappropriate for accurate measurements.

Cephalometric lateral radiography is indicated to evaluate the sagittal interjaw relationship, the soft tissue profile and the anterior bone width.

Tomography

Tomography is the only way to evaluate bone dimensions precisely. Images perpendicular to the dental arch (cross-sectional images) allow measurement of bone width. The absence of deformation and a constant magnification allow direct measurements.

The presence of artifacts with metallic elements affects the quality of images and makes this technique unsuitable for the control of osseointegration.

Conventional tomography (Figure 25.1) can be used for examination of a limited zone, with relatively low radiation dose and cost. It provides thick cross-sectional images, which imply superposition of adjacent structures. Interpretation is not easy without proper training.

A *computed tomography (CT) scan* (Figure 25.2) consists of the acquisition of successive axial images (perpendicular to the long axis of the body), which are reformatted by computer software to obtain cross-sectional views.

The CT scan is the gold standard of tomographic implant bone evaluation. In a very short time (thus limiting patient movement), it provides an accurate examination of the whole mandible and/or maxilla. To limit radiation dose, current scanners use a 'low-dose protocol' sufficient for bone evaluation.

Cone beam computed tomography (CBCT; Figure 25.3) consists of volumetric acquisition of a predefined volume, a computer reconstruction and the possibility of obtaining images in any plane. Compared to a CT scan, the reduction of examined bone volume allows reduction of the radiation dose. The resolution and image quality are quite similar and the cost is lower (small units), but the acquisition time is longer.

Preoperative examination

The following structures must be located:
• *Dental environment*: endodontic and periodontal radiographic examination of adjacent and other remaining teeth.

Table 25.1 Characteristics of different imaging techniques

	Two-dimensional			Three-dimensional		
	Intraoral	Panoramic	Cephalometric	Conventional tomography	CT scan	CBCT
Radiation dose	L	L	L	M	H	H
Accuracy	M	L	M	M	H	H
Distortion	L	H	L	No	No	No
Reproducibility	M	L	H	H	H	H
Magnification	L	H	L	No	No	No
Cost	L	L	L	M	H	M
Patient position	S	ST	ST	ST	SU	ST

CBCT, cone beam computed tomography; CT, computed tomography; H, high; L, low; M, moderate; S, seated; ST, standing; SU, supine.

Table 25.2 Recommendations for radiographic preoperative examination

	Standard radiography	Tomography indication	Tomography technique
MAXILLA Partially edentulous	Panoramic Intraoral Intraoral status (1)	Incisive canal proximity Limited volume/maxillary sinus Ridge alteration	Conventional (2) CBCT/CT scan (3)
MAXILLA Totally edentulous	Panoramic		CT scan
MANDIBLE Partially edentulous	Panoramic Intraoral Intraoral status (1)	Mandibular canal proximity Mandibular foramen proximity	Conventional (2) CBCT/CT scan (3)
MANDIBLE Totally edentulous	Panoramic Cephalometric	Ridge alteration	CT scan

CBCT, cone beam computed tomography; CT, computed tomography; (1) periodontitis patients; (2) small areas; (3) multiple areas.

- *Extraction site*: evaluation of bone surrounding hopeless teeth (particularly for immediate implant protocols).
- *Bone morphology*:
  - height and width of alveolar bone to select the optimum implant size
  - precise location of cortical plates (buccal, lingual, sinus floor, nasal floor) to obtain cortical anchorage if necessary
  - three-dimensional bone orientation, to compare with the prosthetic orientation (radiographic guide).
- *Location of anatomical structures*: essential to avoid damaging them (e.g. inferior alveolar nerve) and to allow adaptation of the surgical approach (e.g. maxillary sinus).
- *Bone quality*: this determines the surgical technique (drilling) and the healing delay. Bone quality evaluation is difficult with imaging techniques. Appreciation during surgical drilling gives a more accurate evaluation.

Specific imaging techniques are recommended, according to the area to explore (Table 25.2).

Radiographic monitoring of implants

Osseointegration is a prerequisite for implant success. It is always associated with a characteristic absence of radiolucency around the implant body on intraoral radiography.

Marginal bone level is measured on periapical radiography, to ensure that no excessive marginal bone loss occurs after implant insertion and prosthetic connection. Implant success requires a maximum of 0.1 mm marginal bone loss per year after the first year of prosthetic loading.

Adjustment of prosthetic components may need to be confirmed by intraoral radiography, to check the absence of any gap between the different components (implant, abutment, prosthesis).

Recommendations for radiographic monitoring of implants

Intraoral radiography with parallel technique is the examination of choice for implant monitoring. Irradiation geometry is crucial to avoid misinterpretation (Figures 25.4–25.6).

Key points

- An intraoral radiograph with a parallel technique is mandatory before implant placement.
- Radiographic examination must be performed with a minimal radiation dose.
- Cone beam computed tomography (CBCT) is the basic 3D imaging technique.
- A computed tomography (CT) scan may be used for specific indications.

26 Patient records

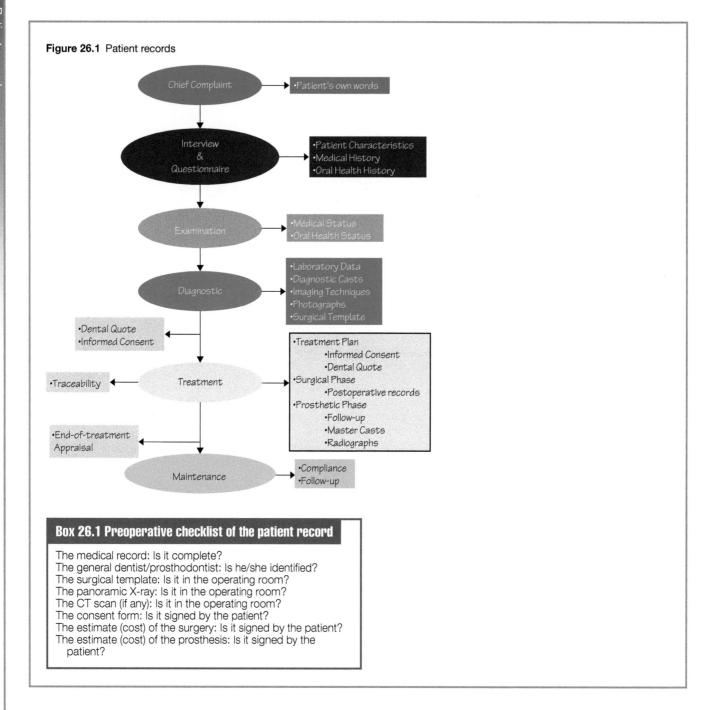

Figure 26.1 Patient records

Box 26.1 Preoperative checklist of the patient record

The medical record: Is it complete?
The general dentist/prosthodontist: Is he/she identified?
The surgical template: Is it in the operating room?
The panoramic X-ray: Is it in the operating room?
The CT scan (if any): Is it in the operating room?
The consent form: Is it signed by the patient?
The estimate (cost) of the surgery: Is it signed by the patient?
The estimate (cost) of the prosthesis: Is it signed by the patient?

The patient record includes the informed consent, the dental quote and the medical records.

Figure 26.1 summarises the documents that should be kept at various stages of treatment. Care must be taken with patients who are having complex care. Patients are considered to have complex care needs if they need ongoing care from a multi-disciplinary team (see Chapter 15). These patients should have separate records from each practitioner involved in the treatment. Each practitioner should be able to provide a copy or summary of the patient's treatment plan to the referring general practitioner before beginning the course of treatment (i.e. following an examination and assessment of the patient).

Implant Dentistry at a Glance, Second Edition. Jacques Malet, Francis Mora and Philippe Bouchard.
© 2018 John Wiley & Sons Ltd. Published 2018 by John Wiley & Sons Ltd.
Companion website: www.wiley.com/go/malet/implant

Figure 26.2 Surgical planning form

SURGICAL PLANNING				General Dentist/Prosthodontist ID						
Patient ID				Surgeon ID					Date	
Implant Brand		One Stage		Two Stage		Immediate Implantation		Immediate Loading	Temporary Implants	
Bone Graft	Bone Substitute	Membrane		Fixation Screw		Sinus Grafting		Specific Comments		

Tooth#	CT Scan		Dental Implants							Specific Comments
	Guide#	Slice#	Type	Length	Diameter	Angle	Head	Neck	Reference	

Informed consent

The surgeon has a legal obligation to provide the patient with information on the planned procedure so that he/she has a clear appreciation and understanding of the surgery, implications and future consequences. Therefore, all patients receiving dental implants and other oral surgeries are asked to sign a consent form. The content of the consent form mainly depends on the relevant country's law. Basically, it is patient centred and based on the standard of care in that country. Ideally, an individual consent form should be created for each patient according to his/her specific condition. However, templates may be used for standard situations (see Appendix E).

Dental quote

The patient must understand the cost of dental implant treatment. Dental practitioners are required to provide a written quote or cost estimate to the patient prior to commencing a course of treatment. The written quote should be signed by both the patient and the practitioner(s). The cost estimate should include the comprehensive range of care related to dental implant therapy, including dental assessments, restorative care such as fillings, crowns and bridges, extractions and other oral surgery, orthodontic treatments and dentures.

Traceability

Dental implants are medical devices. Thus, one must be able to verify the history, location or application of dental implants by means of documented recorded identification. The traceability of dental implants and prosthetic devices such as abutments is mandatory. Stickers and/or labels on the packaging must be included in the patient records.

Medical record

The medical record is a systematic documentation of current and past medical history and care. It can be used as a legal document. The practitioner may use computerised patient record systems or paper-based ones.

The patient's chief complaint – that is, the patient's initial demand – is the cornerstone of the treatment plan. Dental implant therapy may take place over a long time. Further, in complex cases, more than three specialists can be involved in the treatment. There is a risk over time that the patient's demand will be overlooked, due to the complexity of the procedures. Consequently, the patient record should include the patient's own words corresponding to his/her demand, and not the interpretation of the practitioner.

The medical chart should include the following.

Demographics and patient characteristics
- Patient's chief complaint
- Patient's expectation of therapy outcome
- Patient's motivation/ability to provide home care.

Practitioner characterisation

Health conditions/problems

Health history
- Medical history
- Oral/dental history.

Examinations
- Medical status
- Oral health status.

Diagnostic observations
- Laboratory data
- Diagnostic casts
- Imaging techniques
- Surgical template
- Photographs.

Treatment plan

Surgical phase
- *Preoperative checklist.* The surgeon should have the following on the day of the operation:
  - preoperative checklist of the patient record (Box 26.1)
  - a surgical planning form that has been approved, if applicable, by the professional in charge of the prosthetic phase (Figure 26.2).
- *Postoperative records.* The postoperative record depends on national laws. It can be a written narrative of the surgical

procedure or a postoperative form that is completed at the end of the surgical procedure. The electronic postoperative patient records and follow-up that we use are provided in Appendices F and G. They can be modified according to the surgeon's opinion.

Prosthetic phase
- Patient follow-up
- Master cast
- Radiographs.

End-of-treatment appraisal

The surgical procedure and the reconstruction may not be performed by the same professional. The surgeon and the prosthodontist are both responsible for the treatment. Thus, after completion of the prosthetic phase, the patient, before being placed in a maintenance programme, should be re-examined by the surgeon to confirm the dental implant reconstruction.

Key points

- Informed consent to the surgical procedure is a legal obligation.
- An overall cost estimate must be given to the patient before treatment.
- Traceability is mandatory for dental implants.
- The medical record can be used as a legal document.
- The surgical planning form must be approved by the professional in charge of the reconstruction.

27 The pretreatment phase

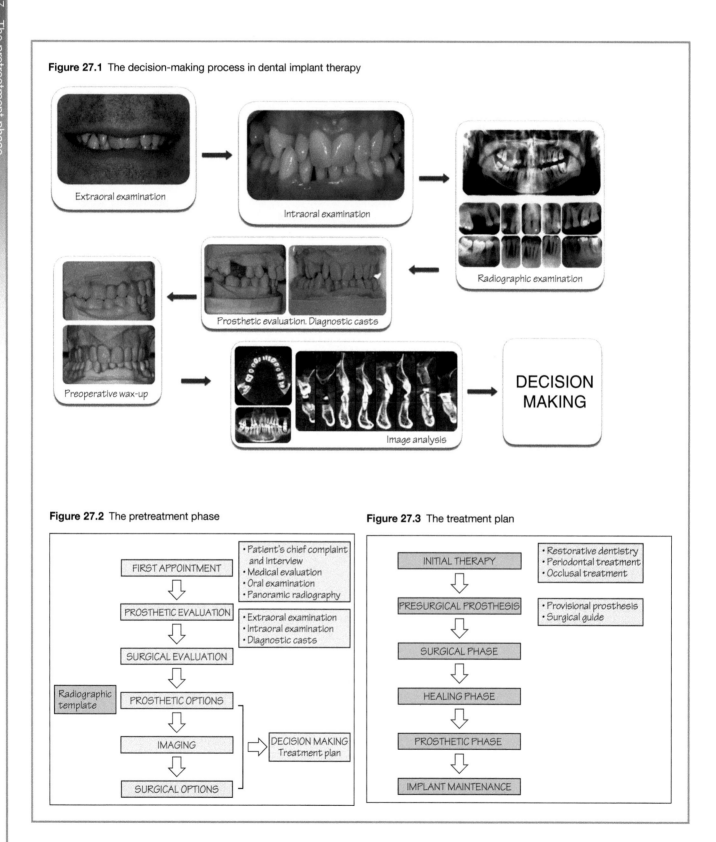

Figure 27.1 The decision-making process in dental implant therapy

Extraoral examination

Intraoral examination

Radiographic examination

Prosthetic evaluation. Diagnostic casts

Preoperative wax-up

Image analysis

DECISION MAKING

Figure 27.2 The pretreatment phase

FIRST APPOINTMENT
- Patient's chief complaint and interview
- Medical evaluation
- Oral examination
- Panoramic radiography

PROSTHETIC EVALUATION
- Extraoral examination
- Intraoral examination
- Diagnostic casts

SURGICAL EVALUATION

Radiographic template

PROSTHETIC OPTIONS

IMAGING

SURGICAL OPTIONS

DECISION MAKING Treatment plan

Figure 27.3 The treatment plan

INITIAL THERAPY
- Restorative dentistry
- Periodontal treatment
- Occlusal treatment

PRESURGICAL PROSTHESIS
- Provisional prosthesis
- Surgical guide

SURGICAL PHASE

HEALING PHASE

PROSTHETIC PHASE

IMPLANT MAINTENANCE

Implant Dentistry at a Glance, Second Edition. Jacques Malet, Francis Mora and Philippe Bouchard.
© 2018 John Wiley & Sons Ltd. Published 2018 by John Wiley & Sons Ltd.
Companion website: www.wiley.com/go/malet/implant

First appointment

The patient's chief complaint determines the main objective of the treatment and is the cornerstone of the prosthetic plan. An in-depth interview is required to identify the patient's profile (see Chapter 26). The functional and aesthetic demands are carefully documented. Patients with unrealistic demands should be excluded from implant therapy. In addition, because some implant procedures are irreversible, time-consuming and expensive, patient compliance is required during and after implant therapy (see Appendix E).

Information is provided to the patient regarding the limitations of dental implant therapy. This information is personalised according to the patient's medical and dental conditions. At this stage, the patient should be made aware of the overall cost of the therapy, including the surgical procedure(s), imaging and restoration fees. The patient should also be verbally informed of the overall length of the treatment.

Panoramic radiography should be sufficient for this preliminary approach. Dental impressions are made in order to obtain diagnostic casts.

Prosthetic evaluation

The prosthetic evaluation should precede the surgical evaluation.

Extraoral examination

The temporomandibular joint status is carefully evaluated. Information is gathered on facial musculature and facial harmony. Attention should be paid to the masticatory muscles (hypertrophy, masticatory forces, bruxism and parafunctions), the loss of occlusal vertical dimension and the lip support in the frontal and sagittal planes. Aesthetic evaluation of the lip–teeth relationship present in the smile, during speech and at rest is mandatory.

Intraoral examination

The clinical examination in dental implant therapy does not differ from the basic preprosthetic examination (Belser *et al.*, 2008a, b). Special attention should be paid to the signs and symptoms of bruxism (tooth wear, indentation of the tongue etc.).

A thorough clinical examination at the implant site evaluates the following features:
• shape of the residual ridge, including the degree of horizontal and vertical alveolar ridge resorption
• thickness of the soft tissues and presence of gingiva
• position/migration of the adjacent teeth
• migration/egression of the antagonist teeth
• width of the edentulous area
• characteristics of the antagonist arch.

During the examination, care must be taken when the arch includes implant-supported fixed partial dentures (FPD) and any type of fixed restoration, especially when the cosmetic reconstruction is made of porcelain. Removable dentures at the opposite arch are at the lowest risk of occlusal stress.

Diagnostic casts

Even if an implant can be surgically placed, this does not mean that the prosthetic envelope is sufficiently large for implant-supported prosthetic restoration. In implant dentistry, the dimensions of the commercially available prosthetic components require a minimum horizontal and vertical space. The diagnostic casts mounted in an articulator are critical to the evaluation of the following parameters:
• The interarch relationship. The interarch distance and the discrepancy between the upper and the lower arches are assessed (Renouard and Rangert, 1999).
• The existing static and dynamic occlusion.
• The interocclusal space. A minimum of 6 mm is required for a fixed restoration. For a removable denture, a minimum of 12 mm is often required.
• The interdental space. For a single implant, a minimum of 7 mm (6 mm for narrow implants) is required. For two implants, the minimum is 14 mm.

Surgical evaluation

The surgical decision-making process is complex and requires a medical approach, an intraoral evaluation and imaging. These points are developed elsewhere in this book (see Chapters 16, 23 and 25).

At the end of the surgical evaluation, a prosthetic option is determined, which enables fabrication of the radiographic template that prefigures the future reconstruction. The final surgical evaluation takes into account the imaging diagnostic, and may confirm or modify the prosthetic option.

Decision-making process

Decision making in dental implant therapy requires a team approach (see Chapter 15). Good decision making integrates the best research evidence with clinical expertise and patient values. Therefore, the final decision leading to the treatment plan combines technical feasibility with the patient's demand. Technical feasibility takes into consideration both the surgical and the prosthetic options (Figures 27.1 and 27.2).

Treatment plan

Normally, the treatment plan should not be modified, because it is the result of the decision-making process. However, a realistic approach allows for changes according to the patient's compliance and complications (Figure 27.3).

The initial therapy aims to control the bacterial load, the occlusal load and the vertical dimension. After the initial therapy, the provisional restoration is prepared and delivered at this stage. The surgical guide is then created from the radiographic template. The dental implants are placed. After the healing phase, a clinical and radiographic evaluation of the integration of the implants to the bone is performed. The prosthetic phase can then begin. At the end of treatment, the patient is enrolled in a maintenance programme.

Key points
• The patient's chief complaint determines the main objective of the treatment.
• A treatment plan is mandatory, even in simple situations.
• The decision-making process requires a team approach.
• The maintenance programme is part of the treatment plan.

28 Treatment planning: Peri-implant environment analysis

Figure 28.1 Minimal interdental space to place a standard-diameter dental implant

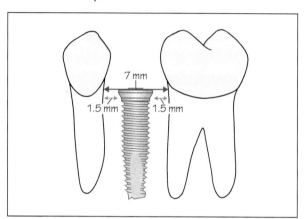

Figure 28.2 Minimal distance between the centres of two standard-diameter dental implants

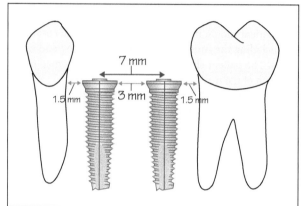

Figure 28.3 Optimal orientation of the implant: the implant axis should emerge in the central fossa and in the direction of the opposing supporting cusps

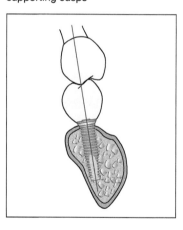

Figure 28.4 Three implants placed in a tripod alignment to minimise stress and torque distribution

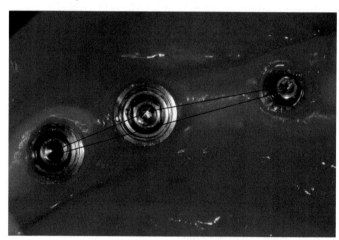

Box 28.1 Checklist of parameters to be evaluated for implant selection

Dimensions of the edentulous area
Adjacent teeth
Biomechanics
Bone volume
Bone quality (loading protocol)
Anatomical structures

Table 28.1 Minimal buccolingual bone volume

Implant diameter	Non-aesthetic areas	Aesthetic areas
3 mm	5 mm	6 mm
4 mm	6 mm	7 mm
5 mm	7 mm	8 mm
6 mm	8 mm	–

Implant selection is performed after prosthetic planning, in order to match implant characteristics with the prosthesis requirements: this is the concept of *prosthetic-driven implant dentistry.*

Guidelines for implant selection are based on several parameters (Box 28.1) and involve clinical examination, radiographic examination and ultimately surgical evaluation.

Implant characteristics include length, diameter, shape, roughness, number and position. In addition, aesthetics may affect the choice of implant (see Chapter 22).

Dimensions of the edentulous area
Ideally, the diameter of the implant platform should be identical to the cervical dimension of the replaced tooth.

Interdental distance: Single-tooth replacement
A 7 mm interdental distance is considered as a routine case; that is, a standard implant can be placed without particular risk (Figure 28.1). For the smallest spaces (5–6 mm), one should consider the use of small-diameter implants to avoid excessive proximal bone loss. For larger spaces, a wide implant may be used if a sufficient thickness of bone is available. For edentulous areas exceeding 14 mm, two implants are required, to avoid horizontal cantilever.

Interdental distance: Multiple-teeth replacement
The number and positions of implants are defined according to the prosthetic planning (see Chapter 27) and with respect to interimplant distances. A minimum of 7 mm is required between the centres of two standard implants (Figure 28.2).

Interocclusal distance
It is important to ensure sufficient space for the prosthetic components of the implant system. Most implant systems require a minimum vertical distance of 6 mm to allow fabrication of the restoration.

Adjacent teeth
For the preservation of alveolar bone and to allow access for hygiene, a minimum of 1.5 mm must separate the implant from the adjacent tooth.

Apical root convergence
The mesiodistal bone volume must be measured over the entire height of the implant site. In cases of apical root convergence, a shorter implant or a conical implant avoids root interference.

Biomechanics
In the posterior area, implant position and implant axis are determined by occlusal force distribution (although it is difficult to prove a correlation between excessive occlusal forces and marginal bone loss or implant failure).

The bone/implant interface is well adapted to axial compressive forces. Shear forces should be avoided. Consequently, for optimal loading, the implant should be placed in the direction of the axial forces (Figure 28.3).

In strong occlusal forces, the use of wide-diameter implants increases the bone-to-implant contact (BIC) and improves the mechanical strength of the implant body (Ivanoff et al., 1999).

Small-diameter implants are contraindicated with high occlusal loading.

For three or more splinted implants, it has been advocated that a tripod configuration improves force distribution (Figure 28.4).

Bone volume
Ideally, the implant should occupy the maximum bone volume and be surrounded by a sufficient bone thickness (1 mm, and 2 mm buccal in aesthetic areas; Table 28.1), while respecting the position (emergence point and axis) guided by the prosthesis (surgical template).

Long implants (>10 mm) may be indicated to achieve primary stability in the following situations: immediate implants, bone defect, tilted implants, poor bone quality.

Small implants (narrow or short) are commercially available for reduced bone dimensions (see Chapters 8 and 9).

Bone quality
Sufficient primary stability is a prerequisite for success for immediate or early loading of implants, while there is no evidence for delayed loading. Nevertheless, primary stability is required if possible.

To improve primary stability in type 3 and type 4 bone, the surgeon may adapt the implant dimensions and select a specific design (see Chapter 7) as well as a rough/bioactive surface (see Chapter 11).

For type 1 and type 2 bone, standard implant designs are preferred to limit bone compression and facilitate insertion. Rough surfaces are not useful either in this indication, except for immediate loading. However, most implant companies offer only relatively rough surfaces.

Key points
- The design of the restoration is a key factor in implant selection.
- A standard implant requires 7 mm mesiodistal distance, 10 mm bone height and 6 mm bone width.
- Wide implants are preferred for molars and when high occlusal loading is expected.
- Long implants (>10 mm) are indicated when poor primary stability is expected with standard implants.
- Limited data are available on the use of short implants as an alternative to bone augmentation surgical procedures.
- Specific implant types are available for type 3 and type 4 bone or for immediate loading.

29 Treatment planning: The provisional phase

Figure 29.1 Single-tooth replacement: removable denture. (a) Extraction of tooth 11. (b) Temporisation with a removable denture. (c) Buccal view after insertion of the provisional denture. Note the lack of artificial gingiva to avoid any buccal compression

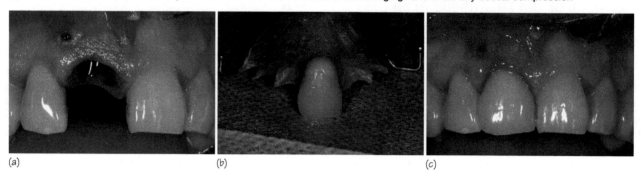

(a)   (b)   (c)

Figure 29.2 Multiple-teeth replacement: removable denture. (a) Modified vacuum-formed clear resin tray (flexible, 0.5 mm thick) replacing the four maxillary incisors during the osseointegration phase. (b) The buccal portion is removed for aesthetics and commercially available artificial teeth are attached to the tray

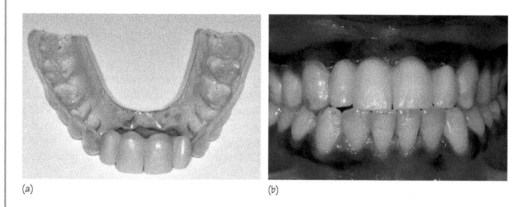

(a)   (b)

Figure 29.3 Multiple-teeth replacement: fixed provisional restoration. (a) Extraction of teeth 11 and 21. (b) Temporisation with a resin-bonded cast metal bridge cemented to the abutment teeth without any tooth preparation (buccal view). (c) Palatal view. Courtesy of Dr Alexandre Sueur, Brussels, Belgium. Reproduced with permission of Alexandre Sueur

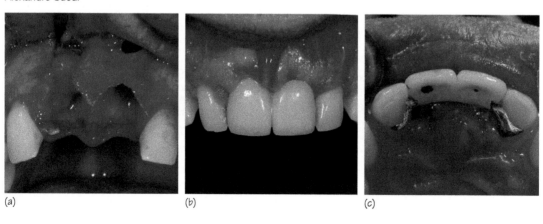

(a)   (b)   (c)

Implant Dentistry at a Glance, Second Edition. Jacques Malet, Francis Mora and Philippe Bouchard.
© 2018 John Wiley & Sons Ltd. Published 2018 by John Wiley & Sons Ltd.
Companion website: www.wiley.com/go/malet/implant

Figure 29.4 Single-tooth replacement: fixed provisional restoration. (a) Tooth-supported provisional bridge on tooth 11, replacing tooth 21 (cantilever). (b) Clinical view without the provisional restoration

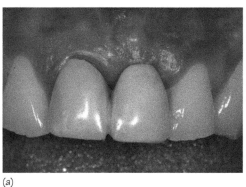
(a)

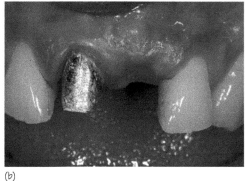
(b)

One critical challenge in implant therapy is the provisional phase. Most patients want a temporary replacement of missing teeth during the period between implant placement and final prosthetic restoration, in particular in aesthetic areas. Temporary solutions may be of three types: removable, tooth supported or implant supported. Their role is to preserve aesthetics and function, and to prevent tooth migration. In non-aesthetic areas and for particularly risky procedures (bone grafts, barrier membranes), clinicians may decide not to place any provisional restoration.

Timing

The decision to use a temporary replacement and the choice of restoration type should be determined during treatment planning. The restoration can be elaborated chairside or in the laboratory. The provisional prosthesis can be elaborated at different steps of the treatment: prior to extraction, before implant placement, after implant placement or after implant osseointegration.

Role of the temporary prosthetic restoration

As in conventional dentistry, the temporary prosthetic restoration in implant dentistry plays a major role during the entire treatment. It maintains aesthetics and provides stabilisation and function.

In the aesthetic area, the provisional restoration is used to maintain soft tissue morphology after tooth extraction and to guide soft tissue healing for the final restoration (see Chapter 31). It is a preview of the future restoration on which all modifications can be tested with the patient and the laboratory.

General specifications of temporary prosthetic restorations

- Not traumatic to adjacent teeth and soft tissues
- No negative interference with osseointegration
- Easy to modify if necessary
- Acceptable aesthetics
- Comfortable
- Easy to clean
- Strong and durable for the duration of the treatment
- Low financial cost.

Removable solutions

A *temporary partial denture* is an inexpensive, simple to elaborate, easy to remove and easily revisable solution. However, a denture may be unstable and compressive on the mucosa, causing indirect loading, marginal bone loss and even loss of osseointegration. This drawback can be particularly obvious with grafted sites.

The denture should be modified for the first weeks, to avoid any contact with the wound, and regular checks and relining are necessary afterwards to avoid hampering the healing process.

In the aesthetic area, the gingival portion of the denture should be reduced or removed to avoid contact with the soft tissue (Figure 29.1).

A *modified clear resin tray* (Figure 29.2) is an alternative to a temporary partial denture, when the clinical situation requires a total lack of compression during the first weeks (bone graft, poor primary stability) or in the case of limited interocclusal space.

Tooth-supported solutions

A *resin-bonded cast metal bridge* is a very reliable, comfortable and stable solution. However, it may not be easy to remove and to reline if necessary. During prosthetic steps, debonding and rebonding procedures can be time-consuming and degrade the bonding strength. In addition, this option has a higher financial cost. It is indicated for long-term temporary placement, particularly in young patients (Figure 29.3).

A *temporary bridge* is an inexpensive, simple to elaborate, easy to remove and easily revisable solution. *Temporary cantilevers* (with low occlusal contact) are possible, but not recommended (Figure 29.4).

However, few clinical situations of this type are encountered, since at least one adjacent tooth must be prepared for a prosthetic reconstruction.

Under a *staged approach*, for extended or complete restorations, it may be possible to elaborate a first temporary bridge on some remaining hopeless teeth. After implant insertion and osseointegration, teeth are extracted, an implant-supported temporary bridge is placed and other implants are inserted if necessary.

Transitional implants

Small screws inserted in some strategic positions and immediately loaded serve to support a provisional fixed restoration or to stabilise a removable denture. Bone volume and cortical anchorage are essential for these devices.

Implant-supported solutions (immediate function)

Modified implant surfaces, evolution of surgical techniques and better understanding of healing processes have led to protocols for the immediate placement of temporary implant prostheses, with acceptable success rates. These *immediate function* devices can be subjected to full occlusal loading (*immediate loading*) or not affected by the occlusal forces (*immediate restoration*; see Chapter 30).

This is a very comfortable and stable solution for the patient, with the added advantage of allowing soft tissue maturation. However, indications are restricted to particular clinical conditions and include, among other parameters, sufficient primary stability of the implants (see Chapter 30).

Key points

- A provisional restoration should replace the missing teeth during the healing phase.
- The design of the provisional restoration must not be detrimental to the osseointegration process.
- In aesthetic areas the provisional restoration should have a design aiming to guide soft tissue healing.

Treatment planning: Immediate, early and delayed loading

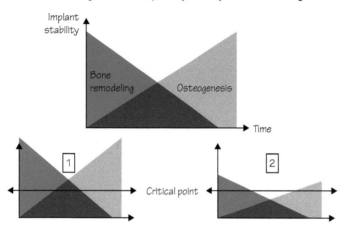

Figure 30.1 Evolution of dental implant stability in time, after surgical placement. 1. Favourable conditions for immediate loading: good primary stability and rapid osteogenesis; 2. unfavourable conditions for immediate loading: insufficient primary stability and slow osteogenesis

Figure 30.2 Immediate loading (edentulous mandible). (a) Four implants are inserted between the mental foramina. An impression is taken at the end of surgery. (b) The fixed restoration (10 teeth and no cantilevers) is delivered within 24 hours. (c) Radiographic control on the day of prosthesis insertion

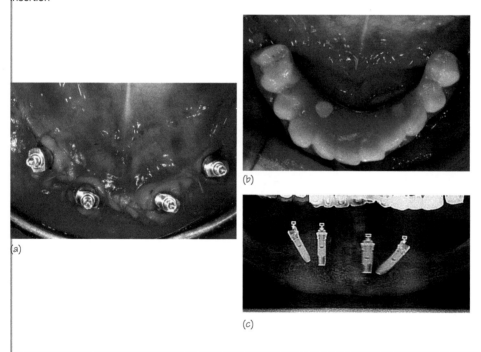

Implant Dentistry at a Glance, Second Edition. Jacques Malet, Francis Mora and Philippe Bouchard.
© 2018 John Wiley & Sons Ltd. Published 2018 by John Wiley & Sons Ltd.
Companion website: www.wiley.com/go/malet/implant

Table 30.1 Loading definitions

Immediate loading	Early loading	Conventional loading	Immediate restoration
Same day to 1 week	1 week to 2 months	After 2–3 months	Within 1 week
			Not in occlusion
In function	In function	In function	

Table 30.2 Different loading protocols: level of scientific evidence (edentulous patient)

		Mandible	Maxilla
Removable prosthesis	Conventional loading	H	M
	Immediate loading	H	L
	Early loading	M	M
Fixed prosthesis	Conventional loading	H	H
	Immediate loading	H	H
	Early loading	M	M
Immediate implants	Immediate loading (fixed prosthesis)	L	M

H, high; M, medium; L, low.
Source: Adapted from Gallucci et al., 2009.

The conventional protocol in dental implant therapy includes a healing period of two to six months during which dental implants are unloaded. Nowadays, this period may be shortened or eliminated.

Rationale

After implant insertion, primary initial stability decreases during the first weeks (*bone remodelling*), while secondary stability (*osteogenesis*) increases during the same period (Figure 30.1). The role of forces transmitted to the implant during this period is not clear: implant *micromotion*, if excessive, can affect osteogenesis and impair osseointegration, but it seems that limited loading may not be detrimental and may even be beneficial. If micromotion is kept under a threshold of about 150 μm during the entire healing process, osseointegration will occur normally. During this period, the control of factors influencing bone remodelling, osteogenesis and micromotion is the biological basis of immediate loading.

Loading is defined as full occlusal contact at least in centric occlusion. Immediate restoration (synonym: non-occlusal loading) means that despite no occlusal contact, some forces are transmitted to the implants by muscles (tongue, lips, cheeks) and food. Other definitions are included in Table 30.1.

Background

Until a few years ago, predictable results with immediate and early loading protocols were only described in the anterior mandible area. Today, more data are available for edentulous maxilla, fixed partial dentures and single-tooth implants.

Although immediate and early loading protocols are viable treatment options, the evidence level is low, and very often clinical studies are characterised by high patient selection and trained operators, both minimising the risk. From a scientific point of view, the more predictable option is still the conventional approach, followed by immediate loading and, finally, the early loading approach (Esposito et al., 2009).

Clinical situations
Edentulous patients (Table 30.2)

Conventional loading of implants for edentulous patients often requires them to wear a complete removable denture, which can compromise implant success (Table 30.2). Consequently, the possibility of an immediate loading protocol must be considered. This is the case for the following well-documented situations:

- Mandibular overdenture supported by four splinted, immediately loading implants in the interforamina area
- Mandibular fixed restoration supported by four, five or six immediately loading implants (Figure 30.2).
- Maxillary fixed restoration supported by six to eight immediately loading implants.

The relatively significant number of implants and the possibility of achieving cross-arch stabilisation explain the good results obtained in these situations. For other situations that are less well documented, a conventional loading protocol is still indicated.

Partially edentulous patients

Although the level of evidence is low, it seems possible to load implants with a fixed partial denture (FPD) immediately or early, even in the posterior maxilla (Roccuzzo et al., 2009). Implant distribution, bone quality, opposite dentition and occlusal schemes are critical parameters for implant success. Furthermore, the possibility of not having the restoration in occlusal contact with the opposite jaw extends the indications of immediate placement of the restoration (Figure 30.3).

Recommendations

Primary stability of implants is essential for immediate loading. It can be measured by the insertion torque value during implant placement. A 30 Ncm insertion torque as a minimum value is generally accepted. However, there is no professional agreement on this value. A modified drilling protocol (underdrilling) can be necessary to improve primary stability.

Prosthesis insertion as soon as possible (within one week) is recommended.

It must be pointed out that not all clinicians will achieve optimal results, as immediate loading requires sufficient training.

Indications for immediate/early loading of implants

See Box 30.1.

Patient benefit

Since conventional loading is still the gold standard, a modified protocol should provide real patient benefit: shortened treatment time, safer provisional restoration and lower financial cost.

Figure 30.3 Immediate restoration (tooth 14). (a) After insertion of the implant, a temporary prosthetic abutment is placed. (b) A temporary crown is elaborated chairside and cemented without occlusal contact. (c) Radiographic control

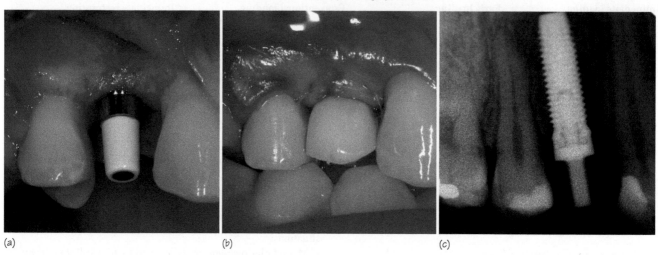

(a)   (b)   (c)

Box 30.1 Parameters involved in immediate loading success

Patient	Implant	Surgery	Prosthesis
Non-bruxing Non-smoker	Osseoconductive surface	Bone quality Bone volume	Lateral load control
	Special design Number/distribution	Drilling protocols	Rigid splinting of implants

Patient selection

Medically compromised patients, bruxism patients and heavy smokers should be excluded.

Site selection

Sufficient good-quality bone allowing placement of implants in optimal conditions is required.

Surgical decision

The decision for immediate loading is validated during surgery, but only if sufficient primary stability of implants is achievable.

Key points

• Immediate/early loading is a technically demanding procedure for experienced clinicians.
• Good primary stability of implants is essential for immediate/early loading.
• Rough implant surfaces play a major role in the success of immediate/early loading.
• The risk–benefit ratio of immediate loading procedures should be considered in the decision-making process.

31 Treatment planning: Single-tooth replacement

Figure 31.1 Replacement of two deciduous incisors retained at the mandible in a 35-year-old adult patient. (a) Preoperative radiograph. (b) Orthodontic treatment aiming to make optimal space for a single dental implant. (c) Clinical view one year after loading. (d) Corresponding radiograph of the tapered narrow implant (diameter 3.25 mm)

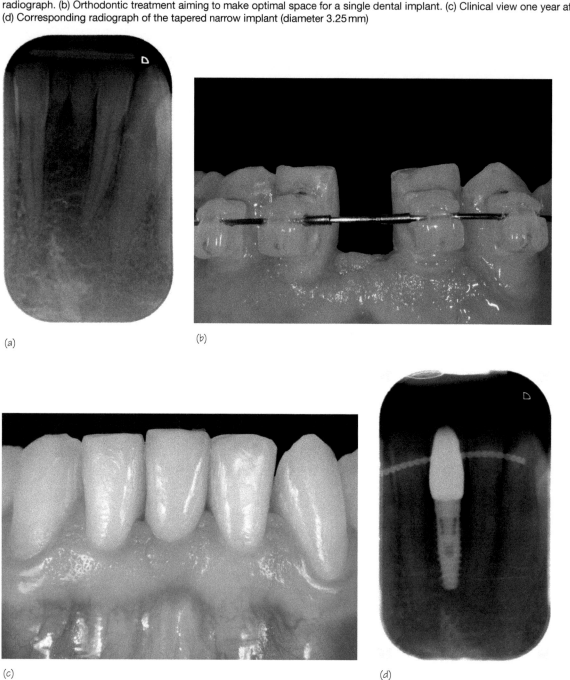

Implant Dentistry at a Glance, Second Edition. Jacques Malet, Francis Mora and Philippe Bouchard.
© 2018 John Wiley & Sons Ltd. Published 2018 by John Wiley & Sons Ltd.
Companion website: www.wiley.com/go/malet/implant

The decision-making process for single-tooth replacement should include all therapeutic options, including tooth-supported fixed partial dentures (FPDs) and resin-bonded bridges. There is limited evidence that implant-supported single crowns perform better than tooth-supported FPDs on a long-term basis. However, taking into account the favourable cost/benefit ratio and the high implant survival rate (ISR), dental implant therapy is the first-line strategy for single-tooth replacement.

Advantages/disadvantages of tooth-supported FPDs

From a biological point of view, preservation of the integrity of the teeth adjacent to the edentulous area is the main advantage. From an economic point of view, it has been shown that dental implant therapy is less costly and more efficient over time than tooth-supported FPDs for the replacement of one missing tooth (Bouchard et al., 2009).

The major disadvantage of dental implant therapy is the need for a surgical procedure. Tissue abnormalities at the implant site may require additional complex surgical procedures. The morbidity of these procedures must be considered in the decision-making process. The risk–benefit ratio with a single implant should be carefully evaluated, and alternative treatment options should be considered.

Indications

Anterior single-tooth replacement

In sites without tissue deficiencies, predictable treatment outcomes, including aesthetics, can be achieved because proximal tissue support is provided by the neighbouring teeth (Belser et al., 2008; Figure 31.1). However, aesthetics in dental implant therapy remains a challenge. Depending on the status of adjacent teeth, tooth-supported FPDs should sometimes be preferred to achieve better aesthetics.

Posterior single-tooth replacement

Aesthetic considerations are less important here than in the anterior area. Therefore, dental implant therapy is the first-line strategy compared to the bridge strategy in the case of intact bordering teeth.

Contraindications

• Interdental space less than 6 mm and/or apical root convergence. This may lead to proximal attachment loss and/or root injury.

• Unpredictable aesthetic achievement in sites with tissue deficiency in anterior areas.

Single-tooth implant in the anterior area

An optimal aesthetic result depends on appropriate patient and implant selection, the correct three-dimensional implant positioning and soft tissue stability. Dental implant therapy in the anterior area is a complex procedure, which is based on a comprehensive perioperative evaluation.

Surgical risk

Evaluation of the implant site should highlight the following high-risk situations:
• buccal bone deficiencies
• soft tissue deficiencies
• distance between the proximal bone and the cemento-enamel junction (CEJ) of the adjacent teeth >2 mm
• buccal cortical bone plate <1 mm.

Optimal implant placement

See Chapter 22, Figure 22.4.

Provisional fixed restoration and soft tissue modelling

The position of soft tissues (papilla preservation and buccal soft tissue margin) is a critical challenge. The provisional restoration plays a major role in the aesthetic outcome. After implant loading, successive modifications of the emergence profile of the provisional restoration are performed, in order to modify the position of the soft tissues and to allow papillae growth within the 'black triangles'. Once an optimal result is obtained, the emergence profile is recorded and transferred to the dental laboratory (see Chapter 36).

Single-tooth implant in the posterior area

In the premolar area, standard-diameter implants are usually used (Figure 31.2).

In the molar area, large-diameter implants are preferred to standard-diameter implants, in order to increase the bone-to-implant contact (BIC) and to improve the mechanical strength of the implant body. A wide platform, which improves the emergence profile, is also recommended in the molar area for better

Figure 31.2 Replacement of a maxillary premolar (no. 25) with a standard dental implant (diameter 4.0 mm). (a) Clinical view five years after loading. (b) Corresponding radiograph

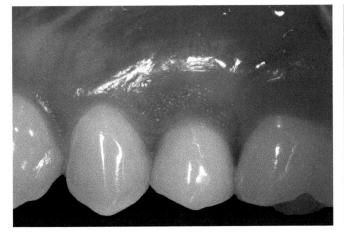

(a)

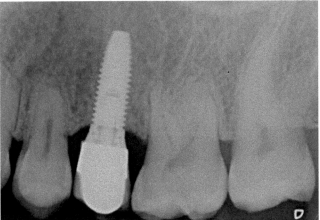

(b)

proximal plaque control. The replacement of a second molar can be a challenging situation.

Masticatory function and patient comfort must be evaluated before deciding to replace a second molar, especially if it requires complex surgical procedures. A passive option (no tooth replacement) may be a simple and viable solution.

Prosthetic considerations

The characteristics of the clinical situation are transferred by a master model to the laboratory technician. The master model is obtained after impression, and contains an analogue of the implant and/or the replica of the abutment. Then the technician folds the crown of the homologous teeth in wax, integrating the same emergence from the labial and interproximal soft tissue margin.

At this stage, selection of the abutment depends on the following factors:
• implant shoulder position in relation to peri-implant gingival margin, with respect to the emergence profile of the suprastructure
• longitudinal implant axis (Belser *et al.*, 2008).

Cemented restorations are normally used due to the simplicity of the technique. However, screw-retained restorations show better marginal precision. In addition, the implant shoulder is often located deep under the mucosa in aesthetic areas. Cement removal may be difficult. Therefore, a screw-retained abutment/restoration interface is advisable, when feasible, for the anterior single-tooth replacement.

Key points

• In non-aesthetic areas, dental implant therapy is the first-line strategy.
• In aesthetic areas, the decision-making process depends on the predictability of aesthetic outcome.
• Screw-retained restorations are generally preferred to cemented restorations.
• In terms of success, there is limited evidence that implant-supported single crowns perform better than tooth-supported fixed partial dentures on a long-term basis.

32 Treatment planning: Implant-supported fixed partial denture

Figure 32.1 (a–d) Anterior area recommendations. The number of implants is reduced to avoid adjacent implants and optimise aesthetics

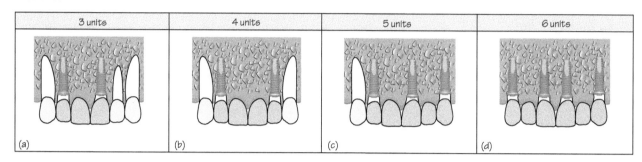

Figure 32.2 Anterior area alternatives. (a) More implants are necessary when the occlusal load is high and/or when the bone volume is reduced. The distance between adjacent implants (red arrow) should be more than 3 mm. (b) Cantilever replacement of a lateral incisor is an alternative to avoid bone augmentation procedures. Excursive tooth contact must be avoided on the cantilever

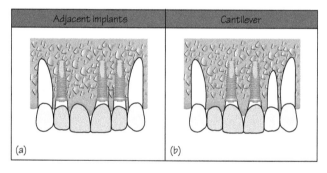

Figure 32.4 Posterior area alternative. Mesial cantilever can avoid bone augmentation procedures. A minimum of two adjacent implants is required

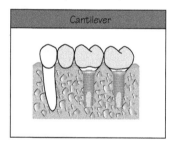

Figure 32.3 Posterior area recommendations. The number of implants depends on biomechanical parameters. (a, c) Short span bridges are preferred for lower financial cost and to avoid implants that are too close. (b) Each molar is replaced by an implant

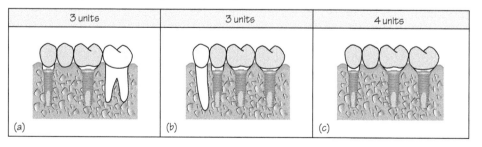

Implant Dentistry at a Glance, Second Edition. Jacques Malet, Francis Mora and Philippe Bouchard.
© 2018 John Wiley & Sons Ltd. Published 2018 by John Wiley & Sons Ltd.
Companion website: www.wiley.com/go/malet/implant

Rationale

Dental implants have become the first treatment option for most edentulous patients and in particular for partial restorations. This is due to the favourable long-term results and the opportunity to deliver a prosthetic restoration with minimal risk, compared to a conventional approach.

Nevertheless, some controversies remain concerning the overall prosthetic decision: distribution of implants, cantilevers, implant/natural tooth connection and screw-retained or cemented restorations.

The general prosthetic goal is to create an overall *reliable* structure consistent with a comfortable *function* (biomechanics), acceptable a*esthetics* and minimum morbidity and cost.

Opinions based on experience with conventional prosthetic treatments are not always reliable, as implant-supported denture concepts follow specific rules, mainly related to the osseointegration process.

Advantages

Compared to most conventional restorations, an implant-supported fixed partial denture (FPD) represents a less invasive prosthetic treatment with a reduction of the overall risk (Pjetursson and Lang, 2008; Table 32.1). This is partly due to the possibility of increasing the number of abutments.

Disadvantages

Financial costs and anatomical limits can represent barriers that are not easy to overcome, and conventional restorations can then be considered.

Indications

Implant-supported FPD, when possible, is the treatment of choice for partially edentulous patients in the following situations:
- healthy adjacent teeth
- intact adjacent tooth restoration
- posterior reduced arch
- extended edentulous segments.

Implant distribution

The number of implants depends on the number of units to be replaced. Other parameters are taken into account, including bone volume, occlusal parameters (antagonist teeth, hyperfunction), dimensions of the edentulous area and adjacent teeth (Figures 32.1–32.4). The implant diameter is selected to best match the replaced tooth.

An optimal number of implants is selected to limit financial cost and improve aesthetics. A prosthetic bridge design with one or two pontics is a reliable option in most cases. However, some clinicians recommend one implant per lost unit in the high-load zone.

Missing second molars are not systematically replaced (shortened arch). The lack of second molar replacement usually has no negative consequences for the masticatory process. However, the individual's chewing capacity should be considered in the decision-making process.

Splinting of implants

In cases of restoration of each lost unit with an implant, there is no scientific evidence to recommend splinting of the implants. While splinting could be justified from a mechanical point of view (better force distribution, fewer technical complications), single units allow a better prosthetic passive fit and easier plaque control.

Indications for splinting of implants include:
- narrow-diameter implants in the posterior area
- short implants
- bruxism
- poor bone quality.

Cantilevers

Although real, the risk associated with cantilevers (abutment fracture, loss of retention) is much lower than with tooth-supported fixed dentures. The option of cantilevers can sometimes avoid bone reconstruction and thus simplify the overall treatment. Mesial cantilevers are considered to be less hazardous than distal ones.

For edentulous patients, cantilevers of limited length are viable for long-span bridges.

Implant/natural tooth connection

Although no data support the hypothesis of a particular risk when connecting implants and natural teeth in an FPD, totally implant-supported FPDs are preferred whenever possible, rather than implant/natural tooth-supported FPDs.

If the only solution is to splint teeth and implants, a rigid connection is preferred, as intrusion of natural abutments has been described in this situation.

Screw-retained or cemented restoration

There is an overall trend to promote cemented restorations over screw-retained FPDs. This is due to the 'similarity' with conventional treatments and the relative expected simplicity. However, better precision is demonstrated with screw-retained FPDs, although it is more difficult to achieve. Both treatment options show good prognosis, with no statistical difference (Table 32.2).

Indications for screw-retained FPDs include:
- reduced interarch distance (<5 mm)
- expected frequent prosthetic modifications in the future
- non-visible areas (maxilla).

Complications

Despite the high survival rates, 38.7% of patients with implant-supported FPDs have some complications during the five-year observation period, as compared to 15.7% for conventional FPDs and 20.6% for cantilever FPDs, respectively (Pjetursson and Lang, 2008).

Compared with tooth-supported FPDs, the incidence of technical complications was significantly higher for implant-supported reconstructions. The most frequent technical

Table 32.1 Survival rate of prosthetic fixed partial dentures

	5 years (%)	10 years (%)
Conventional tooth-supported FPD	93.8	89.2
Cantilever FPD	91.4	80.3
Implant-supported FPD	95.2	86.7
Combined tooth-implant FPD	95.5	77.8
Implant-supported single crown	94.5	89.4
Resin-bonded bridge	87.7	65

FPD, fixed partial denture.
Source: Pjetursson and Lang, 2008.

Table 32.2 Advantages and disadvantages of screw-retained and cemented fixed partial dentures

	Advantages	Disadvantages
Screw-retained FPD	Retrievable	Bacterial colonisation
	Reduced height	More screw loosening
	Margin precision	Cost
		Aesthetics (occlusal holes)
Cemented FPD	Simplicity	Less precise margin
	Cost	Cement removal
	Passive fit	Difficult to retrieve
	Aesthetics	

FPD, fixed partial denture.

complications were fractures of the veneer material (ceramic fractures or chipping), abutment or screw loosening and retention loss.

Key points

- Implant-supported fixed partial dentures (FPDs) is the dominant strategy for partially edentulous patients.
- There is no evidence to support the concept of one tooth, one implant.
- Combined tooth/implant FPDs should be avoided as much as possible.
- There is no evidence that a screw-retained restoration performs better than a cemented restoration.
- Technical complications are frequent with implant-supported FPDs.

33 Treatment planning: Fully edentulous patients

Figure 33.1 Modification of jawbone dimensions in the fully edentulous patient

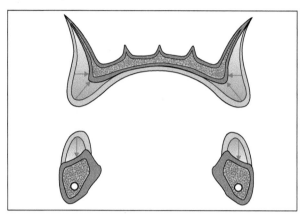

Figure 33.2 Modification of the orofacial support in the fully edentulous patient

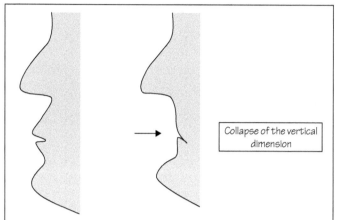

Collapse of the vertical dimension

Figure 33.3 Anatomical areas at the maxilla and at the mandible where dental implants can normally be placed in the native bone (shaded areas)

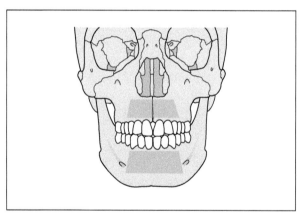

Figure 33.4 Bone resorption in edentulous patients

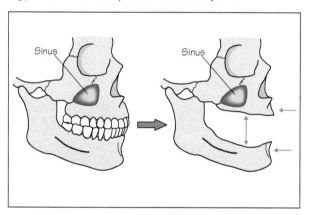

Sinus

Sinus

Figure 33.5 The simplest option: overdenture supported by two dental implants

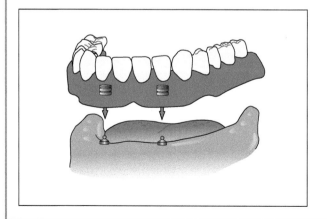

Figure 33.6 A sophisticated option: implant-supported fixed partial denture replacing the entire arch

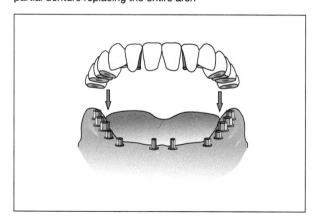

Implant Dentistry at a Glance, Second Edition. Jacques Malet, Francis Mora and Philippe Bouchard.
© 2018 John Wiley & Sons Ltd. Published 2018 by John Wiley & Sons Ltd.
Companion website: www.wiley.com/go/malet/implant

Bone resorption is the major problem in completely edentulous patients (Figure 33.1). The edentulism leads to the loss of orofacial support, facial aesthetics, phonetics and the collapse of vertical dimension (Figure 33.2). Treatment at the maxilla is more complex than at the mandible, and overdentures and fixed restorations show better success at the mandible than at the maxilla.

Surgical specificities

The anatomical areas where dental implants can be placed in the native bone are often limited (Figure 33.3). Bone resorption increases the need for surgical bone compensation (Figure 33.4). Situations where more than six dental implants can be placed in the native bone, either at the mandible or at the maxilla, are rare. Nevertheless, dental implant placement does not differ per se from the standard surgical procedure, except for the fixed prosthesis supported by four implants.

A surgical guide is mandatory because of the lack of benchmarks.

One-stage or two-stage approaches can be used. A two-stage approach may be indicated when it is expected that prostheses could transmit excessive forces onto the dental implants (Esposito *et al.*, 2009).

Number and position of dental implants

There is no evidence to suggest that a minimum number of implants should be placed to achieve a standard clinical level. It cannot be concluded that patient satisfaction, denture function or implant survival improves by increasing the number of implants (Gotfredsen *et al.*, 2008). Restorations can replace the entire arch as long as an appropriate number of implants are able to be placed (see Appendix I, Tables I.1 and I.2).

From a biomechanical point of view, the position of the implants should be symmetrical about the midline. Thus, the number of placed implants should be even. An odd number of implants has been proposed, including the placement of a single implant in the midline. Routine use of these approaches cannot be recommended, except for the five-implant option at the mandible, and specific clinical situations that cannot be detailed in this book.

Prosthetic specificities

The treatment may vary from simple to highly complex (Figures 33.5 and 33.6). The prosthesis may be constructed to be removable by the patient (overdenture) or non-removable if cemented or fixed with screws to the implants (bridge or denture design).

These two main options present both advantages and disadvantages (see Appendix I, Table I.3). Bridge design restorations often necessitate surgical augmentation procedures to achieve good aesthetics and function. Enhancement of aesthetic appearance and facial morphology may be easier with a denture design, possibly with decreased costs and less surgical intervention.

Overdentures or denture design fixed restorations may compensate for defects in the alveolar ridge as well as lip support. In addition, dental implants can be placed according to the bony availability, because there is no need to place the implant at the emergence of a tooth. However, the volume of the acrylic support may vary from a mucosa-borne complete denture to an implant-borne reduced denture, limited to the premolar area, which compensates poorly for bone resorption.

Removable options

Overdentures are implant- and mucosa-borne dentures. The denture base is attached to the dental implants by various commercially available attachment systems. One part of the attachment is connected to the dental implants and the other incorporated within the undersurface of the overdenture.

Attachment systems are adjustable and/or replaceable. They include bar, ball, stud, magnetic and telescopic attachment systems (Preiskel, 1996). Patients prefer bar-clip or ball attachments over magnet attachments (Cune *et al.*, 2005, 2010). The bars can be soldered, cast with milled designs, made using spark erosion or even milled precision bars using non-precious alloys as part of an attachment system (Sadowsky, 2007). The bar can be extended by distal extensions.

It seems that restorations with distal bar extensions up to 12 mm have no influence on crestal bone loss around implants (Semper *et al.*, 2010). The bar may be round, ovoid or parallel sided. The overdenture contains clips, spring pins or other elements that fit onto the bar.

There is no difference in marginal bone loss around implants retaining/supporting mandibular overdentures relative to implant type or attachment design (Cehreli *et al.*, 2010).

Fixed options

According to the number and seating of the dental implants, the restoration may have a denture design (screw retained) or a bridge design (screw or cement retained). These two main options present both advantages and disadvantages (see Appendix I, Table I.4).

Denture design restorations can be implant and mucosa borne or solely implant borne according to the number and position of the implants. A metal framework retains and supports the acrylic resin denture base.

Fixed restorations may have distal extensions. The custom metal framework must seat with no tension on any implants (passive fit).

Key points

- There is no evidence for a single, universally superior treatment modality for the edentulous patient.
- The treatment at the maxilla is more complex than at the mandible.
- Overdentures and fixed restorations demonstrate better success at the mandible than at the maxilla.

34 Treatment planning: Edentulous mandible

Figure 34.1 Removable options: overdentures with attachment systems. (a) Two dental implants. Ball attachment system. (b) Four dental implants. Bar attachment system. Distal bar extensions are possible

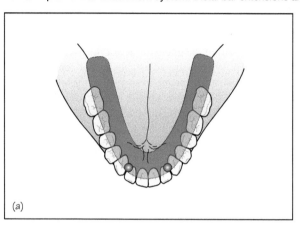

(a)

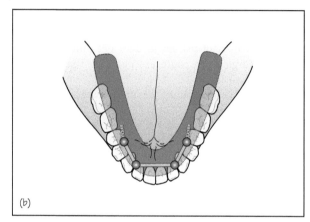

(b)

Figure 34.2 Fixed options: screw-retained denture designs. (a) Four dental implants. The two distal implants are tilted (see Appendix L). (b) Six dental implants. (c) Eight dental implants

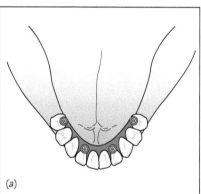

(a)

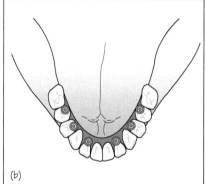

(b)

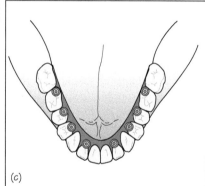

(c)

Figure 34.3 Fixed options: screw-retained or cemented bridge designs. (a) Six dental implants. The second premolar may have a molar shape. (b) Eight dental implants

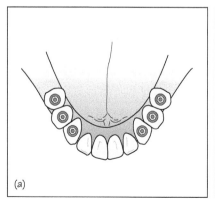

(a)

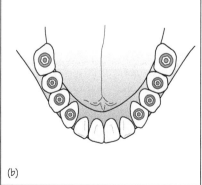

(b)

Implant Dentistry at a Glance, Second Edition. Jacques Malet, Francis Mora and Philippe Bouchard.
© 2018 John Wiley & Sons Ltd. Published 2018 by John Wiley & Sons Ltd.
Companion website: www.wiley.com/go/malet/implant

Removable options
Overdenture supported by two implants: Ball attachment system

See Figure 34.1a. This is the least expensive, shortest and simplest option. Normally, this option is possible in any case, except for severely resorbed mandibles. A bar can also be used. One international consensus has proposed mandibular two-implant overdentures as the minimum standard of care for edentulous patients (Feine *et al.*, 2002).

Treatment plan specificities

Two implants are placed in the anterior mandible between the mental foramina (see Appendix J). Placing the implant in the canine-lateral region is recommended. A minimum of 7 mm of interocclusal distance is necessary. The implants must be parallel with a 10° tolerance. One-stage or two-stage procedures can be used. After the osseointegration process, ball abutments are placed. The existing denture can be used (see Appendix K). If this is not possible for functional or aesthetic reasons, a new denture must be prepared according to the standard principles of complete dentures.

Overdenture supported by four implants: Bar attachment system

See Figure 34.1b.

Fixed options
Fixed prosthesis supported by four implants: Screw-retained prosthesis

This technique is indicated with a minimum bone width of 5 mm and a minimum bone height of 8 mm between the mental foramina (see Appendix L). The posterior implants are tilted to a maximum of 45°. Immediate loading with a provisional restoration is part of the initial description of the technique (Maló *et al.*, 2003). The restoration has a denture design (see below).

The major advantage of this technique, which is technically demanding, is that it may avoid bone transplantation. The restoration is limited to premolars. Molar sites are not replaced.

Fixed prosthesis supported by more than four implants
Denture design restoration: Screw-retained prosthesis
A minimum of four implants is required (Figure 34.2).

Bridge design restoration: Screw- or cement-retained prosthesis
A minimum of six implants is required (Figure 34.3).

Success/survival rates

Overall implant survival ranges from 86% to 100% at five years for fixed prostheses and from 83% to 100% for overdentures (Bryant *et al.*, 2007). Overdentures supported by two implants demonstrate a survival rate of 95.5% after 20 years of loading (Vercruyssen *et al.*, 2010).

Nowadays, immediately and early loaded implants are commonly used in mandibles with good bone quality (Brånemark *et al.*, 1999). Short-term outcomes (24 months) of early or immediate loading protocols for mandibular implant overdentures achieved comparable success to conventional loading ones (Kawai and Taylor, 2007; Alsabeeha *et al.*, 2010). Micro-roughened implants should be preferred to machined implants in this indication.

Key points

- An overdenture supported by two unsplinted implants is an efficient, cheap and simple option. It functions as effectively as four splinted implants.
- Overdentures and denture design fixed restorations can compensate for alveolar bone resorption.
- Bridge design restorations require at least six symmetrical dental implants.
- Eight symmetrical dental implants are necessary to replace all the teeth.

35 Treatment planning: Edentulous maxilla

Figure 35.1 Removable options: overdentures with bar attachment systems. (a) Four parallel dental implants. The denture base has full palatal coverage. Distal bar extensions are possible. (b) Six parallel dental implants. The palatal area of the denture is relieved

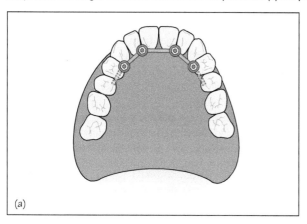

(a)

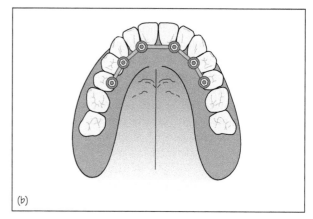

(b)

Figure 35.2 Fixed options: screw-retained denture designs. (a) Four dental implants. The two distal implants are tilted (see Appendix M). (b) Six dental implants. (c) Eight dental implants

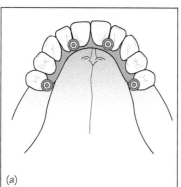

(a)

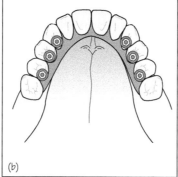

(b)

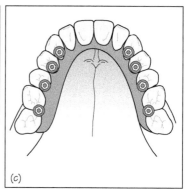

(c)

Figure 35.3 Fixed options: screw-retained or cemented bridge designs. (a) Six dental implants. The second premolar may have a molar shape. (b) Eight dental implants. (c) Ten dental implants

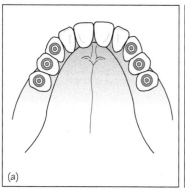

(a)

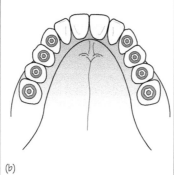

(b)

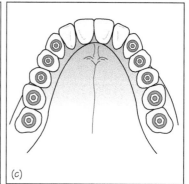

(c)

Implant Dentistry at a Glance, Second Edition. Jacques Malet, Francis Mora and Philippe Bouchard.
© 2018 John Wiley & Sons Ltd. Published 2018 by John Wiley & Sons Ltd.
Companion website: www.wiley.com/go/malet/implant

Bone resorption in the anterior area may jeopardise aesthetic results; and sinus volume following alveolar bone resorption may preclude implant placement in the posterior areas. Consequently, patients who are edentulous at the maxilla are often good candidates for hard and soft tissue augmentation procedures. In addition, the maxillary bone quality is often worse than that of the mandible, making the prognosis for dental implants in the edentulous maxilla less secure than in the mandible.

Thus, the decision-making process depends not only on the surgically available bone volume, but also on the patient's wishes in terms of aesthetics. In other words, treatment choice at the maxilla cannot be reduced to that between removable or fixed options, but should be considered in terms of surgical and aesthetic feasibility.

Removable options
Overdenture supported by four implants: Bar attachment system

The recommended treatment option as the standard of care is at least four splinted implants using a bar attachment system (Mericske-Stern, 2003; Figure 35.1a). The decision to place the implants in the anterior area is mainly due to the reduced volume of bone beneath the sinus floor in the posterior area.

In addition to the improvement of denture stability, the dental implants may also allow for the reduction of prosthesis volume by relieving the palatal area of the overdenture. This advantage is important for patients with gag reflex problems. However, this decision must take into account the number and length of dental implants; removal of the palatal support produces a greater effect and more concentrated stress difference for maxillary overdentures than do differences between the attachment designs (Bueno-Samper et al., 2010).

Care must be taken to evaluate the volume of the bar attachment that is incorporated into the overdenture. An excessive volume of the bar in conjunction with a low-to-moderate bone volume resorption in the anterior area may lead to an overexaggeration of the lip support.

Overdenture supported by six implants: Bar attachment system

From a clinical point of view, it seems that the optimal number of implants to support a bar at the maxilla is six (Figure 35.1b). The stress due to removal of the palatal support seems to be better distributed with six implants than with four.

Fixed options
Fixed prosthesis supported by four implants: Screw-retained prosthesis

This technique is recommended with a minimum bone width of 5 mm and a minimum bone height of 10 mm from canine to canine (see Figure 35.2a and Appendix M). The posterior implants are tilted to a maximum of 45°. Immediate loading with a provisional restoration is part of the initial description of the technique (Maló et al., 2003). The restoration has a denture design.

The major advantage of this technique, which is technically demanding, is that it may avoid bone transplantation. The restoration is limited to premolars. Molar sites are not replaced.

Fixed prosthesis supported by at least six implants

A minimum of six implants is required when the implants are parallel.

Denture design restoration: Screw-retained prosthesis

The implants should be placed as distally as possible in the canine-premolar region (Figure 35.2b). From an aesthetics standpoint, it is preferable to avoid seating the implants in the incisor area in order to facilitate placement of the prosthetic teeth. Sinus lift procedures are often required to place implants in the molar area (Figure 35.2c).

Bridge design restoration: Screw- or cement-retained prosthesis

Surgical augmentation procedures are often needed to compensate for bone loss. They aim not only to increase the vertical dimension of the bone to allow for implant placement, but also to increase the horizontal dimension so as to improve aesthetics and function (Figure 35.3). Thus, complex surgeries are often planned.

Success/survival rates

For removable restorations, implant survival rates (1–10 years) range from 95% to 98%. Prosthodontic survival rate is around 91%. For fixed restorations, implant and prosthodontic survival rates (3–10 years) range from 95.5% to 98%, and from 96% to 100%, respectively.

Overdentures and fixed restorations demonstrate less success at the maxilla than at the mandible. Implant number and distribution along the maxilla seem to influence the prosthodontic survival rate (Lambert et al., 2009).

There is no evidence to support early or immediate loading protocols with removable restorations (Gallucci et al., 2009). There is some evidence to support immediate loading of roughened dental implants with fixed restorations (Weber et al., 2009).

Key points
- The decision-making process depends on the patient's demand in terms of aesthetics.
- Achievements in terms of aesthetics are technically demanding.
- Surgical augmentation procedures are often mandatory.
- A comprehensive view of skeletal maturation, occlusion, facial and dental aesthetics is a key factor in the decision-making process.

36 Treatment planning: Aesthetic zone

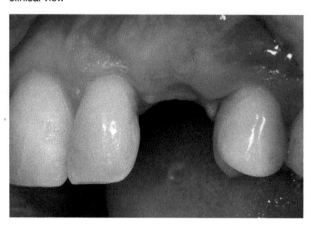

Figure 36.1 Anterior single-tooth replacement. Preoperative clinical view

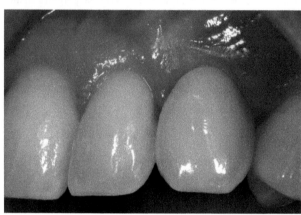

Figure 36.2 Postoperative clinical view (one year)

Although bone resorption is virtually complete 8 weeks post-extraction (Cardaropoli *et al.*, 2006), slow bone resorption has been shown to occur over time (Schropp *et al.*, 2003). Soft tissue stability depends on the supporting bone. Therefore, soft tissue recession around dental implants over time should not be overlooked.

In the aesthetic zone patient expectations are high, and satisfaction is of paramount importance. Consequently, immediate and long-term peri-implant soft tissue stability must be achieved. In other words, clinical management of the biological tissues surrounding dental implants – that is, bone and peri-implant mucosa – is critical, and makes treatment planning in the aesthetic zone specific. There are a few key clinical differences between non-aesthetic and aesthetic areas in terms of treatment planning. These are listed in Table 36.1.

Three-dimensional implant positioning

Three-dimensional surgical insertion of the dental implant is determined by the prosthetic and occlusal design (see Chapter 22). In the aesthetic zone, no compromise is possible regarding the emergence of the dental implant neck. Malpositioning of dental implants precludes any attempt at aesthetic implant restoration (Buser *et al.*, 2004).

Timing of implant placement

It has been suggested that implant placement in a fresh socket may preserve bone and soft tissue more effectively than the delayed or late implantation approach. Recent studies and meta-analyses indicate the significantly higher survival rate of delayed dental implants compared to immediate dental implants (Chrcanovic *et al.*, 2015; Mello *et al.*, 2017). In addition, there are less buccal bone and more

soft tissue recessions with immediate dental implant placement than with other delayed approaches (Chen and Buser, 2014). The quality of the studies conducted to date is not sufficient to provide conclusive evidence on the potential benefits of immediate implant placement (Atieh *et al.*, 2016). Moreover, immediate implant placement is a technically demanding procedure. In the aesthetic zone, the immediate procedure should be limited to areas where the biotype is thick and cortical bone preserved.

In most clinical situations, buccal cortical bone is thin or missing. Consequently, guided bone regeneration (GBR) procedures are recommended. The immediate–delayed (early) option has been proposed to allow soft tissue closure onto the extraction socket (see Chapter 34). In the case of GBR procedure, the dental implant is placed 6 to 8 weeks post-extraction. Thus, the membrane can be covered by the flap without excessive vestibule reduction (see Chapter 47). When socket preservation is used (see Chapter 39), the healing time before dental implant placement is extended to over 6 months.

Bone augmentation procedures

When GBR and/or bone graft procedures are necessary in aesthetic zones, care must be taken with the risk of bone resorption that can lead to soft tissue recession. Nevertheless, there is a paucity of clinical reports on buccal bone stability.

A systematic review indicates an overall stability of peri-implant bone after GBR procedures (Lutz *et al.*, 2015). However, this review indicates little evidence of a correlation between buccal bone stability and soft tissue recession. Consequently, the use of non-resorbable or slow resorbable materials may be advisable in aesthetic zones to prevent buccal bone resorption, and the subsequent soft tissue recession

Implant Dentistry at a Glance, Second Edition. Jacques Malet, Francis Mora and Philippe Bouchard.
© 2018 John Wiley & Sons Ltd. Published 2018 by John Wiley & Sons Ltd.
Companion website: www.wiley.com/go/malet/implant

Figure 36.3 The emergence profile on the provisional restoration is gradually modified. Note the shape of the peri-implant mucosa at the end of this process. The provisional restoration is positioned on the initial cast and the emergence profile is transferred to the laboratory

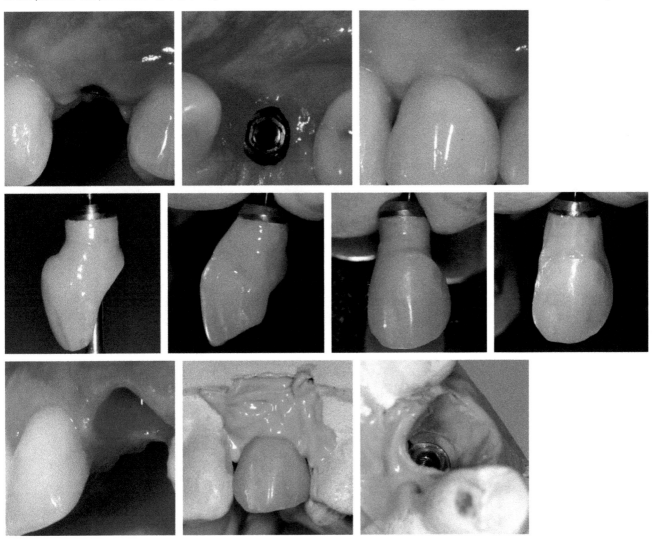

Table 36.1 Guidelines in the aesthetic zone

· Buccal cortical plate preservation at the time of extraction
· Socket preservation techniques when necessary (see Chapter 39)
· Delayed or late implant placement preferred to immediate placement
· Flapless procedure when possible
· Ideal implant position in all three dimensions
· Soft tissue grafting must be considered
· Provisional crown must be implanted as soon as possible

Soft tissue augmentation

A significant association between thin biotypes and peri-implant soft tissue recession have been shown (Kan *et al.*, 2011). Consequently, soft tissue augmentation must be considered to prevent poor aesthetic outcomes. Various graft techniques have been proposed at different time of the procedure (see Chapter 55).

Provisional restoration and soft tissue remodelling

A provisional crown must be placed as soon as possible to support soft tissue maturation. Ideally, it should be screw-retained

to simplify the relining. The emergence profile is gradually modified to reach the ideal soft tissue position, which is then transfered to the laboratory (Figures 36.1–36.3). It has been demonstrated that optimal papillae positioning is achievable after tissue maturation (Jemt, 1999). For immediate single implants, immediate restoration provides optimal soft tissue support for papillae and buccal soft tissue margins (De Rouck *et al.*, 2009). However, immediate restorations have no long-term impact on the buccal soft tissue location, which tends to be biotype related (Kan *et al.*, 2011).

Key points

• Patient satisfaction is the cornerstone of implant dentistry, especially when dealing with aesthetics.
• Extraction must be atraumatic.
• Bone and soft tissue augmentation are often used to ensure 3D positioning.
• Delayed or late dental implant placement is recommended.
• Provisional restoration must be planned as soon as possible.

Dental implants in orthodontic patients

Figure 37.1 Disharmony after passive migration of adjacent teeth surrounding an implant. (a) Clinical view of the final dental implant restoration (no. 11) in a 20-year-old patient. (b) Ten years following implant loading an aesthetic impact due to passive eruption of the teeth is observed. (c) Corresponding radiograph

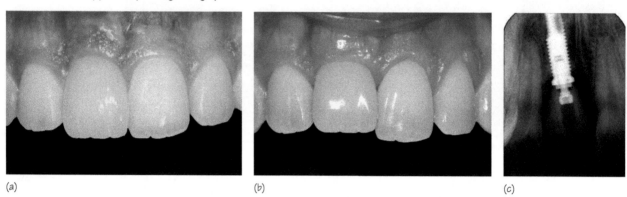

(a)   (b)   (c)

Figure 37.2 Agenesis of teeth 12 and 22. (a) Preoperative clinical view. (b) A horizontal bone deficiency is observed after flap elevation. (c) A block bone graft is adapted to compensate for the alveolar deficiency. (d) Clinical view three years after loading

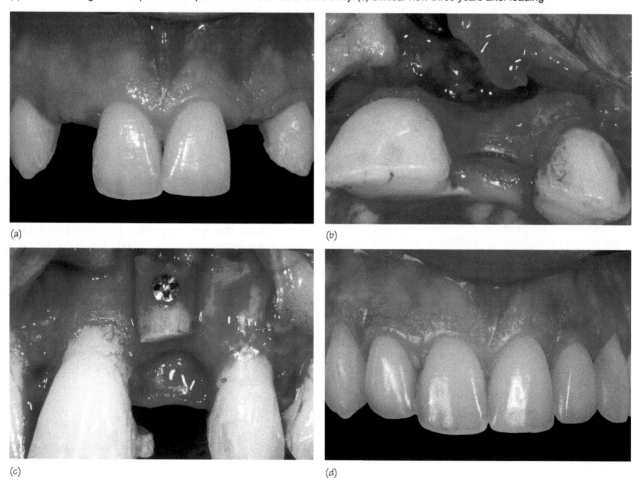

(a)

(b)

(c)

(d)

Implant Dentistry at a Glance, Second Edition. Jacques Malet, Francis Mora and Philippe Bouchard.
© 2018 John Wiley & Sons Ltd. Published 2018 by John Wiley & Sons Ltd.
Companion website: www.wiley.com/go/malet/implant

Orthodontic patients may need dental implants either to replace missing teeth or to facilitate orthodontic movement by providing an additional anchorage point.

Dental implants for patients with tooth agenesis

Congenitally missing teeth can be treated either with prosthesis or with orthodontic treatment only. Prosthesis often needs an orthodontic pre-treatment. Both approaches are effective to compensate for missing teeth. Whatever the treatment, it must be keep in mind that long-term results are mandatory because these patients are usually young.

Decision making

Orthodontics is the first-line strategy when aesthetics and/or function are compatible with this approach. Orthodontics is a less invasive procedure compared with the prosthetic approach. Therefore, it should always be considered first.

The objective of the treatment is to close the space of missing teeth. The indications for orthodontic space closure are the following (Kiliaridis *et al.*, 2016):
• Class 1 molar and mandibular anterior crowding
• End-to-end or class 2 molar without mandibular anterior crowding
• Straight or slightly convex facial profile
• Canine dimension close to the lateral incisor.

In other indications, a *prosthetic option* should be considered. Most of the time, the prosthetic option requires space opening to achieve an adequate aesthetic and/or functional clinical outcome. Among the various prosthetic options, implant-supported fixed partial dentures (FPDs) demonstrate better patient-centred outcomes than conventional FPDs (Terheyden and Wusthoff, 2015). The dental implant option can be performed, provided that skeleton growth is achieved. When craniofacial growth is not complete and an orthodontic option is not indicated (see above), a resin-bonded FPD can be considered as a long-term provisional restoration. Resin-bonded FPDs are also an option if implant-supported FPDs are not indicated.

Optimal time for implantation

The replacement of teeth by implants is usually restricted to patients with completed craniofacial growth. In the last few years, an exception to this restriction was reported in children suffering from extended hypodontia or even anodontia.

In cases of residual facial growth after implant placement, the dental implant will not follow the migration of the alveolar process,

leading to disharmony between implant and adjacent teeth (Figure 37.1). Consequently, it is essential to evaluate completion of *alveolar bone growth* before implant placement in aesthetic areas. In general, this happens around 18 years of age. However, a wide variation is observed among different facial types. Confirmation of no changes by superimposing cephalometric X-rays taken six months apart is an effective evaluation process (Heij *et al.*, 2006).

Orthodontic space opening should allow for adequate intercoronal and inter-radicular space for optimal implant placement. As it is usually performed during the teenage years, an effective provisional retention device must be placed to prevent coronal and apical migration until facial growth is complete. As the latter is difficult to assess, long-term provisional restoration should be favoured to delay implant placement as much as possible.

Resin-bonded FPDs are considered to be the least invasive and most effective long-term provisional restoration method, with a high survival rate in the anterior region, especially when a cantilever design (one retainer) is applied (Karl, 2016).

Mini dental implant-supported crowns have been suggested as a temporary option as an alternative to resin-bonded FPDs (Lambert *et al.*, 2016). These special implants (see Chapter 9) should be used with caution, because there is limited evidence on their space-maintaining ability.

Alveolar bone dimensions

Agenesis is often associated with insufficient bone growth and poor bone density. Bone augmentation procedures are indicated before or during implant placement (Figure 37.2).

When buccal concavity remains after bone augmentation and implant placement, a connective tissue graft can be performed. Adequate buccal soft tissue thickness is recommended to ensure long-term aesthetic outcomes (see Chapter 36).

Dental implants used as 'absolute' orthodontic anchorage
Special implants: Orthodontic mini implants

For more on orthodontic mini implants (OMIs), see Chapter 9.

Partially edentulous patients

For partially edentulous patients, dental implants can be used as orthodontic anchorage during orthodontic treatment and subsequently as prosthetic devices (Figure 37.3). The precise implant location is carefully chosen depending on the orthodontic setup, which is agreed during treatment planning.

After osseointegration, a provisional restoration is placed on the implant and is used as an anchorage point during orthodontic treatment.

Figure 37.3 Dental implants used as orthodontic anchorage. (a) A temporary crown is placed on the osseointegrated implant. The orthodontic appliance is connected to the crown. (b) Straightening and mesial translation of tooth 37. Note the distal bone apposition (red arrows)

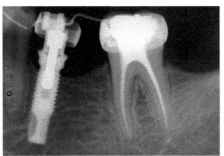
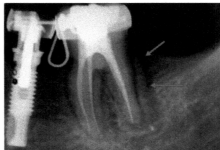

(a) (b)

Orthodontic forces applied to the implants differ from occlusal forces. They are unidirectional and continuous and, below a certain threshold, orthodontic forces positively influence turnover of the bone surrounding the alveolar implant, thereby leading to bone apposition and densification (Melsen and Lang, 2001).

During treatment planning and orthodontic treatment, a team approach is essential to optimise the end result.

Key points

- Preoperative evaluation of facial growth completion is essential before implant placement in aesthetic areas.
- Implant treatment for tooth agenesis often requires a bone augmentation procedure.
- A team approach is required for implant/orthodontic patients.
- Long-term stability is the cornerstone of the decision-making process.

38 Surgical environment and instrumentation

Figure 38.2 Key equipment for the operating room: operating table or dental chair; dental cart; surgical aspirator; over-the-patient stainless steel rolling table adjustable in height to set up instruments; stainless steel rolling dressing cart to set up surgical motors; X-ray viewer; stainless steel bucket on castors; two stools (if the surgeon works seated); containers for disposables.

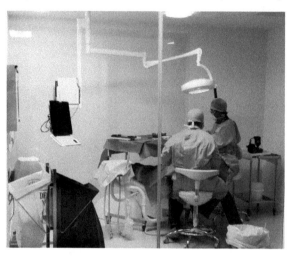

Figure 38.1 A dental practice setting is not adapted for dental implant surgery

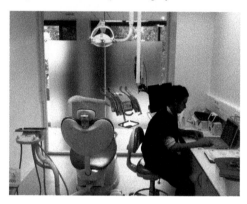

Figure 38.3 Key aspects of the operating suite. (a) Preparation room for the patient; (b) nurses' room, in the storage room of the operating suite; (c) dental X-ray generator; (d) recovery room. Note the monitoring devices and the window where the nurse can provide attention to the patient

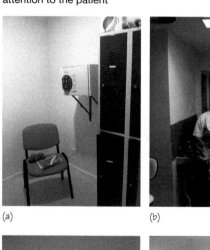

(a)

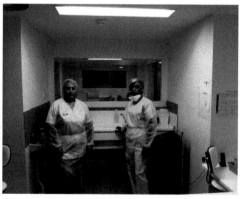

(b)

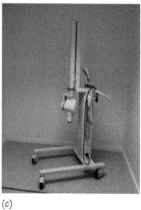

(c)

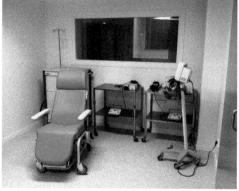

(d)

Implant Dentistry at a Glance, Second Edition. Jacques Malet, Francis Mora and Philippe Bouchard.
© 2018 John Wiley & Sons Ltd. Published 2018 by John Wiley & Sons Ltd.
Companion website: www.wiley.com/go/malet/implant

Dental implants can be placed in an operating room (OR) or in a dental practice. It is imperative that practitioners consider all surgical procedures as potentially infectious. In addition, it has been shown that it is especially important to avoid perioperative infection of the wound during surgery, when foreign bodies are implanted (Haanaes, 1990).

In the oral cavity, several sources of infection during surgery have been identified: instruments, the hands of surgeon and assistants, the air of the OR, patients' nostrils and saliva and the perioral skin (Van Steenberghe et al., 1997).

Thus, the concepts of asepsis and sterility must be adhered to in dental implant surgery, and an OR is by far the most appropriate setting for dental implant surgeries (Figure 38.1). Leaving aside the requirements for an aseptic environment, from an economic point of view, the transformation of a dental setting to an acceptable 'operating room' requires such efforts that the profitability of the surgery is questionable. Consequently, we strongly recommend an aseptic OR being part of the dental setting if the practitioner aims to place implants on a regular basis.

Surgical team

- Surgeon
- Operating room nurse, who assists the surgeon during surgery
- Circulating nurse.

Operating room

Outside the OR is a dedicated scrub area used by surgeons and nurses prior to surgery. There is storage space for common surgical supplies.

The OR is a temperature- and humidity-controlled environment, spacious, easy to clean and without windows. In an OR there are two areas: the sterile operating field and the non-sterile area. The circulating nurse connects the people in the sterile field with the non-sterile area (opens the implant packaging, resupplies the surgical table with disposable material etc.). Operating fields should be cleaned before and after each surgical procedure and at the end of each day.

During surgery, the goal is to keep the operating field totally sterile for patient safety. This involves the following points:
- The door of the OR is closed during the operation.
- Traffic flow and conversation are reduced to a minimum.
- If an instrument or hand touches something outside the sterile field, the instrument or glove should be replaced immediately.

Figure 38.2 indicates the key equipment in the OR. An operating table is more convenient if the surgeon works standing, whereas a dental chair is preferable if the surgeon works seated. We prefer a dental chair because it is more comfortable for the patient and because the patient's head can be easily immobilised.

Operating suite

In large facilities, several operating rooms may be part of an operating suite that forms a distinct section. The operating suite is climate and air controlled and separated from the remainder of the healthcare facility, so that only authorised personnel have access. It contains rooms for personnel to change, wash and rest, preparation and recovery rooms, storage and cleaning facilities, offices and dental X-ray generators (Figure 38.3).

Preparation of the patient

Before surgery, the patient is dressed in a cap, shoe covers and a light gown. Make-up should be removed. The patient's skin is scrubbed with povidone-iodine or chlorhexidine. Scrubbing starts at the lips and moves to the outside in a linear or circular manner.

A sterile fenestrated surgical drape is used to isolate the disinfected area from surrounding areas (covering eyes is preferable).

Preparation of the surgical team (see Appendix C)

The surgeon's hands and arms are scrubbed for three minutes with povidone-iodine or chlorhexidine, rinsed with water and dried prior to gloving.

Hand rubbing with aqueous alcohol solution, preceded by a one-minute non-antiseptic hand wash before each surgical procedure, is as effective as traditional hand scrubbing with antiseptic soap in preventing surgical site infections (Parienti et al., 2002).

Each member of the surgical team wears:
- cap
- face mask
- shoe covers
- sterile gown
- safety glasses or loupes.

Preparation of the surgical table

The surgical table is draped and the instruments are arranged. Various arrangements may be suggested and they vary according to the type of surgery. Appendix B indicates the basic arrangement for dental implant placement. The implant motor and the handpieces are placed on a rolling cart.

Basic instrumentarium (see Appendix B)

This is virtually identical to that used for a standard periodontal flap surgery.

Different surgical trays and instruments are commercially available according to the implant brand. Generally, they include a depth gauge, screwdrivers, a wrench, a ratchet wrench with extensions, implant holders, an implant drill extender and direction indicators.

Disposable single-patient-use drill kits are preferred to reusable drills.

According to the requirements of the surgical procedure, other instruments can be set out on the table (mallet, fixation screw kit, set of trephines, bone crunchers, sinus lift kit, tissue punches etc.).

Key points
- The concepts of asepsis and sterility must be adhered to in dental implant surgery.
- An aseptic operating room is recommended in the dental setting.
- When available, disposable instruments should be preferred to reusable instruments.

39 Surgical techniques: Socket preservation

Figure 39.1 The Bio-Col socket-preservation technique. (a) Soft tissue recession on 22 (hopeless tooth). (b) Intraoral radiography showing an endodontic lesion and root perforation. (c) Stabilisation of a connective tissue graft with mattress sutures. (d) Three months healing, before implant surgery. (e) Three-month CT scan showing bone preservation. (f) Implant bed preparation. (g) Five-year clinical result. (h) Intraoral radiography (five years)

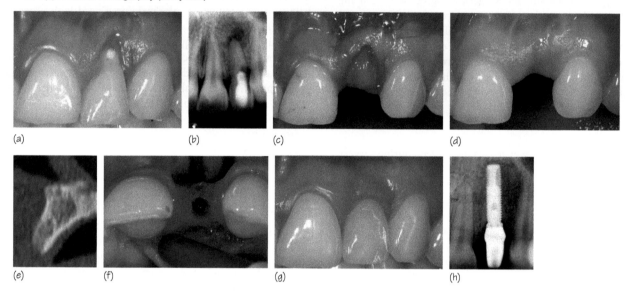

Figure 39.2 Combined surgical protocol (flap elevation). (a) Intraoral radiography showing the complex periodontal lesions in the upper lateral jaw. (b) A flap elevation is combined with teeth extraction. An autologous particulated bone graft associated with xenograft (Bio-Oss® material) filled the fresh alveolar socket extraction. (c) The vestibular mucoperiosteal flap is raised to cover the extraction area. (d) Eight months later, radiography to evaluate the gain of osseous volume. (e) CT scan control at eight months; note the bone gain. (f) The dental implants are placed in the regenerated edentulous area. The bone maturation is partial and Bio-Oss® granules are visible at the top of the alveolar crest (second-stage procedure)

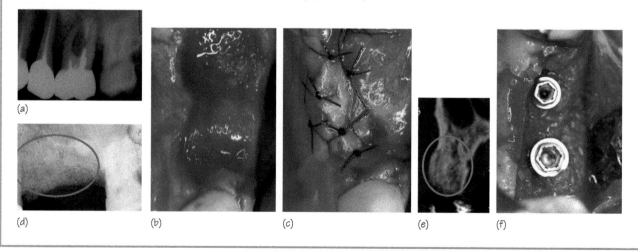

Implant Dentistry at a Glance, Second Edition. Jacques Malet, Francis Mora and Philippe Bouchard.
© 2018 John Wiley & Sons Ltd. Published 2018 by John Wiley & Sons Ltd.
Companion website: www.wiley.com/go/malet/implant

Based on healing events in postextraction sites, socket preservation following tooth extraction seems to be important to prevent ridge resorption, to reduce the need for further augmentation/surgical procedures and to simplify implant placement at a later time (Darby *et al.*, 2009).

Rationale

The healing of an extraction socket results in negative changes in the alveolar bone dimensions. The bundle bone disappears and the height of the buccal wall of the socket is reduced. Tissue loss is more pronounced from the buccal aspect than from the lingual/palatal aspect (Araújo & Lindhe, 2005, 2009a).

Healing is characterised by internal changes (bone formation within the socket) and external changes (three-dimensional resorption of the bony walls). The imbalance between bone formation in the socket and bone resorption of the socket walls results in a net loss of hard tissues. After tooth removal, the extravascular blood cells form a blood clot that fills the socket. Within two to three days, primary granulation tissue infiltrates the clot, beginning at the base and periphery of the socket. After seven days, woven bone, characterised by uncalcified bone spicules, appears and mineralisation is initiated from the base to the coronal part of the socket. Epithelialisation achieves the complete closure of the socket about six weeks after the extraction. Complete healing of the extraction socket is achieved after at least three months, depending on bone destruction following the tooth extraction.

Products and devices

Bone graft materials may be used to limit alveolar bone resorption. Autogenous graft, substitute materials, membrane barriers, collagen sponges and polyglycolide/polylactide (PGA/PLA) sponges can be employed. The true impact of substitute materials on healing periods and regenerative outcomes is unknown (Darby *et al.*, 2009). It is unclear to what extent residual particles of grafting material still present at the time of implant affect the implant survival rate (ISR).

Animal studies indicate that autograft material fails to prevent ridge resorption (Araújo & Lindhe, 2011). Instead, bone substitute (Bio-Oss®) counteracts ridge contraction (Araújo & Lindhe,

2009b). The use of membrane barriers in addition to the graft material can increase the amount of newly formed bone in preserved sockets, but membrane exposure can decrease regenerative benefits.

Clinical studies show little evidence that socket preservation reduces bone loss and prevents the need for additional bone augmentation for implant placement, compared to extraction alone. Human studies also fail to demonstrate any effect of socket preservation on aesthetic and prosthodontic outcomes (Atieh *et al.*, 2015).

Technical procedures
Simplified surgical protocols (flapless)

The blood clot is stabilised with or without a collagen sponge. The extraction socket is either left as is or covered with a connective tissue graft immobilised with mattress sutures (Bio-Col socket preservation technique; Figure 39.1). A bone substitute can be placed within the socket, which may prevent resorption of the facial cortical wall (Carmagnola *et al.*, 2003; Iasella *et al.*, 2003).

Combined surgical protocols (flap elevation)

Either coronally positioned flap techniques or palatal rotation flap techniques are used to fully or partially cover the extraction site (Figure 39.2). A bone substitute is placed within the socket. A barrier membrane is used to protect the particulate bone graft and to prevent contact between the graft material and the inner portion of the flap.

There is no evidence to support the superiority of one technique over another (flapless or flap elevation).

Antibiotics are usually prescribed, but no conclusions can be drawn regarding their influence on ISR (Esposito *et al.*, 2010).

Indications

The indication is to prevent the occurrence of three-dimensional alveolar bone resorption following tooth extraction, with special attention to the buccal portion of the alveolar crest (Figure 39.3). It has been shown that dental implants inserted in fresh alveolar extraction sockets have not prevented the resorption of the buccal aspect of the ridge (Araujo *et al.*, 2006). Consequently, adjunctive augmentation procedures are often required *prior* to implant

Figure 39.3 Decision making in socket-preservation procedures

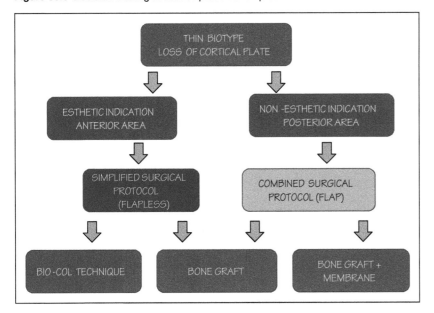

placement, especially in the anterior region of the maxilla with thin periodontal biotypes. In grafted sites, the mean ISR is high (94%; Darby *et al.*, 2009).

Complications

There is no evidence in humans on the optimal healing time for implant placement when graft materials have been placed in the sockets. Consequently, the implant can be inserted even if socket bone regeneration is not completely achieved. The poor quality of the immature new bone and/or the presence of non-integrated graft particles may compromise the primary stability of the implant and may lead to implant failure. Consequently, implant placement should be delayed to six months, or more, after socket preservation.

Infections have been described in the literature (Kim *et al.*, 2017). They are mainly due to membrane exposure. No other adverse effects have been documented.

Key points

- Socket-preservation procedures are effective in preventing alveolar bone resorption.
- Despite socket preservation, additional bone augmentation could be required for implant placement.
- Long-term data on ridge stability and implant survival are limited.

40 Surgical techniques: The standard protocol

Figure 40.1 Standard protocol: surgical technique. (a) Mid-crestal incision in the keratinised tissue. (b) Mucoperiosteal flap elevation. (c) Alveolar ridge preparation to obtain a flat surface (if necessary) followed by perforation of the cortical bone at the exact implant location. (d) Drilling (2 mm diameter) to the appropriate depth and direction. (e) The depth gauge is inserted in the implant bed to check the drilling depth. (f) The direction indicators are placed in the sites to verify the parallelism and direction of the implants. (g) Drilling is continued to the desired final diameter (pilot drills may be used). (h) Before implant placement, direction indicators confirm the final implant bed

Figure 40.2 Dental implant installation (speed: 25 rpm; torque: 35 Ncm)

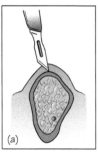 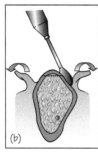 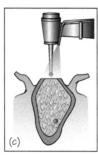 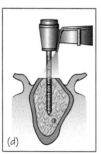
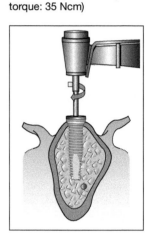
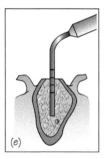 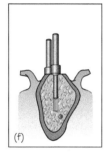 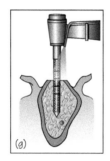 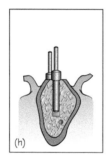

Figure 40.3 One-stage procedure. (a) Healing abutment tightened with light finger force. (b) Flap adaptation around healing abutment (mattress sutures)

Figure 40.4 Two-stage procedure. (a) Cover screw tightened with light finger force. (b) Flap carefully closed over cover screw (mattress sutures)

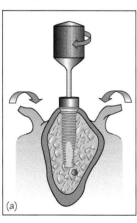 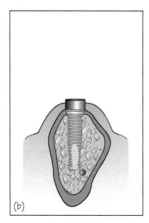 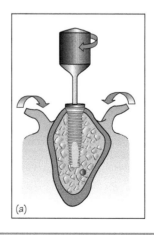 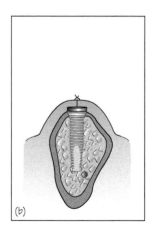

Implant Dentistry at a Glance, Second Edition. Jacques Malet, Francis Mora and Philippe Bouchard.
© 2018 John Wiley & Sons Ltd. Published 2018 by John Wiley & Sons Ltd.
Companion website: www.wiley.com/go/malet/implant

Rationale

The rationale for dental implant placement is based on the osseointegration process as defined in Chapter 2. Various dental implant systems are commercially available. Surgical techniques may vary according to the implant brand. However, some basic surgical guidelines can be set to define a standard protocol corresponding to a late implantation procedure.

Products and devices

An implant system should be selected according to the available scientific background, ease of use in surgical practice, cost–benefit ratio and the ability of the company to ensure follow-up on the products. Not all commercially available implant systems meet the basic selection criteria.

Generally, the dental implant tray includes the following:
- disposable drilling kit
- screw-taps
- screwdrivers
- drill extension
- handpiece connectors or implant drivers
- ratchet extension
- direction indicators
- depth gauge
- ratchet wrench.

In addition to these implant instruments, the surgical equipment includes a basic surgical kit (see Appendix B) and a surgical drilling unit.

Technical procedure
Soft tissue elevation and preparation of the alveolar ridge

A mid-crestal incision is made in the keratinised tissue (Figure 40.1a). A mucoperiosteal flap is elevated without releasing the incision (Figure 40.1b). After opening the gingiva, the alveolar ridge is prepared with a large round burr or a bone chisel in order to obtain a flat bone surface (Figure 40.1c). The surgical template is placed.

Preparation of the implant bed

All drilling should be performed under profuse saline irrigation at a speed around 1000 rpm, according to the instructions of the manufacturer and considering the bone density (Quirynen and Lekholm, 2008).

The planned position of the implant bed is marked with a round burr through the surgical template (Figure 40.1c). The first step consists of drilling with a 2 mm drill to the appropriate depth in the planned direction (Figure 40.1d). The depth gauge enables checking of the drilling depth (Figure 40.1e). The direction indicator is placed in the site (Figure 40.1f). The patient is asked to bite. The tip of the direction indicator must be oriented to the occlusal surface of the antagonist tooth. When more than one implant is placed, the direction indicator is left in place to verify the parallelism of the other implants.

Once the direction and depth of the implant bed are validated, drilling is continued with drills of increasing diameter to the desired final diameter (Figure 40.1 g,h). Depending on the selection of the implant system, pilot drills may be used to facilitate the penetration of a subsequent drill.

With *high bone density (type 1)*, an extra-wide drill may be used in conjunction with a screw-tap to prevent high compressive strengths.

With *low bone density (type 4)*, the diameter of the final drill may be reduced to prevent the lack of primary stability.

Implant installation

The dental implant is removed from the sterile package and connected to the implant driver. The implant is installed with a contra angle at low speed (25 rpm) and the torque is set (35 Ncm; Figure 40.2). When the bed is adequately prepared, the implant should work its way into the site without any pressure. If an overly high insertion torque is necessary, the implant should be retrieved for additional drilling.

The implant shoulder is positioned at the marginal bone level. Adequate primary stability should be obtained at this stage.

Wound closure
One-stage procedure

A healing abutment corresponding to the implant diameter and the soft tissue thickness is tightened with a manual screwdriver (light finger force; Figure 40.3a). The flap is adapted and tightly sealed around the healing abutment using mattress sutures (Figure 40.3b).

Two-stage procedure

A cover screw is inserted into the implant (Figure 40.4a). The flap is carefully closed over the cover screw using mattress sutures (Figure 40.4b). The height of the cover screws may prevent complete adaptation of flap edges. Consequently, a periosteal fenestration of the buccal flap may be performed to facilitate the wound closure, and to avoid excessive tensions during the contraction phase of wound healing.

After an adequate healing phase, the cover screws are removed. In the standard protocol, when soft tissue management is not required, a minimally invasive approach is recommended. When the keratinised tissue is sufficient, a gingivectomy is performed above the cover screw using a tissue punch. Otherwise, a mini-flap is recommended to maintain a band of keratinised tissue around the healing abutment.

Healing duration

The mean healing time is three to four months in the maxilla and two to three months in the mandible.

Indications

The standard protocol is indicated when the vertical and horizontal bone volume is sufficient, and when the amount of soft tissue allows adequate oral hygiene procedures and aesthetics.

Contraindications

An implant site requiring soft and/or hard tissue augmentation is a contraindication.

Complications

Leaving aside the classic complications of any surgical procedure, the major complication of the standard protocol is the lack of primary stability of the implant. This complication can be prevented by thorough patient examination and treatment planning.

Key points
- Implant placement is a demanding procedure.
- However, implant placement is not difficult in standard situations if the surgeon adheres to a strict protocol.
- Surgical training is mandatory to achieve the success rates indicated in the literature.

41 Surgical techniques: Implants placed in postextraction sites

Figure 41.1 Relationship between healing events and time of implant placement

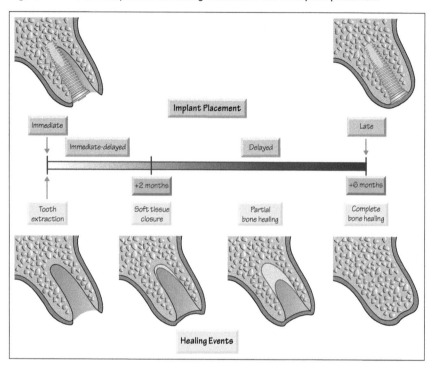

Figure 41.2 Immediate implant placement in anterior site at the maxilla. (a) Drilling palatal to the axis of the socket. Note the gap with buccal native bone. (b) A bone substitute is placed between the implant and the native bone

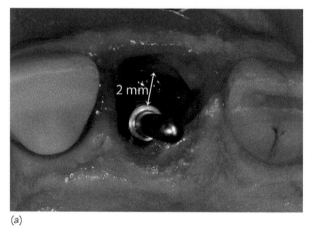

(a)

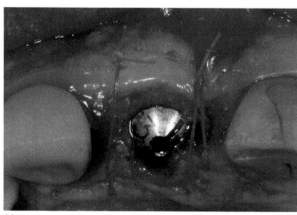

(b)

The standard dental implant protocol corresponds to a late implantation; that is, implant placement after complete bone healing of the extraction site. This means that the postextraction phase is no less than 24 weeks in standard clinical situations. Surgical alternatives have been explored to reduce the length of the treatment, leading to immediate, immediate–delayed and delayed implantation procedures, the background to which is now documented (Chen and Buser, 2008). All the postextraction procedures shorten the treatment time. In addition, the immediate implantation procedure improves

Implant Dentistry at a Glance, Second Edition. Jacques Malet, Francis Mora and Philippe Bouchard.
© 2018 John Wiley & Sons Ltd. Published 2018 by John Wiley & Sons Ltd.
Companion website: www.wiley.com/go/malet/implant

Figure 41.3 Immediate implant placement in molar site at the mandible. The inter-radicular septum is used to drill the implant bed and to ensure primary stability

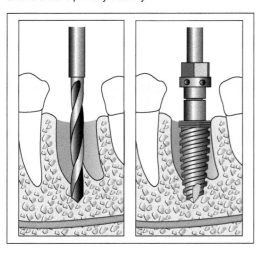

patient comfort, because only one surgical procedure is required for both tooth extraction and implant placement.

Definitions

Figure 41.1 indicates the time of implant placement (Esposito *et al.*, 2010):

• *Immediate implantation*: implant placement within the extraction socket at the time of extraction.

• *Immediate–delayed implantation*: any implant placed in an extraction socket within eight weeks after tooth extraction; that is, after soft tissue closure of the extraction site.

• *Delayed implantation*: implant placement at least two months after tooth extraction; that is, after soft tissue closure and partial bone healing.

Outcomes

It has been shown that the implant survival rates (ISRs) with postextraction procedures are comparable to those of the standard procedure (Chen and Buser, 2009). Immediate and immediate–delayed implants may be at higher risk for implant failures and complications than delayed implants (Esposito *et al.*, 2010).

Rationale

From a biological point of view, the fresh extraction socket does not preclude the osseointegration process. However, following implant installation in fresh extraction sockets, the resorption

process of the buccal and lingual bony walls still continues to a level similar to that of an edentulous site (Botticelli *et al.*, 2004; Araújo *et al.*, 2006; Sanz *et al.*, 2010).

Products and devices

Periotomes and piezoelectric devices should be used for the extraction procedure.

Bone regeneration is recommended to compensate for bone modelling and to optimise aesthetic results. It should combine the use of bone substitute and barrier membrane. However, there is no reliable evidence that supports the need for augmentation procedures or the superiority of one augmentation technique over another.

Specific dental implants may be used. They have various trunco-conical shapes and different diameters, and are designed to be used as immediate implants in sockets of varying dimensions. They aim to reduce the gap between the socket walls and the dental implant.

Technical procedures

Postextraction procedures are time-saving approaches. It is therefore not surprising that the one-stage implantation procedure is preferred. The necessity of raising a flap for covering the implant, if a two-stage procedure is performed, calls into question the advantages of the postextraction protocol.

Meticulous tooth extraction is essential to the success of the technique. Socket-wall preservation is critical. Atraumatic manoeuvres should be implemented by using periotomes, root-section technique and ultrasonic devices. The operator should pay particular attention to weak osseous walls in order to avoid fractures.

After removal of the granulation tissue, the socket is carefully evaluated. If the primary stability of the implant seems doubtful, implant placement is postponed for delayed or late implantation. When soft tissue closure is mandatory (membrane barriers) or when aesthetics is a priority, implant placement is postponed for immediate–delayed implantation.

The implant is then placed. In single-root sites, the drilling is palatal/lingual to the axis of the socket (Figure 41.2). In multi-rooted sites, the implant is placed in the inter-radicular septum, when possible (Figures 41.3 and 41.4). The implant shoulder is positioned slightly beneath the coronal border of the socket (about 1–2 mm).

If the gap exceeds 2 mm, a regenerative material is placed between the implant and the native bone (Figure 41.2). This has been shown to improve the level of marginal bone-to-implant contact (BIC). Otherwise, there is no need to fill the gap, because complete defect resolution is achieved with a gap of less than

Figure 41.4 Immediate implant placement in molar site at the maxilla (one-stage procedure). (a) Preoperative X-ray of a hopeless first molar (pulp floor perforation). (b) Perioperative view of the extraction: root separation to preserve the inter-radicular septum. (c) Clinical view of the healing abutment after completion of the surgical procedure. (d) Postoperative X-ray four months after surgery

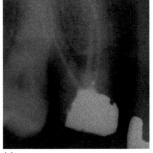
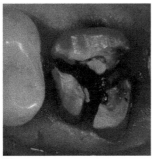
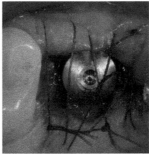
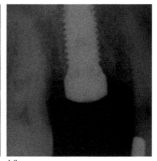

(a)   (b)   (c)   (d)

2 mm with intact socket walls. Two- or three-wall defects are favourable for bone augmentation.

The soft tissues are closely tightened to the implant neck.

Indications

All healthy extraction sockets with completely or partially preserved bony walls allow primary stability.

Aesthetics

It has been suggested that ridge dimensions can be preserved if implants are placed in the fresh extraction socket. Animal studies and clinical trials have demonstrated that implant placement in fresh extraction sockets fails to preserve the hard-tissue dimension of the ridge following tooth extraction. Immediate implantation procedure in aesthetic areas should be carefully planned. A thick periodontal biotype preventing osseous/gingival recession is recommended. The amount of bone resorption and soft tissue recession following immediate implant placement is unpredictable.

Contraindications

- Presence of an acute infection
- Periapical infections
- High aesthetic risk profile
- High risk of lack of primary stability.

Complications

Postoperative complications, including infection at the socket site and soft tissue recession, are common with immediate implantation.

Key points

- The postextraction procedures shorten the treatment time.
- In cases without complications, the implant survival rate is comparable to that of the standard procedure.
- Following immediate implant placement, the edentulous site undergoes substantial resorption, in particular at the buccal aspect.
- Immediate implantation procedures in aesthetic areas should be carefully planned.
- Postoperative complications are common with immediate implantation.

42 Surgical techniques: Computer-guided surgery

Figure 42.1 Edentulous maxilla: computer-guided surgery and immediate loading protocol. Radiopaque markers (white spots) are inserted in the denture, which serves as a radiographic template

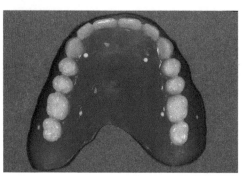

Figure 42.2 During radiographic examination, the template is stabilised with an occlusal index to avoid incorrect positioning

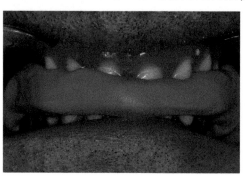

Figure 42.3 Implant positions and stabilising pins are planned virtually. The data are transferred to the implant company that will fabricate the template

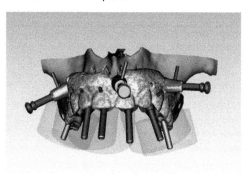

Figure 42.4 End of the surgery. Six implants are placed. Note that the surgical template is stabilised on the maxilla with three pins

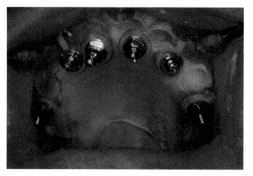

Figure 42.5 An immediate provisional implant-supported fixed partial denture, fabricated from the surgical template

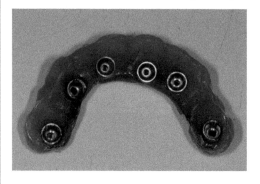

Figure 42.6 The provisional implant-supported fixed partial denture is screwed on the implants at the end of the surgery

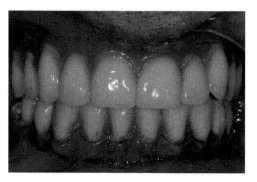

Implant Dentistry at a Glance, Second Edition. Jacques Malet, Francis Mora and Philippe Bouchard.
© 2018 John Wiley & Sons Ltd. Published 2018 by John Wiley & Sons Ltd.
Companion website: www.wiley.com/go/malet/implant

Rationale

The general principle is to create a virtual image of the jaws through a computed tomography (CT) imaging technique (CT scan or cone beam computed tomography, CBCT) and 3D reconstruction software. Radiopaque landmarks, included in the images through a radiographic template, allow the simulation of a prosthetic-driven virtual surgery.

A surgical tool (solid guide or live navigation images) is produced and used during the actual surgery, so that the clinician is guided to comply with the virtual planning.

Definitions

The following definitions have been proposed (Hammerle et al., 2009):
- *Computer-assisted surgery* consists of the use of 3D imaging software, to combine prosthetic planning with the anatomical structures.
- *Computer-guided surgery* is the use of a static surgical template that reproduces the virtual implant position directly from computed tomographic data and does not allow for intraoperative modification of the implant position.
- *Computer-navigated surgery* is the use of a surgical navigation system that reproduces the virtual implant position directly from computed tomographic data and allows for intraoperative changes in implant position. This is also called real-time navigation.

Products and devices

Computer-guided surgery

The CT scan or CBCT data are processed with specific software, allowing the production of a precise 3D reconstruction of the jaw, including prosthetic information from the radiographic template. After virtual surgery, planned implant positions are transferred to a precise surgical template by a stereolithographic process. The template includes fixation devices and drill guides. It can be used by the laboratory before surgery to elaborate a provisional implant-supported fixed partial denture (FPD), which will be placed at the end of the surgery.

Computer-navigated surgery

Special devices are securely attached:
- to the patient (during CT radiographic examination and during surgery)
- to the clinician's handpiece.

During implant surgery, the system records the position of the handpiece and the position of the patient (by infra-red camera, laser or tactile device) and reproduces a real-time 3D image of the situation in progress.

Accuracy

Accuracy is a critical factor that may limit the technique. Accuracy is evaluated by comparing the planned position of the implants with the result after actual implant placement (Table 42.1). Some deviation can occur between the two positions for the entry point, the apex, the axis and the vertical position of the implant.

It seems that navigated surgery is, on average, more accurate than guided surgery (Jung et al., 2009). Nevertheless, if the range of error (and not only the mean) is taken into account, the values are inconstant.

Technical procedures

- *Prosthetic planning*: as in conventional procedures, the future prosthetic teeth positions are planned via a wax-up or set-up.
- *Radiographic template* (see Chapter 24): for edentulous patients, the denture (if sufficiently stable) can be used for the radiographic template. Insertion of specific markers on the template could be necessary before radiographic examination (Figure 42.1).
- *Radiographic examination*: CT scan or CBCT, with the radiographic template. Stability of the template is mandatory to assure accuracy (Figure 42.2). Some companies require an additional CT scan of the template alone.
- *Virtual surgery*: implants are placed according to the prosthetic planning. Optimal length and diameter are selected to respect anatomical structures (Figure 42.3). Different implant libraries are available for each company.
- *Surgical template*: once achieved, the simulation is sent to the company, which produces a customised surgical template (Figure 42.4).
- *Anticipation of the prosthesis (immediate loading)*: the laboratory can use the surgical template to prepare an immediate fixed prosthesis according to the planned positions of the implants (Figure 42.5).
- *Actual surgery*: the surgical template is precisely secured to the jawbone, with either tooth retention or bone-stabilising pins. It contains metallic sleeves in which successive drill guides are inserted (to assure precise guidance of each drill diameter) and through which implants are installed in the planned 3D position. Then the surgical template is removed.

For the immediate loading protocol, the prosthesis is inserted at the end of the surgery (Figure 42.6). A radiographic control is mandatory (Figure 42.7).

Figure 42.7 Radiographic control

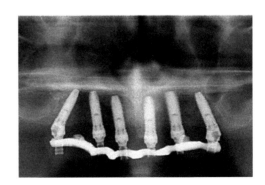

Table 42.1 Deviation (error) between computer-assisted planning and actual surgery

	Entry point (mm)	Apex (mm)	Angulation (°)	Vertical (mm)
Computer-guided surgery	0.82–1.42	0.87–1.52	1 to 12°	No data
Computer-navigated surgery	0.58–0.90	0.55–0.80	1 to 20°	0 to 1.4

Computer-guided versus computer-navigated surgery

Computer-navigated surgery provides real-time observation and allows modifications of the implant position during surgery. The visibility is compatible with all surgical procedures. The financial cost is still high.

Computer-guided surgery does not permit any modification once the virtual surgery is validated. It allows for the preparation of an immediate prosthesis for immediate loading protocols. The financial cost is acceptable for complex cases.

Indications

- Adequate bone volume
- Anatomical complexity
- Need for a less invasive or flapless surgery
- Complex aesthetic cases, to optimise implant placement
- Anticipation of the prosthesis for immediate loading (Vercruyssen *et al.*, 2015).

Limitations

Because the surgeon must anticipate all surgical events and integrate the error range before actual surgery, computer-guided surgery is reserved for experienced clinicians, and is indicated for favourable bone and soft tissue cases.

Key points

- A high level of clinical expertise is required for the use of computer-guided surgery.
- Deviation between virtual and actual surgery must be anticipated.
- Flapless procedures require ideal soft and hard tissue conditions.
- Indications are still limited.

43 CAD/CAM and implant prosthodontics: Background

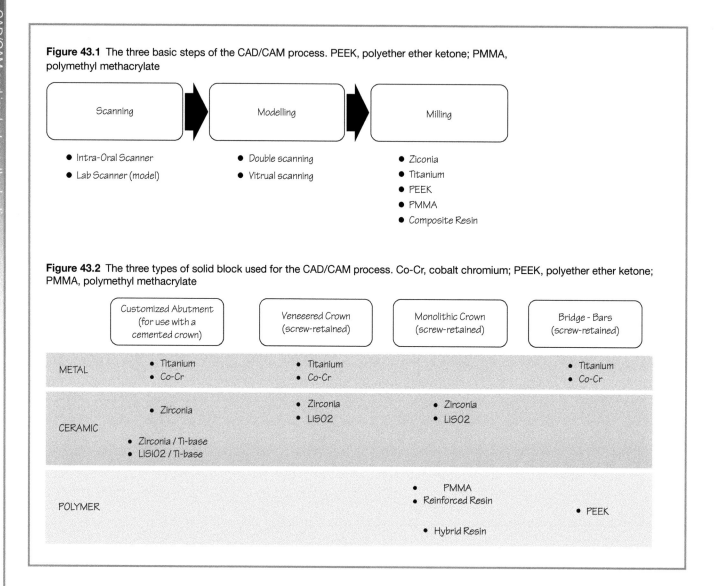

Figure 43.1 The three basic steps of the CAD/CAM process. PEEK, polyether ether ketone; PMMA, polymethyl methacrylate

Scanning
- Intra-Oral Scanner
- Lab Scanner (model)

Modelling
- Double scanning
- Virtual scanning

Milling
- Ziconia
- Titanium
- PEEK
- PMMA
- Composite Resin

Figure 43.2 The three types of solid block used for the CAD/CAM process. Co-Cr, cobalt chromium; PEEK, polyether ether ketone; PMMA, polymethyl methacrylate

	Customized Abutment (for use with a cemented crown)	Veneeered Crown (screw-retained)	Monolithic Crown (screw-retained)	Bridge - Bars (screw-retained)
METAL	• Titanium • Co-Cr	• Titanium • Co-Cr		• Titanium • Co-Cr
CERAMIC	• Zirconia • Zirconia / Ti-base • LiSiO2 / Ti-base	• Zirconia • LiSO2	• Zirconia • LiSO2	
POLYMER			• PMMA • Reinforced Resin • Hybrid Resin	• PEEK

The traditional approach for implant prosthodontics uses stock or cast abutments and cast crowns or bridges. Another technology is available called computer-aided design and computer-aided manufacturing (CAD/CAM). The CAD/CAM approach was formerly used for tooth-supported fixed prosthodontics, such as inlays/onlays, crowns or bridges. The technology has also been used for several years to produce implant abutments, monolithic crowns or frameworks (Abduo and Lyons, 2013). These pieces can be made of metal, ceramic or polymer materials depending on the clinical indication.

General process

The CAD/CAM process involves three consecutive steps: scanning, modelling and milling (Figure 43.1; Appendix N). The entire process is often referred to as the digital workflow. The scanner records 3D geometry to precisely locate the implant(s) and the surrounding soft tissues and teeth. This scan is taken either intraorally in the dental surgery (chair-side option) or using a laboratory scanner and a plaster model created from a conventional impression (lab-side option). In both cases, the

Implant Dentistry at a Glance, Second Edition. Jacques Malet, Francis Mora and Philippe Bouchard.
© 2018 John Wiley & Sons Ltd. Published 2018 by John Wiley & Sons Ltd.
Companion website: www.wiley.com/go/malet/implant

Figure 43.3 Comparison between intraoral and laboratory scanning

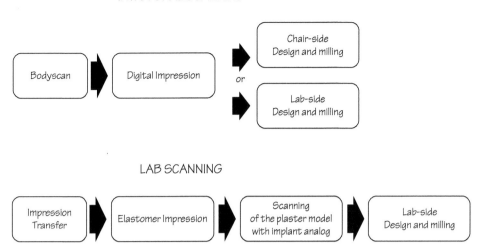

image produced is called a digital impression. Through reverse engineering of oral implant(s), dedicated software is used to design the virtual prosthetic component(s). The computer then sends these data to a machine, where the piece is milled out of a solid block of metal, ceramic or polymer (Figure 43.2). In implant dentistry, the milling step is mostly carried out in a central production facility. Typical systems include Procera® (Nobel Biocare), Etkon® (Straumann) and Atlantis® (Dentsply Sirona). More recently, a chair-side process has also become available for single units (abutments or monolithic crowns) in particular (Figure 43.3).

Advantages and indications

CAD/CAM-customised components are manufactured with similar accuracy to that obtained with industrial workpieces (Kapos et al., 2009; van Noort, 2012) while allowing all the other morphological parameters to be changed. In fact, for the abutment, the rapid milling process is limited to the external surfaces. The fitting surfaces, including the engaging connection, are obtained either by precise industrial milling (central production; Glauser et al., 2004) or through a bonded component called a 'Ti-Base' (chair-side production). Studies on the accuracy of CAD/CAM implant abutments have reported a vertical gap ranging from $2.5\,\mu m$ to $3.2\,\mu m$ (Yuzugullu and Avci, 2008) for both titanium and zirconia. These values are comparable to stock implant abutments. A major advantage of customised abutments is that the thickness, shape of the emergence profile and location of the finish line can be anticipated.

For screw-retained implant frameworks, the CAD/CAM process should be compared to the traditional lost wax/casting process. In the CAD/CAM process, the non-engaging fitting surfaces are produced by milling. The accuracy of the non-engaging fitting surfaces ranges from 1 to $27\,\mu m$, which is significantly better than that observed with cast frameworks (Abduo et al., 2012; Ortorp et al., 2003; Takahashi and Gunne, 2003). Moreover, compared to cast frameworks, this accuracy does not seem to be affected by the span of the framework (Abduo et al., 2012; Ortorp et al., 2003; Takahashi and Gunne, 2003).

Another advantage of CAD/CAM production is the option to use various materials. Whereas a traditional approach is available exclusively for castable alloys, CAD/CAM is the only technique for producing components from high-strength ceramics such as glass-ceramic, densely sintered alumina or partially stabilised zirconia. These options are of interest for abutments in the aesthetic area, as well as for monolithic crowns.

Titanium-based frameworks are more easily managed with a milling process than a cast process. In fact, titanium alloys must be cast in specially designed casting machines using a different technology than that used for conventional dental alloys. Despite these inert atmosphere casting machines, porosity and inadequate mould filling are frequently observed.

Limitations and contraindications

The limitations of CAD/CAM technology in implant prosthodontics are directly linked to the scanning process. Laboratory scanners may be used to provide full-arch or short-arch screw-retained frameworks, whereas intraoral scanners should be restricted to single crowns or small bridges. This is mainly due to the 3D deformation of the digital impression currently obtained with the intraoral scanning process (Joda et al., 2017).

Note

This chapter was written by guest author Olivier Etienne, Strasbourg, France.

Key points
- The computer-aided design/manufacturing (CAD/CAM) approach is more accurate than the traditional approach.
- CAD/CAM components display accuracy similar to that of industrial workpieces.
- The design of customised abutments can be anticipated.
- CAD/CAM technology allows a wide range of materials to be used.

CAD/CAM and implant prosthodontics: Technical procedure

Figure 44.1 Single-implant scanning: intraoral abutments. (a) Clinical view; (b) digital view

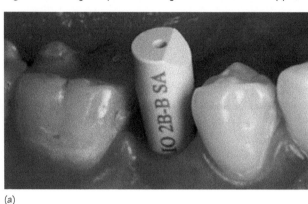

(a)

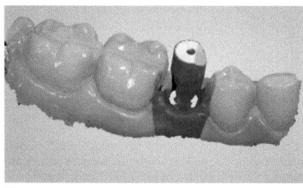

(b)

Figure 44.2 Multiple implant scanning: scanning abutments fixed on the model

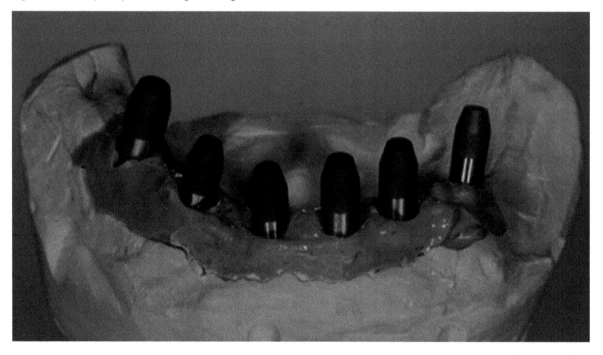

Scanning

Intraoral scanning has been reported as a validated option only for partially edentulous patients (Papaspyridakos *et al.*, 2014). It has not yet been validated for complete edentulism. The latest studies report better results when using the newest devices (Amin *et al.*, 2017; Vandeweghe *et al.*, 2017). The method requires the placement of intraoral scanning abutments (Figure 44.1), also called body scans or scan bodies, preferentially screwed on the implant.

Some companies, such as Biomet 3i, propose another approach using a coded healing abutment that indicates the implant depth, diameter, hex orientation, location of gingival tissues and orientation of the implant. The main advantage of this option is the absence of the impression step and of its potential deformation.

A traditional impression scanned with a laboratory scanner is usually recommended for multiple implant scanning (Flugge *et al.*, 2016). The accuracy of the work model should be verified

Implant Dentistry at a Glance, Second Edition. Jacques Malet, Francis Mora and Philippe Bouchard.
© 2018 John Wiley & Sons Ltd. Published 2018 by John Wiley & Sons Ltd.
Companion website: www.wiley.com/go/malet/implant

Figure 44.3 Tooth positioning at the maxilla. (a) Digital view of the emergence of the dental implants; (b) virtual positioning of the tooth onto the dental implants

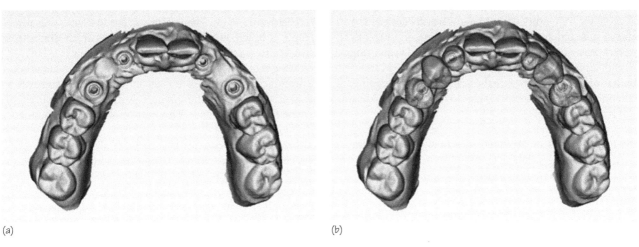

(a) (b)

Figure 44.4 Implant-retained bar at the mandible. (a, b) Preset design; (c) cast metal framework

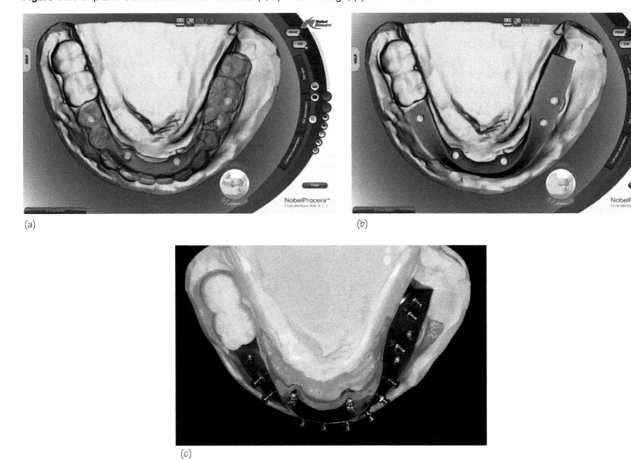

(a) (b)

(c)

intraorally with a verification jig before engaging the CAD/CAM process. This model should include a gingival mask and be made from high-quality plaster (preferably scannable plaster). The scanning abutments are then fixed on the model by screws or clips. This ensures that the position of the implants remains stable and precise during the entire laboratory scanning process (Figure 44.2). They define the position of the implants in the 3D space, while any remaining teeth are also scanned and positioned.

Modelling

Two different modelling methods are usually available: double scanning (Appendix O) and virtual modelling (Appendix P). The first method involves a wax-up of the abutment or framework. This wax-up is built on the master model and scanned separately. The second method is software driven and proposes standard morphology to the lab technician. Modelling of the abutment, framework or bar is highly dependent on the software tools.

Various solutions are feasible. Generally, the preparation limit as well as the abutment emergence profile are configured by dragging dots to the desired location. To create space for the veneered ceramic layer, the framework of the bridge is usually designed by homothetic subtraction of the final restoration morphology (Figure 44.3; Parpaiola *et al.*, 2013). Such anatomical contouring reduces and homogenises the thickness of the veneering ceramics. This has been found to reduce the risk of ceramic chipping, especially in the case of zirconia (Guess *et al.*, 2013; Kokubo *et al.*, 2011; Silva *et al.*, 2011).

Finally, implant-retained bars can easily be designed by dragging dots to a preset design. This preset design is proposed by the software using a double-scanning process that includes the wax-up or the provisional denture as a reference (Figure 44.4).

Milling

Various materials are available for the milling process. However, chair-side fabrication does not allow titanium or any other metal alloys to be milled.

The choice of the milled material depends on the kind of restoration required. Temporary restorations can be milled out of polymethyl methacrylate (PMMA) blocks or PMMA disks. Definitive restorations can be milled using titanium, zirconia or, more recently, polyether ether ketone (PEEK).

To date, low-quality clinical studies have revealed comparable outcomes between zirconia and titanium abutments (Ekfeldt *et al.*, 2011; Sailer *et al.*, 2009). Aesthetic areas with a thin gingival phenotype should take advantage of the zirconia option.

Regarding the clinical performance of zirconia frameworks, the percentage of ceramic chipping is relatively high, ranging from 50% to 90% (Larsson and Vult von Steyern, 2010; Larsson *et al.*, 2010). The main reasons to explain zirconia failures are linked to the design of the frameworks (not homothetic) and the veneering process (cooling temperature and speed; (Guess *et al.*, 2012; Selz *et al.*, 2015). The framework per se usually fails when zirconia is modified using a diamond burr, which diminishes resistance to fracture (Kohal *et al.*, 2010). Thus, CAD/CAM modelling should be carefully considered when producing zirconia workpieces sensitive to further modifications. Moreover, a maximal thickness of the zirconia workpiece is required to increase fracture resistance. This may conflict with the aesthetic indication of zirconia.

More recently, chair-side fabrication of single-implant abutments or monolithic crowns can be achieved using CAD/CAM. A pre-holed block is milled to obtain an optimal contour. Available block materials are limited to PMMA, reinforced composite, high-strength glass-ceramic (LiSiO2) and zirconia. After milling, the crown needs to be adhesively bonded on a pre-fabricated titanium cylinder called a 'Ti-Base', generating a so-called hybrid abutment (Brown and Payne, 2011; Rauscher, 2011).

Note

This chapter was written by guest author Olivier Etienne, Strasbourg, France.

Key points

- Intraoral scanning is limited to partially edentulous patients.
- The modelling phase can either be achieved by scanning a wax-up or completely designed using software.
- Aesthetic areas with a thin gingival phenotype should take advantage of the zirconia option.
- Zirconia chips easily.

45 Bone augmentation: One-stage/simultaneous approach versus two-stage/staged approach

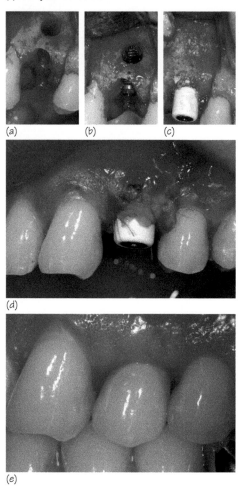

Figure 45.1 The simultaneous approach. (a) Tooth extraction; (b) implant insertion; (c) bone grafting (Bio-Oss®) – the final prosthetic abutment is screwed; (d) clinical view after suturing; (e) four-year outcome

(a) (b) (c)

(d)

(e)

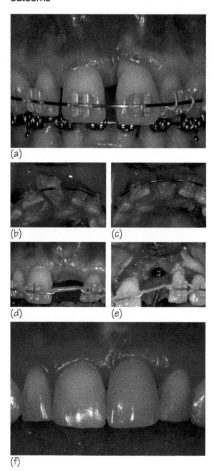

Figure 45.3 The staged approach. (a) Tooth 21 must be extracted for periodontal reasons; (b) extraction and socket preservation (Bio-Oss®); (c) bone substitute covered by connective tissue graft; (d) four-month clinical view; (e) implant placement; (f) two-year outcome

(a)

(b) (c)

(d) (e)

(f)

All bone augmentation techniques, except alveolar distraction, can be performed in a one-stage approach (bone augmentation and implant placement simultaneously) or a two-stage approach (bone augmentation in a first stage and implant placement in a second stage, four to six months later).

The choice between simultaneous and staged approaches depends on the following clinical parameters: treatment duration, morbidity, risk–benefit ratio and implant outcome.

Optimal timing for bone augmentation

Bone augmentation procedures (simultaneous or staged approach) can be performed at different times after tooth extraction. The later the procedure is performed, the more bone resorption occurs. Consequently, bone augmentation procedures must be performed as soon as possible.

For most bone augmentation procedures, soft tissue primary closure is recommended to prevent material exposure. In these

Implant Dentistry at a Glance, Second Edition. Jacques Malet, Francis Mora and Philippe Bouchard.
© 2018 John Wiley & Sons Ltd. Published 2018 by John Wiley & Sons Ltd.
Companion website: www.wiley.com/go/malet/implant

Table 45.1 Risk of complication with bone augmentation procedures

Time after extraction	Resorbable membrane	Non-resorbable membrane	Graft materials	Block bone grafts	Split osteotomy	Sinus floor elevation
Immediate	H		M	H	M	M
2 months		H				
>4 months	M		L	M	L	L

H, high risk; L, low risk; M, medium risk.

cases, a healing period of six to eight weeks after tooth extraction is considered as the optimal timing.

Optimal timing for implant placement

The decision to place the implant at the time of the augmentation procedure depends on the ability to obtain the primary stability of the implant and to achieve soft tissue closure. One must keep in mind that immediate implantation usually increases the risk of complication of the bone augmentation procedure (Table 45.1).

Risk of complication with bone augmentation procedures

Complications may result in inflammation, infection or reduction of new bone gain.

The *quality of the risk* depends on the procedure itself and on the soft tissue healing at the time of the surgery (Table 45.1). Soft tissue covering is mandatory for membranes and block bone grafts. Complications are frequent with non-resorbable membranes.

One-stage/simultaneous approach

See Figures 45.1 and 45.2.

Implant configuration

There must not be any material exposure during the healing period after bone augmentation procedures. This involves the use of a submerged implant configuration in order to achieve complete soft tissue covering. For immediate implantation, flap advancement or a soft tissue graft can be required.

An augmentation procedure concomitant with a transmucosal implant configuration is also possible (Hammerle and Lang, 2001). However, a high level of clinician experience is required.

Advantages
• The global healing time is reduced to the osseointegration period.
• There is low morbidity.

Disadvantages
• In cases of partial bone augmentation, implant success may be compromised.
• In cases of failure, implant and augmentation material are lost.

Indications
• Low-risk procedures: two- and three-wall defects, split osteotomy, sinus floor elevation with residual bone ≥5 mm.
• Implant primary stability achieved with a correct implant position.
• Low healing risk: thick biotype, non-smoker.

Recommendations
• Block bone grafts are not recommended, since the survival rate is lower with a simultaneous approach (Chiapasco et al., 2009).
• Membrane barriers are not recommended for inexperienced clinicians.

Two-stage/staged approach

See Figures 45.3 and 45.4.

Figure 45.2 One-stage/simultaneous approach (maxilla)

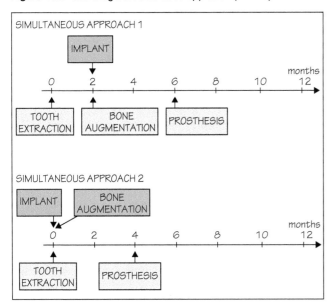

Figure 45.4 Two-stage/staged approach (maxilla)

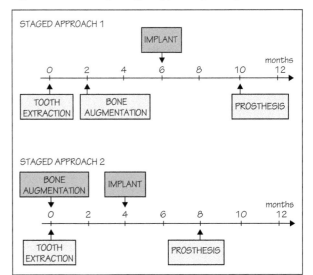

Advantages

• Primary stability of the implant is easier to achieve.
• Optimal positioning of the implant into the regenerated/grafted bone can be achieved.
• In cases of complication or failure, the implant is not affected.

Disadvantages

• The global healing time before prosthetic procedures is higher.
• There is higher morbidity.

Indications

• Medium- and high-risk procedures: zero- and one-wall defect, vertical augmentation, sinus floor elevation with residual bone <5 mm, block bone grafts.
• No primary stability of the implant.
• High healing risk: thin biotype, heavy smokers.

Implant survival, marginal bone loss and implant complications

When the augmentation procedure is uneventful, implant survival rate, marginal bone loss and implant complications are similar with simultaneous and staged approaches. However, in cases of complication or failure of the augmentation procedure during a simultaneous approach, the implant can be compromised or even lost.

Key points

• The choice between simultaneous and staged approaches is first based on a risk evaluation.
• With block bone grafts, implant survival is lower with the simultaneous approach compared to the staged approach.
• For other procedures, implant survival is similar when healing is uneventful.
• Implant primary stability is mandatory for a simultaneous approach.
• For low-risk situations, the simultaneous approach is preferred.
• For high-risk situations, the staged approach is preferred.

46 Bone augmentation: Guided bone regeneration – product and devices

Figure 46.1 Configuration of membranes used for bone augmentation procedures. (a) Titanium-reinforced e-PTFE membrane (Gore-Tex®). (b) Titanium-reinforced high-density PTFE membrane (Cytoplast®). (c) Polyglycolic acid membrane (Resolut Adapt LT®). (d) Collagen porcine membrane (Biogide®). (e) Polylactic acid membrane (GUIDOR® bioresorbable matrix barrier. Courtesy of Sunstar Suisse SA, www.sunstar.com)

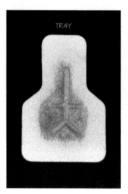 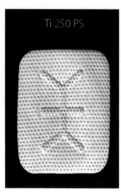 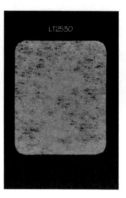 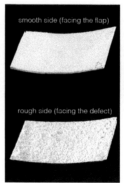 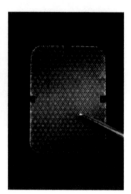

Table 46.1 Impact of the resorbability of the membrane on GBR outcomes and procedures

	Bone formation	Surgical removal	Time control of membrane effect	Need for additional supporting material	Membrane exposure
Consequences	Success improvement	Increased risk of stress, morbidity, tissue damage and cost	Allows control of risk of undesirable inflammation process	Increased risk of inflammation and cost	Inflammation or infection, reduction of average gain of new bone
Non-resorbable	More than resorbable	Yes	Yes	No (titanium-reinforced membranes)	High
Resorbable	Less than non-resorbable	No	No	Yes	Medium

Table 46.2 Biological characteristics of collagen membranes

- Excellent tissue integration
- Biocompatibility
- Rapid vascularisation
- Biodegradation without foreign-body reaction
- Chemotactic for fibroblasts
- Haemostatic
- Weak immunogenicity
- Osteoblastic adhesion

Implant Dentistry at a Glance, Second Edition. Jacques Malet, Francis Mora and Philippe Bouchard.
© 2018 John Wiley & Sons Ltd. Published 2018 by John Wiley & Sons Ltd.
Companion website: www.wiley.com/go/malet/implant

A guided bone regeneration (GBR) membrane (synonym: barrier) material must be (i) biocompatible; (ii) cell occlusive to prevent soft connective tissue contact with the adjacent bone; (iii) able to maintain space for the blood clot to provide a regeneration chamber for osseous formation; (iv) capable of integrating to the host tissues to optimise the stabilisation of the blood clot; and (v) clinically manageable to facilitate the surgical procedures. In other words, an ideal GBR membrane not only has biological properties such as (i), (ii), and (iv), but also physical characteristics such as (iii) and (iv).

All membranes are commercially available in different sizes and design. They must function as a barrier for two weeks and must not be removed – when necessary – before three to four weeks have passed. Most membranes are designed with a rough surface towards the bone and a smooth surface towards the soft tissues.

A wide range of non-resorbable and resorbable materials has been used in GBR membrane engineering. There is no evidence to support or refute the superiority of a specific membrane. Some advantages and disadvantages of the membrane can be outlined according to whether they are resorbable or not (Table 46.1). In short, the main drawback of non-resorbable membranes is that they require an additional surgical procedure for removal, leading to increased morbidity and cost. The major disadvantage of resorbable membranes is that they cannot be used without a supportive material, except when the defect is space-making by itself.

Non-resorbable membranes

The non-resorbable membranes category includes expanded polytetrafluoroethylene (e-PTFE; Gore-Tex® – the W.L. Gore Co. discontinued the production of Gore-Tex regenerative membrane in 2011), high-density polytetrafluoroethylene (d-PTFE; Cytoplast™ TXT; OsteoShield™ OSNRM; TefGen FD™; Nonresorbable ACE) and titanium-reinforced high-density polytetrafluoroethylene (Ti-d-PTFE; Cytoplast™ Ti; OsteoShield™ OSTRNRM) membranes.

From a historical perspective, e-PTFE membranes were the first commercialised in the 1980s. Thus, these correspond to the longest clinical experience. However, the porosity of e-PTFE (0.5–30 µm) was high enough to allow bacterial penetration through the pores when the membrane was exposed in the mouth. In addition, excessive soft tissue ingrowth within the membrane rendered its surgical removal difficult. Microporous

dense PTFE membranes (d-PTFE) were then developed. The lower porosity of these membranes (0.2–1.36 µm) makes them more impervious to bacteria. Thus, the risk of infection in case of membrane exposure is reduced. Moreover, the membrane is easy to detach during the removal procedure. It is recommended that the membrane stay in place for three to four weeks and that it is then removed to allow good revascularisation of the soft tissues.

In theory, these membranes are space-maintaining; that is, they do not require the use of a supportive material. However, to ensure tenting and space maintenance, their physical characteristics have been reinforced by a titanium frame (Ti-d-PTFE). Titanium-reinforced d-PTFE membranes are now the non-resorbable gold standard, especially for ridge augmentation and defects of one or more walls, because they adequately fulfil all the biological and physical requirements for GBR. (Titanium mesh – that is, pure titanium membranes – have sometimes been advocated for GBR procedures, but they are not cell occlusive and thus do not fulfil the biological principles of GBR.)

Resorbable membranes

The resorbable membranes category (synonym: bioresorbable or bioabsorbable membrane) includes natural polymers and synthetic polymers.

Natural polymers

Various chemicals based on chitosan, gelatin and silk fibroin have been experimented with in GBR research (Wang et al., 2016). However, xenogeneic-derived collagen, mostly type I and type III, has shown the best-adapted characteristics to the biological properties of GBR (Table 46.2).

The major advantage of natural polymer membranes is their bioactivity (Table 46.1). Collagen membranes have been extensively used and numerous types are commercially available in different sizes (Table 46.3). The choice between collagen membranes should be based on the required resorption rate, clinical manageability and cost. The cultural preferences of patients may also influence the choice between a bovine or porcine origin for the membrane. The major drawback of natural polymers is that they have poor mechanical properties and a short function time due to their short degradation cycle. (The function time, which is the period during which the membrane keeps its GBR properties, must be differentiated from the resorption rate, which is the time the product takes to biodegrade.)

Table 46.3 Characteristics of commercially available collagen membranes

Commercial name	Native (N) or cross-linked (C-l)	Origin	Collagen type	Resorption rate (weeks)
Bio-Gide®	N	Porcine skin	I and III	24
Periogen	N	Bovine dermis	I and III	4–8
Tutodent	N	Bovine pericardium	I	8–16
BioMend®	C-l	Bovine tendon	I	8
BioMendExtend®	C-l	Bovine tendon	I	18
BioSorb™	C-l	Bovine	I	26–38
Neomem™	C-l	Bovine tendon	I	26–38
OsseoGuard®	C-l	Bovine tendon	I	24–36
OsseoGuard Flex®	C-l	Bovine dermis	I	24–36
Ossix Plus®	C-l	Porcine tendon	I	16–24

Table 46.4 Characteristics of commercially available synthetic membranes

Commercial name	Origin	Resorption rate (weeks)
Atrisorb®	Poly-D,L-lactide	36–48
Biofix®	Polyglycolic acid	24–48
Epiguide®	Poly-D,L-lactic acid	24–48
Resolut Adapt™	Poly-D,L-lactide/co-glycolide	20–24
Resolut Adapt LT™	Poly-D,L-lactide/co-glycolide	20–24
OsseoQuest®	Hydrolysable polyester	16–24
Vicryl®	Polyglactin 910 mesh	8
Guidor®	Poly-D,L-lactide + poly-L-lactide, blended with acetyl tri-n-butyl citrate	52
Vivosorb®	Poly-D,L-lactide-Є-caprolactone)	96

Synthetic polymers

Polylactic acid (PLA) and polylactic acid/polyglycolic acid copolymer (PLGA) are most commonly used as GBR membrane components because of their suitable mechanical properties and their biocompatibility (Table 46.4). Other polymers, polymer blends, composites of polymer and bioactive components are promising chemical options and are in a development phase. Among these products, synthetic hydrogel made of polyethylene glycol exhibits prospective potential for horizontal bone augmentation and ridge preservation.

It must be noted that the bioactivity of synthetic polymers is poor. Furthermore, the degradation of the polymer within the tissues is associated with an inflammatory foreign-body reaction. However, the biocompatibility of synthetic polymer membranes is excellent and they can be used as carriers for drug delivery. Research programmes are being implemented to explore polymers loaded with antibacterial agents or growth factors. Another advantage of polymer membranes compared with collagen membranes is their non-animal origin, which eliminates the potential risk of disease due to animal-to-human transmission, and which does not raise ethical or cultural issues for clinical use.

Key points

- A guided bone regeneration membrane must stay in place a minimum of three to four weeks.
- Non-resorbable membranes require an additional surgical procedure for removal.
- Resorbable membranes require the use of a supportive material.
- There is no evidence to support or refute the superiority of a specific membrane.
- The choice of a membrane product depends not only on technical considerations but also on the patient's preference.

47

Bone augmentation: Guided bone regeneration – technical procedures

Figure 47.1 Staged approach without bone grafting

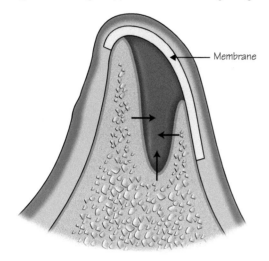

Membrane

Figure 47.2 Staged approach with bone grafting

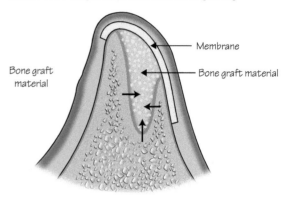

Membrane

Bone graft material

Bone graft material

Figure 47.3 Combined approach with bone grafting

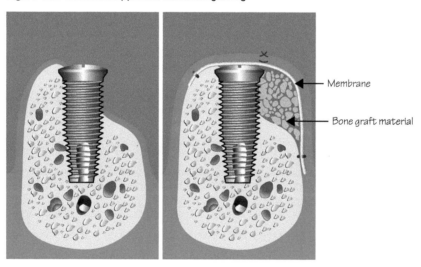

Membrane

Bone graft material

Guided bone regeneration (GBR) has been investigated extensively from both a biological and a clinical standpoint (Esposito *et al.*, 2009). It is one of the most common techniques for bone regeneration around dental implants and bone preservation after tooth extraction. However, the impact of GBR on implant survival and success rates, and the long-term stability of the augmented bone, is still unknown (Benic and Hammerle, 2014).

Rationale

Guided regeneration procedures, also called membrane techniques, aim to use barrier membranes to allow spaces to be filled with bone. The physical separation between soft tissues and areas of bone formation – that is, guided tissue regeneration (GTR) – was first described in the spine in the late 1950s (Hurley *et al.*, 1959). It was shown that soft tissue ingrowth might disturb

Implant Dentistry at a Glance, Second Edition. Jacques Malet, Francis Mora and Philippe Bouchard.
© 2018 John Wiley & Sons Ltd. Published 2018 by John Wiley & Sons Ltd.
Companion website: www.wiley.com/go/malet/implant

Figure 47.4 Combined approach with bone grafting. Clinical case. (a) Initial clinical view; (b) clinical view six weeks after extraction; (c) implant; (d) graft material (BioOss®); (e) collagen membrane (Osseoguard®); (f) soft tissue closure; (g) final result (two years)

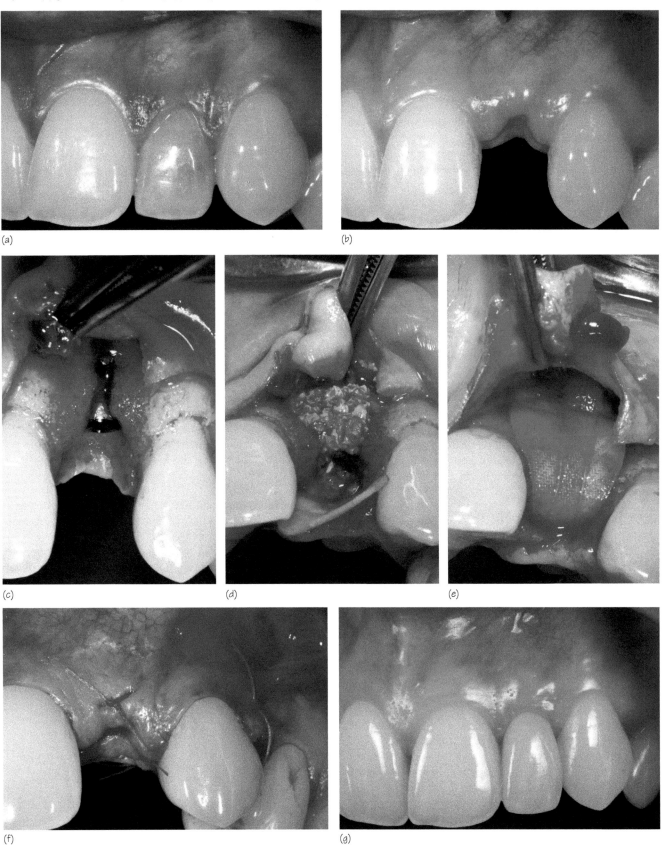

(a)

(b)

(c)

(d)

(e)

(f)

(g)

or totally prevent osteogenesis in a defect or wound. The GTR biological principle was then described for periodontal regeneration around teeth (Gottlow *et al.*, 1984). When dental implants became clinically available, the same biological principle was advocated, not only to generate new bone around implants, but also to prevent alveolar bone loss after tooth extraction. The biological principle was subsequently referred to as guided bone regeneration (Dahlin *et al.*, 1989).

Basically, membrane barriers are employed to make sufficient bone available for dental implant placement. The procedure aims to:

- stabilise the blood clot
- prevent the growth of soft tissue cells (connective tissue and epithelium) into the bone defect
- allow spaces maintained over the defect to be filled with bone progenitor cells that may develop bone.

Membrane barriers are often supported by bone graft materials, but they can be used without a space maintainer when they are reinforced with titanium and/or the defect is compatible with a stable clot (Figure 47.1). In all cases, the membrane must be fixed onto the bone surface. It can be stabilised with titanium tacks. Care must be taken with absorbable tacks due to their poor mechanical properties.

Technical procedures

Guided bone regeneration procedures are difficult to perform. The skills and experience of the clinician are critical factors in treatment success. Various combined procedures have been proposed, but it is unclear which are the most efficient. However, some clinical recommendations can be made (Appendix Q, Box Q.1).

A bone defect may be treated prior to (staged approach; Figures 47.1 and 47.2), during (combined approach; Figure 47.3) or after implant placement (peri-implantitis therapy). Compared to the staged approach, the combined approach reduces the lag between implant surgery and the beginning of the prosthetic phase by one to three months (Appendix Q, Figure Q1). However, with the combined approach, the consequences of complications during initial surgery may not only impair the amount of bone regenerated, but can also lead to primary implant failure.

Any membrane should remain in place for at least three to four weeks.

Indications
Transmucosal implants

Evidence for the use of the GBR technique combined with transmucosal implants is scant (Chiapasco and Zaniboni, 2009). In other words, one-stage approaches are not good candidates for GBR procedures. The membrane should only be employed in this specific indication by highly experienced clinicians.

Vertical and horizontal bone augmentation

The GBR technique is a predictable procedure for lateral ridge augmentation. The technique has also been successfully performed for vertical augmentation, but there is less documented evidence compared to that for horizontal augmentation (Esposito et al., 2009). GBR reports indicate a range of 2–8 mm in terms of vertical bone gain (Tonetti and Hammerle, 2008).

Extensive alveolar ridge defects require a grafting material to support the membrane. These large bone defects are often augmented with autogenous block grafts and membranes (von Arx et al., 2001). The use of expanded polytetrafluoroethylene (e-PTFE) membranes covering onlay bone grafts for lateral ridge augmentations seems to reduce resorption of the bone graft (Antoun et al., 2001).

Immediate and delayed implantation

The lack of soft tissue for primary healing is a frequent problem when placing implants directly into extraction sockets. The GBR technique cannot be recommended for direct implantation given the high risk of membrane exposure. It may be recommended for delayed implantation, since it can compensate for the small loss of bone volume that occurs over the six to eight weeks required for soft tissue closure (Figure 47.4).

Dehiscences and fenestrations

The placement of oral implants into alveolar ridges of inadequate dimensions may result in dehiscence or fenestration. These types of defect can be successfully treated with GBR using non-resorbable membranes, either alone or in combination with a graft (Klinge and Flemmig, 2009).

Peri-implantitis

The use of a bone substitute with a resorbable membrane may improve some clinical parameters, but there is very little reliable evidence to indicate that the GBR technique is beneficial in the surgical treatment of peri-implantitis (Esposito et al., 2010).

Contraindications

- Lack of patient compliance
- Lack of individual plaque control
- Heavy smoker (more than 10 cigarettes per day)
- Untreated periodontitis
- Infection at the surgical site.

Complications

Membrane exposure and infection are frequent complications. Premature exposure of the membrane does not always preclude success if closely monitored (Appendix Q, Box Q2).

Regarding resorbable membranes, exposure may often be managed and monitored over time. The physical qualities of the material are affected by the hydrolysis/resorption process. Thus, when the membranes have to be removed (because of infection), care must be taken to avoid tearing the membrane remnants.

Key points

- Guided bone regeneration (GBR) is a difficult procedure to perform.
- GBR procedures may be successfully considered for horizontal bone augmentation, delayed implantation, dehiscence and fenestration. Further studies are needed for the other indications.
- Better bone formation is observed with non-resorbable membranes compared to resorbable membranes.
- There are more exposures with non-resorbable membranes than with resorbable membranes.

48 Bone augmentation: Graft materials

Figure 48.1 Autogenous bone. (a, b) Bone is harvested at the donor site with a trephine. (c, d) Bone is ground in a bone mill

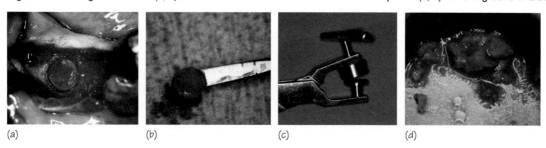

(a)   (b)   (c)   (d)

Figure 48.2 Autogenous bone plus xenograft. (a–c) Bone is harvested with a trephine mill system. (d, e) The retrieved bone is collected and may be blended with a bone substitute

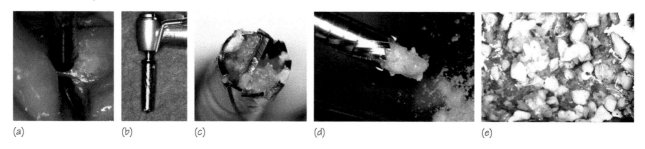

(a)   (b)   (c)   (d)   (e)

Figure 48.3 Xenograft. (a) Implant placement with two important bone dehiscences requiring horizontal bone augmentation. (b) The bone substitute is soaked with blood. (c) The xenograft covers the defects. (d) A collagen barrier membrane is secured with mattress sutures over the bone material. (e) Periosteal fenestration is performed to achieve soft tissue closure

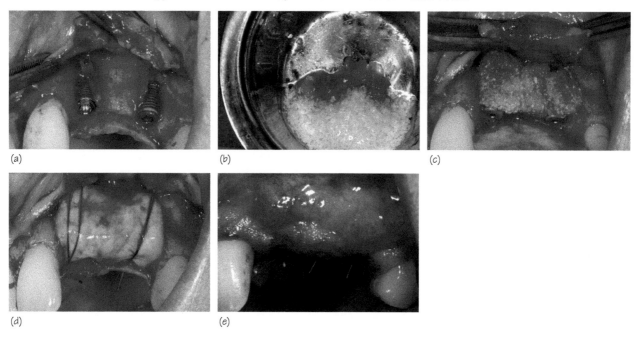

(a)   (b)   (c)

(d)   (e)

Implant Dentistry at a Glance, Second Edition. Jacques Malet, Francis Mora and Philippe Bouchard.
© 2018 John Wiley & Sons Ltd. Published 2018 by John Wiley & Sons Ltd.
Companion website: www.wiley.com/go/malet/implant

The autogenous bone graft with its biological properties (osteogenicity, inductivity, conductivity) has long been considered the ideal grafting material in bone reconstructive surgery. Recent advances in biotechnology have provided the surgeon with access to a great variety of bone grafting materials – that is, osteobiologics – in order to reduce the morbidity and unpredictable resorption of autogenous bone graft (Hallman and Thor, 2008). Graft materials are commercially available in blocks or particles of different sizes. Trends suggest that the survival rate of dental implants in grafted zones may be slightly lower than the survival rate of implants placed in native bone (Tonetti and Hâmmerle, 2008; Esposito et al., 2009).

Autografts (grafts from a donor who is the also the recipient)

Autogenous bone grafts are the patient's own tissue and can be intraorally or extraorally harvested. The grafted bone can be regarded as a scaffold that serves later in new bone formation. The vascular supply of cortico-cancellous bone graft enables the survival of cells, the diffusion of nutrients and revascularisation (Davies and Hosseini, 2000). The healing events describe osteoconduction (new bone is gradually formed around the resorbed graft) and osteoinduction (releasing of proteins stimulating osteoblasts to form new bone).

Positive outcomes have been reported in sinus floor augmentation (Boyne and James, 1980). Rigid fixation of block bone graft is a prerequisite for stimulating the progenitor cells. Ground bone grafts particulate or chip with/without substitutes and non-resorbable membranes are available alternatives (Figure 48.1).

Autogenous bone grafts can be mixed with any of the bone graft materials listed below (Figure 48.2).

Allografts (graft from a donor of the same species as the recipient)

These are bone grafts harvested from cadavers and processed by methods such as freezing or demineralising and freezing. Freeze-dried bone and demineralised freeze-dried bone allografts are reported to be less immunogenic than fresh-frozen bone allografts (because of the risk of transfection). These materials are frequently used in mixtures with autogenous bone or bone substitutes.

Xenografts (graft from a donor of a different species to the recipient)

Xenografts consist of either animal bone mineral from various origins, such as bovine, porcine and equine, or bone-like minerals (calcium carbonate) derived from corals or algae. Deproteinised bovine bone (DBB) is widely used because of its similarity to human bone and its osteoconductive properties (Berglundh and Lindhe, 1997; Figure 48.3). The proteins in DBB are extracted to avoid immunological rejection.

In human studies of maxillary sinus alveolar ridge augmentations (Carmagnola et al., 2000), DBB and autogenous bone have histologically been associated with active bone formation. Biopsies harvested after a 6–9-month healing period of sinuses grafted with DBB showed 30% newly formed bone, 30% DBB and 40% bone marrow. Increased mineralisation was detected after 14 months and osteoclastic resorption of DBB particles was found after 4 years (Piatelli et al., 1999; Valentini et al., 1998). It has been shown that there is no benefit to adjunct autogenous bone in maxillary sinus procedures (Yildirim et al., 2001).

Alloplast (synthetic material)

Alloplastic bone substitutes represent synthetic calcium-based biomaterials. Calcium phosphate, calcium sulfate and bioactive glasses have been used in dental implant surgery for bone augmentation. Alloplasts provide a physical framework for bone ingrowth. Pore size greater than 300 µm (similar to bone structure) shows enhanced formation of new capillaries and bone.

Calcium phosphates can be bound to collagen carriers to form a network on which minerals can crystallise. Biphasic tricalcium phosphate, produced by sintering hydroxyapatite, has been shown to be effective in repairing skeletal defects (Daculsi, 1998). Calcium sulfate resorbs quickly and must be used carefully in aesthetic areas because of the lack of control of the resorption process.

Bioglass is a commercially available family of bioactive glasses. Bioglass (particle size of 300 µm) releases in the biological fluids calcium ions, which can stimulate stem cells to produce bone-building cells. Bioglass is slowly resorbed (12–16 months) before the graft is replaced by newly formed bone. Biopsies of a mixture of autogenous bone and bioactive glass particles (300–355 µm in size) have shown new bone after 16 months. Biopsies harvested after two years have revealed similar bone-forming outcomes (Turunen et al., 2004).

Growth factors and platelet-rich plasma

These may be incorporated into any of the graft types.

Growth factors, which are present at low concentrations in bone matrix and plasma, induce bone formation, growth, migration and differentiation of cells. They play a regulatory role in homeostasis as well as in tissue repair. Recombinant bone morphogenetic proteins (BMPs) are associated with carriers or scaffolds such as substitute materials. They are released on the repaired site to increase tissue reconstruction (Terheyden et al., 1999).

Platelets are non-nucleated bone marrow fragments, abundant in blood. They act in haemostasis, wound healing and inflammation, and are activated by collagen, thrombin, thromboxane A_2, adenosine phosphate and P-selectin. By using a common centrifugation technique, platelet-rich plasma (PRP) can be prepared in the operating room during surgery (Anitua, 1999). Before implant installation, positive effects with or without allografts have been reported (Merkx et al., 2004). However, these benefits are controversial. The association of PRP with β-tricalcium phosphate has not enhanced bone formation in sinus augmentation procedures in the absence of osteoblasts or osteocytes (Thor et al., 2005; Wiltfang et al., 2003).

Key points

- Autogenous bone grafting and osteobiologics are predictable materials for the correction of edentulous ridge defects.
- Various bone graft substitutes can augment bone horizontally and vertically, but it is unclear which is the most efficient.
- Some bone substitutes could be a preferable alternative to autogenous bone, since they are associated with less postoperative morbidity.

49 Bone augmentation: Block bone grafts

Figure 49.1 Intraoral autogenous bone block grafts: anatomical areas (shaded) at the mandible where cortical bone can be harvested

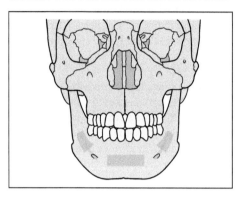

Figure 49.2 Bone block graft harvested from the chin. (a) Donor site after harvesting; (b) adaptation and fixation of the blocks in the anterior area of the maxilla

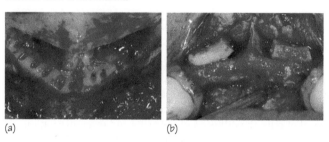

(a) (b)

Figure 49.3 Horizontal bone augmentation. (a) Preparation of the recipient site; (b) bone block graft harvested from the ramus; (c) graft fixation with a titanium screw; (d) a bone graft substitute (Bio-Oss®) is placed to fill the spaces and a resorbable membrane is adapted on the site; (e) soft tissue covering and sutures without any tension; (f) second-stage surgery four months later and implant placement

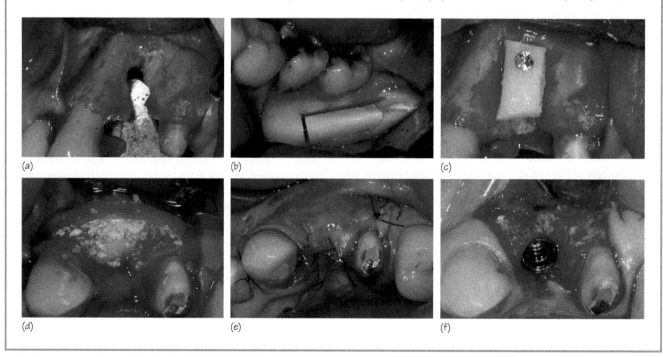

(a) (b) (c)

(d) (e) (f)

Rationale

Bone grafts taken from patient themselves are the 'gold standard' in bone reconstruction. Autogenous bone grafts can be harvested from intraoral sites (Figure 49.1) for small defects, or from extraoral sites (calvaria, iliac crest, tibia) for larger defects.

We will focus on intraoral sites for harvesting performed under local anaesthesia; that is, mental symphysis (chin; Figure 49.2), retromolar mandible region (ramus; Figure 49.3) and maxillary tuberosity.

Results
Bone augmentation

During the healing process, block bone grafts provide a scaffold for new bone growth and simultaneously undergo a resorption process. This resorption is greatest in the first year

Implant Dentistry at a Glance, Second Edition. Jacques Malet, Francis Mora and Philippe Bouchard.
© 2018 John Wiley & Sons Ltd. Published 2018 by John Wiley & Sons Ltd.
Companion website: www.wiley.com/go/malet/implant

Table 49.1 Harvesting sites of autogenous bone block grafts

	Intraoral		Extraoral	
	Symphysis	Ramus	Iliac crest	Calvarium
Bone quantity	Low	Medium	High	High
Graft resorption	Low	Low	High	Low
Morbidity	Medium	Low	High	Low
Indication	Small defect	Small to medium-sized defect	Large defect	Large defect
	Ramus unavailable		Calvarium unavailable	

after grafting and stabilises after one year of implant loading (Chiapasco *et al.*, 2009).

Implant survival

Survival rates of dental implants inserted into block bone grafts are lower than those for implants placed in native bone. Furthermore, a two-stage approach (implant placement after four months of healing) is associated with better survival rates than a one-stage approach (simultaneous implant placement).

Rough-surface implants have a better survival rate than machined-surface implants when placed into bone block grafts.

Limited data are available in the literature.

Technical procedures
Preoperative examination

Cone beam computed tomography (CBCT) or a CT scan is performed to visualise the alveolar ridge defect precisely and to explore the donor site.

Recipient site

A full-thickness flap with good visibility of the bone plate is mandatory. Bone is freed from all soft tissues (Figure 49.3a) and small perforations of the buccal plate are performed to improve blood supply.

Graft harvesting

Bone is harvested with a handpiece saw, an oscillating saw or a piezoelectric surgical device (Figure 49.3b). The latter is the easiest to use and allows better visibility. It is recommended to harvest enough bone to overbuild the defect and to anticipate graft resorption. Bone chips are collected for filling spaces. The donor site is sutured.

Graft adaptation

The bone block is modified to fit perfectly into the defect. For vertical defects, part of the bone block is placed on top of the ridge. The contact surface between the bone graft and the recipient site must be as intimate as possible.

Graft fixation

Bone blocks must be locked onto the recipient site to avoid any movement that could impair healing. Usually, titanium screws are used to secure the bone graft (Figure 49.3c).

Additional procedures

Graft materials can be used to fill the spaces and augment the final bone volume. The use of regenerative resorbable membranes is recommended to prevent the resorption process and to secure the graft materials (Figure 49.3d).

Simultaneous implant placement is not recommended with bone block grafts.

Soft tissue covering

Sutures without any soft tissue tension are a prerequisite to avoid bone graft exposure and complications (Figure 49.3e).

Second-stage surgery

A four- to six-month period is required before second-stage surgery. Fixation screw removal and implant placement are performed during the same surgery (Figure 49.3f).

Advantages

Bone block grafting is a relatively well-documented technique (except for maxillary tuberosity) and gives predictable results for horizontal defects. Usually, the healing phase is uneventful and allows the placement of implants in good-quality bone.

Disadvantages

Compared to other techniques, the presence of a donor site (particularly if extraoral) leads to greater morbidity. However, this biological cost is limited with intraoral harvesting, in particular with ramus sites.

Bone block grafting is a technically sensitive technique and there is a limited quantity of bone (intraoral).

The correction of vertical defects shows poorly predictable results and more complications.

It is a two-stage procedure and, consequently, a time-consuming technique involving a high financial cost.

Indications

It is difficult to choose this technique over another, on a scientific basis, because of the lack of comparative studies. However, situations where the bone volume is insufficient to allow implant stabilisation in the residual ridge (horizontal or vertical severe resorption) or placement in the optimal implant position (aesthetic) are good indications (Chen *et al.*, 2009).

Intraoral harvesting is preferred for small and moderate defects, while extraoral harvesting is indicated for extended defects (Table 49.1).

Bone block grafts can be performed whatever the defect morphology: horizontal, vertical or a combination of vertical and horizontal. However, horizontal defects are the indication of choice.

Complications
Bone augmentation

For horizontal defects, block bone grafts allow higher gains and lower complications compared to guided bone regeneration (GBR) techniques with graft materials. For vertical defects, there are more complications than with horizontal defects (Esposito *et al.*, 2009).

Harvesting site

During harvesting at the mental symphysis site, injury of the incisal nerve can occur, leading to permanent paraesthesia of anterior mandibular teeth (prevalence 10%).

Complications are uncommon with the ramus site.

Iliac crest harvesting is associated with pain and gait disturbances (prevalence 2%), as well as a higher bone resorption (cancellous bone).

Key points

- Bone block grafting is indicated when implant stabilisation in the correct position is not possible in native bone.
- Horizontal augmentation is more predictable than vertical augmentation.
- The use of additional membranes and/or graft material may prevent graft resorption.
- Intraoral harvesting is the technique of choice for small or moderate defects.
- For extended defects, extraoral harvesting must be considered.

Bone augmentation: Split osteotomy (split ridge technique)

50

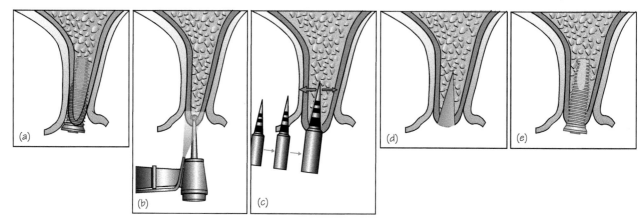

Figure 50.1 Split ridge technique for single dental implant placement at the maxilla. (a) The dental implant cannot be placed due to the knife-edge alveolar bone morphology. (b) Lamellar cortical splitting is initiated by using a burr. (c) A set of chisels of increasing width is used to split the alveolar ridge. (d) The gap created by splitting is left empty. (e) Transverse expansion allows for immediate dental implant installation

(a) (b) (c) (d) (e)

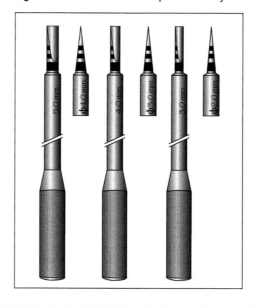

Figure 50.2 Set of chisels for split osteotomy

Rationale

Split ridge and expansion techniques are effective for the correction of moderately resorbed edentulous ridges in selected cases. Transverse expansion is based on osseous plasticity obtained by corticotomy. It progressively allows for an adequate transversal intercortical diameter large enough to insert one or several dental implants. The gap created by sagittal osteotomy expansion undergoes spontaneous ossification, following a mechanism similar to that occurring in fractures (Figure 50.1).

Products and devices

Various ridge splitting/expanding chisels (from 3 mm to 6 mm) are designed to define the appropriate shape and size of the osteotomy (Figure 50.2). Ultrasonic units may facilitate and improve the safety of the procedure.

Implant Dentistry at a Glance, Second Edition. Jacques Malet, Francis Mora and Philippe Bouchard.
© 2018 John Wiley & Sons Ltd. Published 2018 by John Wiley & Sons Ltd.
Companion website: www.wiley.com/go/malet/implant

Figure 50.3 Split osteotomy at the mandible. (a) Lamellar cortical splitting with a 3 mm chisel. (b) The gap is progressively created by the use of different chisels. (c) The dental implants are placed and the gap is filled with a bone substitute. (d, e) A resorbable membrane is trimmed and adapted over the implants before closure. (f) Three months later, the uncovering procedure can be performed. The regenerated tissue has filled the gap. (g) The prosthetic phase can begin one month after the uncovering procedure

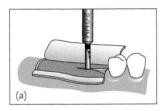 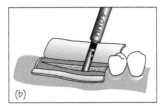
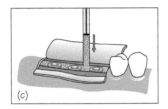 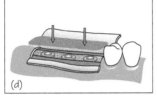
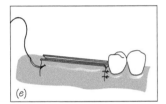 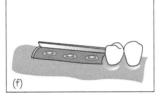
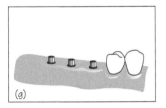

Technical procedure

See Figure 50.3.

• *Full-thickness crestal incision* with vertical releasing incisions one tooth further than the site being treated.

• *Elevation of a mucoperiosteal flap* palatally and buccally to expose the bone ridge.

• *Lamellar cortical splitting* initiated by one horizontal crestal osteotomy using a diamond disk, a burr or, preferably, a piezosurgery tip. The longitudinal split can be limited by placing transverse cuts in the bone. Two additional vertical cuts, 2 mm distal to the site of implantation and 1 mm mesial to the adjacent teeth, can be performed to facilitate the expansion.

• *Longitudinal splitting* of the alveolar ridge performed using a set of chisels of increasing width. They are optimally used by pressing the instrument manually into the bone or by gently tapping the chisels with a hammer. Normally the chisels are extended to a depth of 5–7 mm, but the penetration depends on the width of the ridge. The direction of chisel force should be aimed palatally to decrease the damage exerted on fragile and thin buccal plates. The chisel should be removed by movement in a mesial-distal direction. Facial-lingual movement should be avoided so as not to further deform the buccal plate.

• *The gap created by splitting* can either be left empty or filled with different materials, such as collagen sponge, autogenous bone chips or bone substitute. The split ridge can be covered with membranes. However, there is a lack of evidence concerning the split ridge technique with interpositional graft materials or with covering membranes.

• *Dental implant placement* at the same time or later, according to a standard procedure. There is a lack of evidence for delayed implant placement when using the split ridge technique. When placed immediately, primary implant stability is achieved by placing the implants at the most apical non-fractured portion of the jawbone. To improve primary stability of the implants and to prevent fracture of the buccal plate, the use of osteotomes to prepare the implant bed is recommended.

• *Wound closure* with vertical mattress sutures.

• *Dental rehabilitation* may be started three to six months afterwards.

Indications and advantages

The split ridge/ridge expansion technique is indicated in selected situations where atrophy of the edentulous ridge has developed horizontally and cancellous bone is present between the oral and facial cortical plates, and adequate residual height exists. This technique is mainly indicated in the maxilla.

The procedure results in a significant increase (range 87.5–100%) in the width of the alveolar ridge (Donos *et al.*, 2008) and allows a gain of 4–5.5 mm of thickness. Survival rates of implants placed at sites augmented using these techniques are similar to those of implants inserted in native bone; that is ranging from 98% to 100% at eight months post-loading (Chen *et al.* 2009).

Contraindication and limitations
Unfavourable bone angularity

Excessive facial inclination of the alveolar ridge may contraindicate this procedure, as it may worsen the initial situation from a prosthetic and aesthetic point of view. When excessive buccal inclination of the implants creates problems, guided bone regeneration (GBR) or bone grafting techniques seem more suitable.

Severe horizontal atrophy

The technique can only be applied when the buccal and palate/lingual plates are separated by spongy bone. Therefore, the indications are more limited compared to onlay bone grafts and GBR, which can also be applied in cases presenting severe horizontal atrophy.

Ridge expansion in the mandible

Although possible, ridge expansion in the mandible is frequently difficult due to the rigidity of the bone. The risk of fracture of the osteotomised fragment is higher than at the maxilla.

Complications

• *Basal greenstick fracture of the segments* during widening has not been controllable to date. Thus, fracture of the buccal plate is the most common complication. Care must be taken in the presence of undercuts that may increase the risk of bone fracture. A minimum width of 2–3 mm of the coronal alveolar crest is necessary to avoid bone fracture.

• *Loosening or fracture of microscrews* may happen.
• *A labyrinthine concussion* may occur during tapping of an osteotome.
• The patient may experience a *benign positional vertigo*.

Key points

• Bone splitting/expansion seems to be a reliable and relatively non-invasive technique to correct narrow residual edentulous ridges.
• It is mainly indicated at the maxilla.
• Bone fracture is the most frequent complication.
• The procedure is technically demanding.
• Piezosurgery facilitates and improves the safety of the procedure.

51 Bone augmentation: Sinus floor elevation – lateral approach

Figure 51.1 Lateral approach, two-stage technique. (a) A mucoperiosteal flap is reflected to expose the buccal wall of bone. (b) The osteotomy is prepared with a piezo tip (or round burr). (c) The osteotomy is complete. The osseous window is reflected medially and superiorly using a spoon elevator. (d) The sinus membrane is elevated with blunt sinus curettes. At the end of this stage, the Valsalva manoeuvre indicates that the sinus membrane is intact. (e) The compartment is filled with the grafting material through the window. (f) The bone graft material is extended to the osteotomy border and packed into the osteotomy site. A resorbable membrane is trimmed and adapted to the lateral window (at least 3 mm beyond the osteotomy lines). (g) The window is completely covered with the resorbable membrane. Care is taken not to leave graft material particles outside the sinus cavity. (h) Soft tissues are closed with mattress sutures and the graft material is used as a scaffold for new bone formation. (i) The dental implants are inserted about four months after sinus elevation

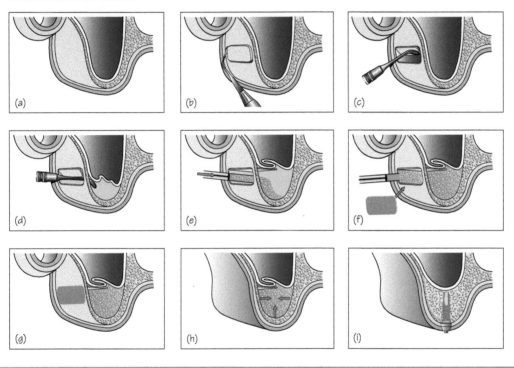

Due to a limited residual bone height following dental extraction in the maxillary posterior area, standard dental implants cannot generally be placed. Sinus floor elevation techniques therefore allow standard dental implant placement. These procedures are performed frequently, regardless of the approach, be it lateral or transalveolar. The implant survival rate (ISR) following sinus floor elevation is greater than 90% after three years (Graziani *et al.*, 2004; Pjetursson *et al.*, 2008; Wallace and Froum, 2003).

Rationale

The biological rationale for this procedure is based on the ability of a graft material to promote bone formation in a compartment that is surgically created between the Schneiderian membrane and the sinus walls (Esposito *et al.*, 2014). In the lateral approach, a bone window is prepared on the lateral sinus wall, to lift the sinus membrane. The major advantage of this traditional open procedure is that it allows direct vision of the sinus membrane and control of its integrity. However, this procedure is more invasive than the transalveolar approach (Chapter 52), against which it must be balanced.

Products and devices
Specific instrumentation

- Round carbide and diamond burrs
- Piezoelectric surgical device (optional)
- Sinus curettes.

Graft materials

Bone substitutes are now preferred to autogenous bone because of the lack of donor site morbidity. Allografts, alloplasts and xenografts can be used alone or in combination with autogenous bone. Xenografts (Bio-Oss®) are now extensively used and well documented. No relevant differences between grafting materials

Implant Dentistry at a Glance, Second Edition. Jacques Malet, Francis Mora and Philippe Bouchard.
© 2018 John Wiley & Sons Ltd. Published 2018 by John Wiley & Sons Ltd.
Companion website: www.wiley.com/go/malet/implant

Figure 51.2 Surgical complication: perforation of the sinus membrane. (a) Clinical view of the perforation, which occurred during membrane elevation. The membrane contours around the perforation are in the operator's field of view. (b) A collagen membrane is used to obliterate the perforation

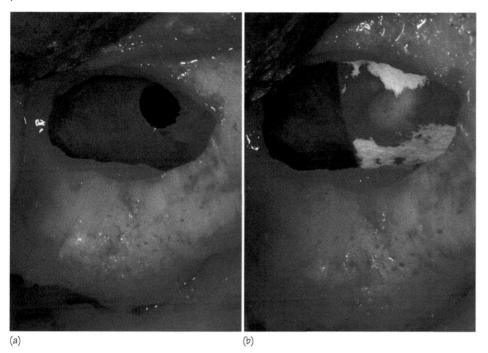

(a)   (b)

in terms of ISR (96.3% to 99.8%) are found for rough-surface dental implants (Chiapasco *et al.*, 2009; Lutz *et al.*, 2015; Nkenke and Stelzle, 2009; Schmitt *et al.*, 2013). Autogenous bone may be added to the xenograft. This can potentially reduce the healing time (Del Fabbro *et al.*, 2004).

Barrier membranes

A resorbable barrier membrane can be applied to cover the lateral window after grafting (Chapter 46). Procedures performed with a membrane show a higher ISR than when no membranes are used (Tonetti and Hammerle, 2008).

Implants

Nowadays, only rough-surface implants are used in sinus floor elevation procedures, regardless of graft material or technical procedure.

Technical procedures

See Figure 51.1. The lateral approach is technically demanding. A mid-crestal incision is performed and a buccal-releasing incision is extended into the buccal vestibulum. A mucoperiosteal flap is elevated. The outline of the window is marked onto the lateral sinus wall with a small round carbide burr or with the saw of the piezoelectric device.

The osteotomy is performed with a no. 6 round diamond until the transparency of the sinus membrane appears as a blue/grey line. Piezoelectric osteotomy is time-consuming but safer than the burr technique. Diamond-coated tips are used for the window cut and minimise damage to the sinus membrane.

The sinus membrane is elevated with blunt sinus curettes. The bone attached to the membrane forms the roof of the grafting space. The bone window attached to the membrane can be removed to facilitate access for membrane elevation, and thus avoid tearing.

If the sinus membrane is damaged, the implant placement is postponed to allow re-epithelialisation of the sinus membrane over the following two months.

One-stage technique

Before implant insertion, the medial part of the compartment is filled with the grafting material, the implants are inserted and the remaining space is filled to the bone surface. The window is then covered with a resorbable membrane and the flap is closed with tension-free sutures.

Two-stage technique

The compartment is filled to the bone surface with the grafting material and covered with a resorbable membrane. The dental implants are inserted four to six months after sinus elevation.

Indications

The lateral approach is used when short dental implants and/or a transalveolar approach are not indicated.

Contraindications

• Untreated maxillary sinus pathology.
• Cigarette smoking has a negative effect on ISR. There are no data supporting the fact that smoking is a contraindication. However, smokers must be informed that (i) postoperative complications are more frequent and severe; and (ii) the ISR is lower than in non-smokers.

Complications

Although infrequent, these can nevertheless significantly affect outcome and patient morbidity.

Membrane perforation

The most frequent complication is perforation of the sinus membrane, which occurs in about 20% of procedures. Small perforations can be managed by careful elevation of the sinus membrane around the perforation, which is covered within the sinus by a resorbable membrane (Figure 51.2). Implant survival is generally not affected by perforation of the sinus membrane, irrespective

Figure 51.3 Identification of the alveolar antral artery. (a) The artery adheres to the sinus membrane. (b) The artery is carefully separated by dissection from the outer portion of the membrane with a sinus curette, before elevation. Care is taken to avoid any artery injury during filling with the graft material

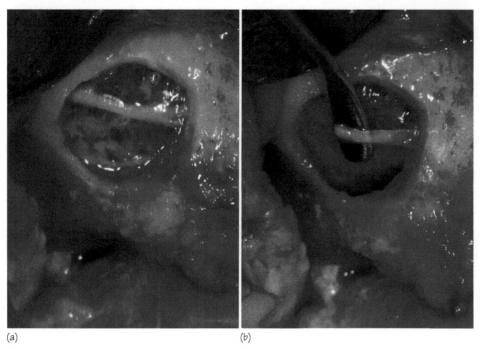

(a)   (b)

of the technique. If there is a large tear of the sinus membrane, the procedure is stopped and a second attempt can be performed six to nine months later.

Perioperative haemorrhage

As with any sinus surgery a nosebleed can occur. The alveolar antral artery sometimes follows an intrabony pathway into the lateral sinus wall. This location can interfere with the osteotomy, resulting in extensive bleeding when the artery is damaged. The precise location should be confirmed during pre-surgical X-rays to avoid arterial injury. Large arteries are sometimes easy to identify (Figure 51.3). They should be dissected. A piezoelectric device is useful in this instance.

Infection

Infections following sinus elevation are rather uncommon (occurring in approximately 3% of cases). They are generally associated with membrane perforation. Sinusitis tends to occur in previously unhealthy sinuses. Graft loss is caused by severe complications, and occurs at a rate of approximately 2%.

Key points

- Sinus floor elevation procedures are predictable treatment methods.
- Perforation of the sinus membrane is the main complication.
- The lateral approach is demanding and requires adequate training to perform the procedure, as well as clinical expertise to manage the complications.

52 Bone augmentation: Sinus floor elevation – transalveolar approach

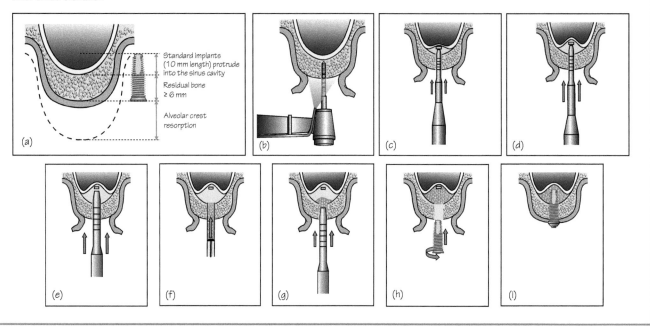

Figure 52.1 Transalveolar approach. (a) Depending on bone quality, a minimum residual bone height of 4–6 mm is necessary to ensure primary stability of the implant. (b) The alveolar bone is drilled (diameter 2 mm) to within 2 mm of the sinus floor. Care is taken not to drill the sinus floor. (c) The sinus floor is carefully fractured with the tip of the first osteotome (diameter >2 mm). (d, e) Osteotomes of wider diameters are used to compress and expand the bone opening. (f) The sinus is filled with a bone substitute through the canal created by the osteotomes. (g) Prior to implant placement, the bone graft material is packed with the tip of the wider-diameter osteotome into the osteotomy site. (h, i) The implants are inserted immediately. The prosthetic phase can begin about four months after sinus elevation

This technique was first introduced in 1994 by Robert Summers (Summers, 1994) and has been slightly modified over time (Fugazzotto and De, 2002; Trombelli *et al.*, 2010). However, the transalveolar approach is less documented than the lateral approach.

Rationale

The biological rationale for this procedure is the same as for the lateral approach (Chapter 51). With the transalveolar approach, osteotomy is performed on the alveolar crest at the surgical site of the implants. The sinus membrane is carefully lifted by osteotomes inserted through the implant bed. The compartment created beneath the Schneiderian membrane is supported by the apex of the dental implant body and/or graft material, which not only acts as a space-maker but also aims to stimulate new bone formation.

Advantages and disadvantages of the transalveolar technique

There is insufficient evidence to conclude whether one specific sinus lift procedure leads to fewer implants or prosthetic failure than another in bone with a residual height of 4–9 mm (Esposito *et al.*, 2014). A systematic review indicates an estimated implant survival rate (ISR) of 92.8% at three years (Tan *et al.*, 2008). This value corresponds to the ISR of the lateral approach.

The transalveolar approach (synonym: crestal approach) is a very popular sinus lift procedure because it is a minimally invasive technique, which is time-saving compared to the lateral approach. Consequently, morbidity and postoperative discomfort are very limited. In the absence of specific complications, patient-reported outcomes are comparable to those achieved with implants placed in native bone (Franceschetti *et al.*, 2017). However, some perioperative discomfort may be occasionally induced through the use of hand mallets in osteotomy procedures. It has been shown that patients may prefer rotary instruments over hand malleting (Esposito *et al.*, 2014).

Compared to the lateral approach, the transalveolar procedure is less invasive but is performed blind. Thus, it requires advanced surgical skills, especially during the sinus floor fracture. Furthermore, the extent of bone augmentation within the maxillary sinus seems to be surgeon dependent (Franceschetti *et al.*, 2015).

Implant Dentistry at a Glance, Second Edition. Jacques Malet, Francis Mora and Philippe Bouchard.
© 2018 John Wiley & Sons Ltd. Published 2018 by John Wiley & Sons Ltd.
Companion website: www.wiley.com/go/malet/implant

Figure 52.2 (a) Replacement of tooth #26. Preoperative radiograph showing a 4 mm bone height that does not allow dental implant placement. (b) The osteotomy is gradually performed with tapered osteotomes with different diameters. The figure shows a 3.9 mm diameter osteotome, which corresponds to the placement of a 4.1 mm implant. (c) The integrity of the sinus membrane can be checked through the implant bed using the Valsalva's maneuver. (d) Graft material is placed in the osteotomy and pushed with the osteotome within the sinus cavity. (e) An 8 mm long dental implant is selected and placed into the osteotomy. (f) Postoperative radiograph. Courtesy of Dr Eric Maujean, Rothschild hospital, AP-HP, Paris France

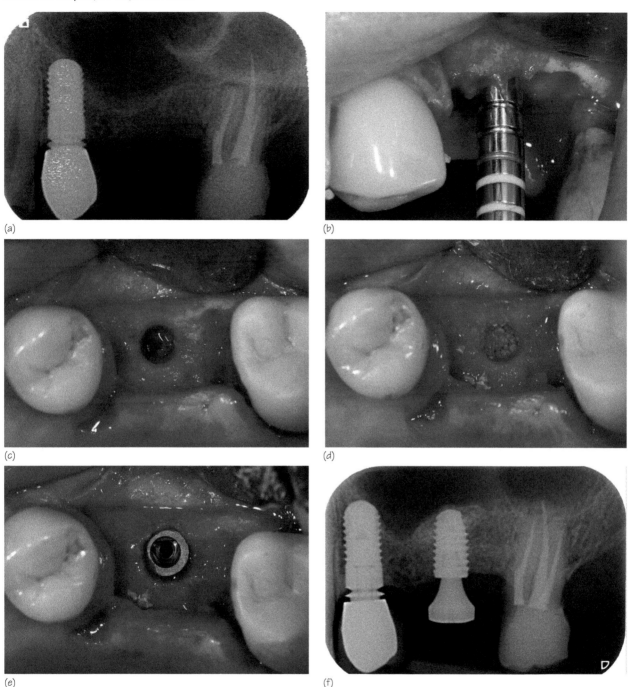

(a) (b) (c) (d) (e) (f)

Products and devices
Specific instrumentation

- Sinus osteotomes
- Mallet.

Optional

- Graft material (see Chapter 51).

Technical procedures

See Figure 52.1 and Figure 52.2. The implant bed is drilled to the sinus floor. A microfracture of the sinus floor is carefully per-

formed by hand malleting with the osteotome tip from 1 to 2 mm into the sinus. The implant bed is then enlarged manually with the osteotomes. At this stage, care is taken to avoid sinus membrane perforation. Indeed, it is not the tip of the osteotome that elevates the membrane but the graft material, which is gently packed into the implant bed and carefully inserted within the sinus. The sinus floor can be elevated up to 5 mm without membrane perforations (Engelke and Deckwer, 1997). The implant is then inserted. Intraoperative radiographic controls are recommended.

There is no need for additional graft material when sinus floor elevation does not exceed 2 mm. In such cases, bone formation has been shown around the apex without any graft material (Sohn *et al.*, 2008).

In soft bone (types III and IV), the implant bed can be prepared solely through the use of osteotomes (Fig 52.2). When primary stability is not achieved, implant placement must be postponed.

Indication

Residual bone height of 4–6 mm in the maxillary posterior area (Tan *et al.*, 2008).

Contraindications

For surgical procedure: residual bone height less than 4 mm. (Chapter 51).
For dental implant placement: questionable primary stability.

Complications

Although complications are rare, they are more difficult to diagnose and manage during the surgical procedure because, as previously mentioned, a blind approach is used. Basically, the types of complication are similar to those documented with the lateral approach (Chapter 51). However, the complications specified below are specific to the transalveolar approach.

Membrane perforation

This may occur during the drilling phase beneath the sinus floor or because the fracture of the sinus floor with the tip of the oste-otome is too rough. Membrane perforation can be checked with the Valsalva manoeuvre. If the sinus membrane is damaged, the implant placement is postponed to allow re-epithelialisation of the sinus membrane over the following two months.

Perioperative haemorrhage

This complication is rare, and caused by damage to the posterior superior alveolar artery or the alveolar antral artery by the oste-otomes, on their lateral sinus wall or intrasinusal pathway. As this is a blind procedure, graft material and implant placement should be postponed in case of peroperative haemorrhage.

Benign paroxysmal positional vertigo (BPPV)

This is an occasional consequence of the osteotome/mallet action and of the hyperextended head position that favours the displacement of otoliths in the inner ear. Referral to an ear, nose and throat specialist (ENT) is recommended.

Key points

- Sinus floor elevation with transalveolar approach is indicated for a residual bone height of 4–6 mm.
- The implant survival rate with a transalveolar approach is similar to that for the lateral approach.
- Perforation of the sinus membrane is the main complication.
- The transalveolar approach is a demanding procedure.

53 Bone augmentation: Alveolar distraction osteogenesis

Figure 53.1 The three components of a miniature intraoral distraction device

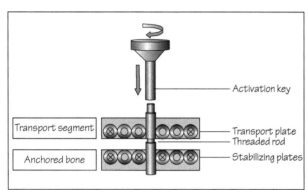

Activation key

Transport segment

Transport plate
Threaded rod

Anchored bone

Stabilizing plates

Figure 53.3 Traditional time schedule of the distraction protocol

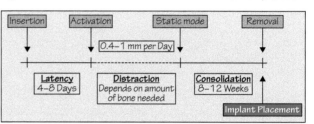

Insertion | Activation | Static mode | Removal

0.4–1 mm per Day

Latency 4–8 Days | Distraction Depends on amount of bone needed | Consolidation 8–12 Weeks

Implant Placement

Figure 53.2 Alveolar distraction technique at the mandible. (a) Osteotomy is performed. (b) The stabilising plate is fixed to the jawbone and the transport plate is secured to the transport fragment. (c) The activation key is slightly turned to ensure the mobility of the transport fragment. (d) The distractor is activated with the key by the patient or a family member. (e) The transport segment is slowly mobilised in a coronal direction. (f) A consolidation period in static mode allows calcification of the regeneration chamber. (g) The distractor is removed. (h) The implants are inserted at the same time. (i) The flap is secured around the implant neck. A two-stage procedure can be also performed

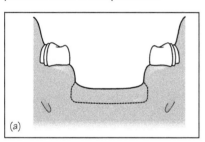

(a)

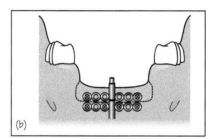

(b)

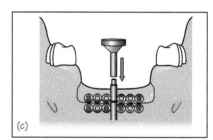

(c)

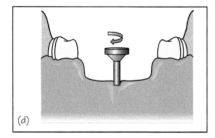

(d)

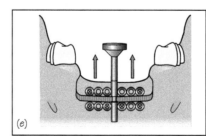

(e)

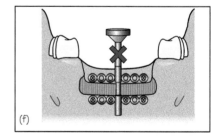

(f)

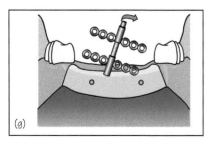

(g)

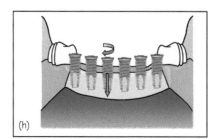

(h)

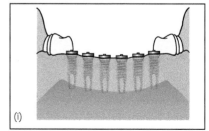

(i)

Implant Dentistry at a Glance, Second Edition. Jacques Malet, Francis Mora and Philippe Bouchard.
© 2018 John Wiley & Sons Ltd. Published 2018 by John Wiley & Sons Ltd.
Companion website: www.wiley.com/go/malet/implant

Rationale

Distraction osteogenesis involves gradual, controlled displacement of surgically created fractures, which results in simultaneous expansion of soft tissue and bone volume. The regeneration chamber created by the displacement of the bone segment is gradually filled with immature non-calcified bone that calcifies during a subsequent fixation period.

The principles of distraction osteogenesis have been adapted to implant surgery to increase alveolar bone volume (Chin, 1999).

Products and devices

Various distraction devices are commercially available (Figure 53.1). Basically, the device consists of three components (Figure 53.2):
• a threaded rod, which activates the device by turning the hexagonal head
• a transport plate, which is attached to the transport segment
• a stabilising plate, which is attached to the bone bordering the horizontal osteotomy.

Technical procedures

The segment to be distracted has to be at least 3 mm in height.
• *Buccal full-thickness flap* reflections to allow proper visualisation of the ridge during the osteotomy.
• Intimate *adaptation of the fixation plates* to the cortical bone.
• *Transient fixation of the distractor* in its planned position by self-tapping miniscrews.
• Osteotomy site scribed using a small round burr or a piezosurgery device.
• Removal of the distractor.
• *Osteotomies* using an oscillating saw or a piezosurgery device. Care is taken to ensure the cuts do not protrude beyond the lingual cortex, which is the only source of vascular supply.
• *Mobilisation of the transport segment* by placing an osteotome within the osteotomy lines.
• Final *fixation of the distractor*. Plates are secured to the bone using self-tapping microscrews. Care is taken that the threaded rod does not interfere with the occlusion.
• Transient activation of the distractor (screwing) to ensure the mobility of the transport segment and to return to its passive state (unscrewing).
• Soft tissue closure.
• *Activation of the distractor* after four to eight days. An instructed family member turns the threaded rod 0.5 mm every half day by using a wrench.
• Periapical radiographs can be used to follow the consolidation and maturation of the regeneration chamber.
• After the *consolidation period* (Figure 53.3), the distractor is removed and two-stage implants can be placed at the same time. An osseointegration period of four to six months is recommended.

Indications

Distraction osteogenesis is a technique-sensitive procedure and is only recommended for well-trained surgeons (Chen *et al.*, 2009).

Expansion occurs only in the direction of transport. Horizontal distractors have recently been proposed, but have not yet been fully evaluated. The technique performs better at the mandible than at the maxillary.

Alveolar distraction osteogenesis allows for more vertical bone augmentation than other regenerative techniques (Esposito *et al.*, 2009). Alveolar distraction procedures report a range of bone gain of 5–15 mm (Tonetti *et al.*, 2008).

This technique is more expensive than guided bone regeneration (GBR) and bone grafting, but may reduce treatment time. When horizontal augmentation is necessary at the same time, it can be combined with other techniques. These situations make the use of the alveolar distraction technique questionable, compared with GBR and onlay bone grafting that allow for a three-dimensional bone augmentation.

Contraindications

• Insufficient bone quantity to allow adequate anchorage of the plates. The use of the technique is not indicated in severely deficient mandibles, which are at risk of neural damage and/or fracture. Similarly, the presence of maxillary sinus and/or nasal cavities may be a contraindication.
• Presence of a thin knife-edge bone.
• Lack of patient cooperation during the activation process.

Nevertheless, the procedure seems well accepted by patients (Allais *et al.*, 2007).

Complications

Complications are frequent (27%), but total failure of the procedure is only reported in 1.1% of patients (Chiapasco *et al.*, 2009). Corrections with prosthetic/orthodontic appliances or further minor augmentation procedures are often needed to allow dental implant placement. Complications include the following:
• Change of the distraction vector. This is the most frequent complication, varying from 13% to 35.4% (Chiapasco *et al.*, 2009). The bone fragment may incline during the distraction phase due to the traction on the osteotomised segment by muscle forces, in particular in the anterior area of the lower jaw, where traction by the muscles of the floor of the mouth is important (Chiapasco *et al.*, 2007). Similarly, the inelastic palatal mucosa may negatively influence the distraction vector.
• Incomplete distraction.
• Premature consolidation.
• Inability to move the distracted fragment.
• Fracture of the distracting device.
• Partial relapse of the initial bone gain.
• Marginal bone loss of the most coronal part of the distracted segment is frequent and may lead to a slight overcorrection at the completion of transport.
• Transient paraesthesia at the mandible.
• Fractures of the basal bone or the distracted segment.

Key points
• Expansion occurs only in one direction (vertical or horizontal).
• The technique performs better at the mandible than at the maxilla.
• Complications after distraction are frequent.
• The advantages of the technique are lost when additional corrective procedures are needed.
• Distraction osteogenesis is only recommended for well-trained surgeons.

54 Soft tissue integration

Figure 54.1 Transmucosal implant. Note the lack of inflammation of the soft tissues surrounding the dental implant neck

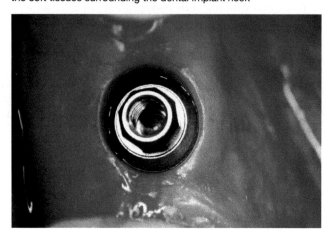

Table 54.1 Recommendations for soft tissue integration

- Use one-piece transmucosal implants
- Place the implant–abutment interface ≥1mm above the bone level (≥1 mm)
- Avoid repeated abutment disconnection with two-piece implants
- Place the abutment as soon as possible
- Avoid micromotion at the implant–abutment interface

Figure 54.2 Bone-level implant. (a) Clinical view (tooth #11). (b) Clinical view after crown removal showing the non inflammatory aspect of the soft tissues after epithelial downgrowth

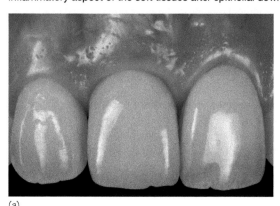

(a)

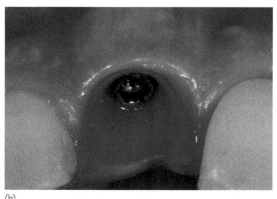

(b)

The osseointegrated portion of dental implants is protected from the oral environment by the adhesion of soft tissue to the transmucosal part of the implant (see Chapter 2). The soft tissue barrier is made of a peri-implant epithelium sealed to the implant surface via hemidesmosomes and connective tissue adhesion. This soft tissue interface is weaker than the tooth–gingiva interface because the connective tissue fibres run parallel to the implant collar, and are not inserted into the dental implant surface.

The quality and stability of the soft tissue seal around the dental implant neck promote healthy peri-implant tissue. Thus, soft tissue integration (STI), which refers to the implant–soft tissue interface, guarantees marginal bone-level stability as well as an optimal aesthetic outcome (Figures 54.1 and 54.2). Consequently, STI is now deemed fundamental to implant success, and some recommendations are suggested (Table 54.1).

Soft tissue integration evaluation

The following measurements are used in animal and clinical studies to assess STI:

- *Clinical parameters*: probing depth, gingival inflammation, plaque index, soft tissue papilla fill, soft tissue recession, keratinised mucosa
- *Radiographic parameter*: marginal bone level
- *Histological parameters*: biological width, junctional epithelial length, connective tissue characteristics.

Implant Dentistry at a Glance, Second Edition. Jacques Malet, Francis Mora and Philippe Bouchard.
© 2018 John Wiley & Sons Ltd. Published 2018 by John Wiley & Sons Ltd.
Companion website: www.wiley.com/go/malet/implant

Figure 54.3 Clinical view of two transmucosal dental implants after abutment placement. Note the excellent soft tissue integration

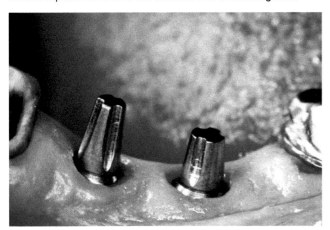

Figure 54.4 Zyrconium abutment

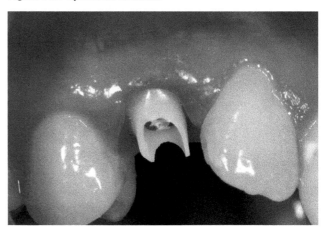

Influence of dental implant materials

Soft tissue integration depends on the characteristics of the different *materials* facing the mucosa.

Surface topography (roughness)

Most studies show that the biological width is similar for the implants with turned or moderately rough surfaces (Abrahamsson *et al.*, 2001). Changes to the topography of the transmucosal part of the implant or the abutment may have a positive impact on biological width. For instance, the junctional epithelium is shorter on transmucosal rough surfaces (Glauser *et al.*, 2005), and the use of laser microgrooved abutments generates a dense network of perpendicular collagen fibres that prevents apical migration of the epithelial barrier on a canine model (Nevins *et al.*, 2010). However, increased surface roughness may have a negative impact on the bacterial biofilm/plaque formation and on inflammation (Degidi *et al.*, 2012). In vitro studies show that smooth titanium implant surfaces provide optimum conditions for a soft tissue seal on bacterially contaminated implant surfaces (Zhao *et al.*, 2014). Consequently, a smooth (turned) surface is recommended at the transmucosal portion of the dental implant (Figures 54.1 and 54.3).

Chemical composition (biocompatibility)

The soft tissue interface is optimal with commercially pure (CP) titanium oxide, aluminium oxide and zirconium oxide abutments (Figure 54.4; Abrahamsson *et al.*, 1998). No statistical difference has been shown between titanium and zirconia abutments (Linkevicius and Vaitelis, 2015). The quality of the STI onto gold or porcelain appears to be worst than with other materials. (Abrahamsson *et al.*, 1998).

Chemical and bacterial contamination

Chemical and bacterial contamination of customised abutments during laboratory procedures modifies the surface properties. Therefore, proper cleaning procedures and sterilisation of the abutments are recommended to manaqe a biocompatible surface conducive to soft tissue adhesion prior to implant-abutment connection. Chemical agents, steaming and plasma are suggested methods for decontamination. Positive long-term outcomes have been reported with plasma argon cleaning (Canullo *et al.*, 2016). An agreed standard cleaning protocol has not yet been established. The use of standard sterile non-customised abutments may prevent contamination.

Influence of surgical techniques

Functional maturation of the soft tissue barrier is achieved 6 to 8 weeks after placement of the dental implant (Sculean *et al.*, 2014). The biological width is stable at 12 systems and surgical protocols on the dimension and quality of STI. The reader must keep in mind that the biological investigation of STI requires biopsies. Consequently, most of the outcomes discussed below are based on animal studies. Hence the results of the studies must be carefully interpreted on a clinical standpoint.

One-piece vs two-piece implants

Animal studies have shown that one-piece (transmucosal) implants and two-piece (bone-level) implants have a similar biological width (Berglundh *et al.*, 1991). In dogs, when two-piece implants are placed on a healed ridge, the biological width is around 4 mm corresponding to 60% junctional epithelium, and 40% connective tissue (Berglundh *et al.*, 2007). One study shows a longer junctional epithelium for submerged implants compared to intentionally non-submerged implants (Weber *et al.*, 1996). Irrespective of the surgical protocol (submerged or non-submerged), the gingival margin is located more coronally for one-piece implants than for two-piece implants (Hermann *et al.*, 2001; Pontes *et al.*, 2008).

Immediate implants vs implants on healed sites

The epithelium dimension seems longer (±3 mm) with immediate implants than with implants placed in healed sites, regardless of the implant system used (de Sanctis *et al.*, 2009; Vignoletti *et al.*, 2009).

Flapless vs flap surgery

After flapless surgery on a healed site, the epithelium dimension is smaller than with a conventional procedure using a traditional flap access (You *et al.*, 2009).

Immediate loading vs delayed loading

Soft tissue dimensions are comparable for dental implants placed into fresh extraction sockets or on healed sites, regardless of whether or not immediate restorations are placed (Blanco *et al.*, 2012; Glauser *et al.*, 2006).

Influence of abutment connection

An inflammatory cell infiltrate is described with two-piece implant systems between the implant neck and the abutment. In the event of STI disruption, the extension of this infiltrate after bacterial contamination could be detrimental by increasing marginal bone remodelling (Tallarico *et al.*, 2017).

Key points

- Soft tissue integration is one of the pivotal features required for long term dental implant success.
- A smooth surface is recommended at the transmucosal portion of the dental implant.
- There is little evidence in humans to indicate that a specific surgical techniques modify soft tissue integration.

55 Soft tissue augmentation

Figure 55.1 Connective tissue graft. Thin biotype. (a) The deciduous tooth must be replaced by a dental implant. Note the thin biotype. (b) A connective tissue graft is performed during implant surgery, to thicken the buccal mucosa. (c) Clinical view after six years

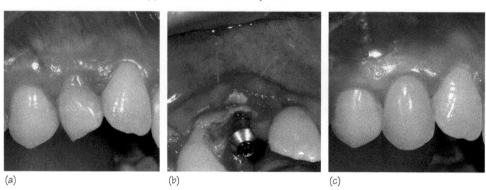

(a)   (b)   (c)

Figure 55.2 Soft tissue ridge augmentation. (a) Horizontal and vertical defect. A three-unit bridge supported by two dental implants (teeth 12 and 14) is planned. (b) A connective tissue graft increases the soft tissue volume in the area of ridge defect to improve the shape of the pontic (tooth 13). (c) Clinical view after five years showing the aesthetic improvement due to the soft tissue augmentation

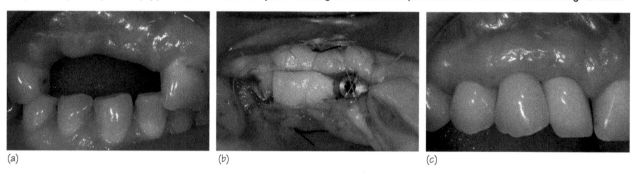

(a)   (b)   (c)

Figure 55.3 Peri-implant soft tissue recession coverage. (a) Peri-implant soft tissue recession. (b) Connective tissue graft before suturing. (c) Sutures (tunnel technique). (d) Clinical view after one year showing aesthetic improvement

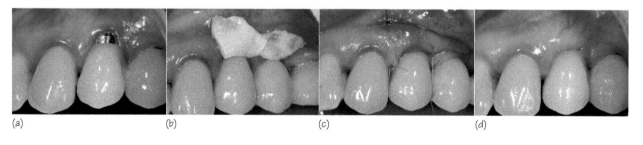

(a)   (b)   (c)   (d)

Rationale

Peri-implant soft tissues differ from periodontal tissues in terms of structure (more collagen fibres in a parallel arrangement) and defence capacity (fewer cells; see Chapter 3). The role of soft tissue in implant success is still questionable.

Although the presence of keratinised tissue is not essential for peri-implant tissue health and implant survival (Wennstrom *et al.*, 1994), it can certainly facilitate plaque control, which is a crucial prerequisite for long-term implant success. Moreover, soft tissue quality and quantity around implants can have implications for aesthetic results and soft tissue margin stability.

Implant Dentistry at a Glance, Second Edition. Jacques Malet, Francis Mora and Philippe Bouchard.
© 2018 John Wiley & Sons Ltd. Published 2018 by John Wiley & Sons Ltd.
Companion website: www.wiley.com/go/malet/implant

Table 55.1 Guidelines for soft tissue augmentation procedures

	Aesthetic	Keratinised augmentation	Volume augmentation	Morbidity
Apically positioned flap	Moderate	Moderate	Low	Low
Rotational flap	High	Moderate	Low	Low
Free gingival graft	Low	**High**	Moderate	**High**
Allogenic graft	Moderate	Moderate	Moderate	Low
Subepithelial connective tissue graft	**High**	Low	**High**	Moderate

Soft tissue augmentation techniques aim to create an optimum soft tissue environment around implants, in order to improve implant prognosis and/or prosthetic cosmetic integration.

However, it should be noted that the recommendations that follow are essentially based on clinicians' opinions, as scientific data regarding indications or technique selection (Klinge and Flemmig, 2009) are very limited in the literature.

Although soft tissue grafts may improve soft tissue thickness and aesthetics (Esposito *et al.*, 2012), the scientific evidence on the marginal stability of the peri-implant mucosa over time is poor (Rotundo *et al.*, 2015). Similarly, the impact of soft tissue augmentation on peri-implant bone level needs to be confirmed.

Indications

The indications for soft tissue augmentation procedures can be divided into three groups.

Keratinised tissue augmentation

This is required when:
• a *reduced keratinised tissue* height (less than 2 mm) or width (less than 1 mm) is associated with insufficient plaque control
• a *shallow vestibule* prevents access to oral hygiene originally or after tissue displacement (bone regenerative procedures)
• soft tissue quantity is too small to assure covering of augmented bone areas.

Soft tissue volume augmentation

This is performed in the following situations:
• a *thin biotype* when long-term soft tissue margin stability is required (aesthetic)
• *ridge defect* correction to improve pontic design for aesthetic or plaque control (Seibert and Salama, 1996)
• primary *soft tissue closure* on fresh extraction socket for ridge preservation (see Chapter 39, Figure 39.1) or covering of guided bone regeneration (GBR) material (Jung *et al.*, 2004).

The decision to perform a soft tissue augmentation is based on *risk assessment* (implant survival or aesthetics) and the *morbidity* of the surgery. These two parameters should be evaluated at the beginning of the treatment, as additional surgery is not always well received by the patient.

Soft tissue recession at implants

There are limited data showing aesthetic improvement or plaque control following subepithelial connective tissue graft in shallow peri-implant soft tissue recessions (Sculean *et al.*, 2017; Figure 55.3).

Technical procedures

All the techniques described here (see also Table 55.1) are derived from periodontal plastic surgery (Bouchard *et al.*, 2001).

Technique selection depends on the quantity of residual keratinised mucosa and the type of indication. The first choice is the least invasive one (low morbidity).

Apically positioned flap (APF) is a simple technique that can be applied during implant placement or at second-stage surgery. The initial incision is displaced on the lingual/palatal side to manage a band of keratinised tissue on the vestibule. It is the technique of choice for non-aesthetic areas. APF is performed when the keratinised mucosa quantity is limited, at the time of implant placement (one-stage implant) or at second-stage surgery.

Rotational flap (RF) techniques have been developed to augment soft tissue volume for aesthetics (small defects; Scharf and Tarnow, 1992) or to allow adequate closure after GBR procedures. Tissue manipulation can be delicate and requires sufficient skill. The presence of a pedicle allows good vascular nutrition of the displaced tissue.

Free gingival graft (FGG) allows a better keratinised tissue augmentation than all other procedures (Thoma *et al.*, 2009). The aesthetic result is generally bad, therefore this technique is not recommended in aesthetic areas.

Allogenic graft, freeze-dried skin allograft or acellular dermal matrix graft, could be an alternative to free gingival graft for tissue stabilisation, with less morbidity. Clinical documentation is limited.

Subepithelial connective tissue graft (SECTG) is the technique of choice when soft tissue volume augmentation is required (Thoma *et al.*, 2009), especially in aesthetic areas: thin biotype (Figure 55.1), extraction socket closure or ridge defects (Figure 55.2). As for FGG, quantity is limited by anatomical parameters (donor site).

Timing for soft tissue augmentation

From a clinical point of view, evaluation of peri-implant mucosa should be done at each treatment step. The global approach is to prevent soft tissue loss and to limit the number of surgeries.

Two-stage implants

Decision making for soft tissue augmentation can be performed at second-stage surgery (except for aesthetic cases).

One-stage implants

Soft tissue quality has to be adequate at the time of implant placement. In compromised cases, a soft tissue augmentation must be performed six weeks before implant placement.

Bone augmentation areas

A good soft tissue environment is required for GBR and bone graft procedures. In cases of limited keratinised tissue, soft tissue augmentation can be performed six weeks before bone surgery, to improve soft tissue manipulation and site covering.

However, the vascular supply can be decreased (scar tissue) by this first surgery, which is thus indicated only for compromised cases.

Demanding aesthetic cases

As several soft tissue augmentations could be indicated, they should be performed as soon as possible: at the time of tooth extraction (FGG, SECTG), at the time of implant placement (RF, SECTG) or at second-stage surgery (RF, SECTG).

Key points

- Keratinised mucosa around implants is not a prerequisite for the survival of dental implants, but may improve plaque control and aesthetics in some situations.
- The flap design should preserve the keratinised tissues around the implants.
- In an aesthetic area, subepithelial connective tissue graft (SECTG) is the gold standard.

56 Prescriptions in standard procedure

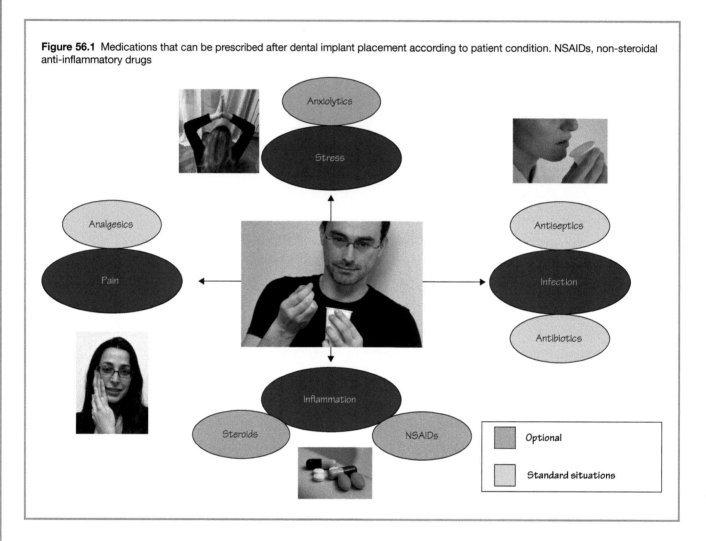

Figure 56.1 Medications that can be prescribed after dental implant placement according to patient condition. NSAIDs, non-steroidal anti-inflammatory drugs

In ordinary conditions – when the patient is not medically compromised, and dental implant placement does not imply bone augmentation procedures and/or sinus penetration – dental implant placement is at low risk of postoperative infection and is not painful. A standard pharmacological protocol is hard to define after dental implant placement, not only because the guidelines are different from country to country, but also because many general and local variables need to be considered. Basically, all preoperative and postoperative prescriptions aim to reduce surgical discomfort and the risk of infection.

The following medications must be considered after dental implant placement in ordinary conditions (Figure 56.1):
- anxiolytic premedication
- local antiseptics
- systemic antibiotics
- analgesics
- non-steroidal anti-inflammatory drugs (NSAIDs)
- steroids.

The prescription of these drugs should always take into account the possibility of an allergy to prescribed medicines.

Anxiolytic premedication

Anxiolytic premedication may prevent an increase of preoperative anxiety levels and may reduce pain levels during dental implant placement, but it is often associated with moderate/severe drowsiness in the postoperative period. Many types of anxiolytics, including certain herbs, are available. *There is no specific indication for this type of premedication* in ordinary conditions, unless the psychological profile of the patient suggests their use.

Local antiseptics

There is no evidence that use of a mouth rinse will prevent the risk of infective complications after dental implant placement. However, the use of 0.2% chlorhexidine gluconate alone (not in combination with alcohol) is still a reference for mouth rinse

Implant Dentistry at a Glance, Second Edition. Jacques Malet, Francis Mora and Philippe Bouchard.
© 2018 John Wiley & Sons Ltd. Published 2018 by John Wiley & Sons Ltd.
Companion website: www.wiley.com/go/malet/implant

before and after dental implant placement. A three-minute pre-surgical rinse reduces the bacterial load (good level of evidence). A postsurgical rinse twice daily for two weeks is effective in preventing bacterial colonisation of the wound (low level of evidence).

Systemic antibiotics

Antibiotic prophylaxis in surgery is only indicated for patients at risk of infectious endocarditis, for patients with reduced host response, when surgery is performed in infected sites, in cases of extensive and prolonged surgical interventions, and when large foreign bodies are implanted. Thus, the use of prophylactic antibiotics in dental implant surgery has been controversial so far. However, recent data indicate that there is some evidence that 2 g or 3 g of amoxicillin given orally one hour preoperatively significantly reduces failures of dental implants placed in ordinary conditions, with no significant adverse events reported (Esposito *et al.*, 2013). It is still unclear whether postoperative antibiotics are of any additional benefit, and which antibiotic is the most effective to avoid the risk of postoperative infection.

Analgesics

The severity and response to other medication determine the choice of agent.

Paracetamol (synonym: acetaminophen)

Paracetamol is a safe, effective drug for the treatment of postoperative pain following implant placement. It is one of the most commonly used over-the-counter analgesics and is widely available around the world. It is most effective at 1000 mg dose, and can be taken at six-hourly intervals without compromising safety. To maintain freedom from pain, drugs should be given 'by the clock' – that is, every six hours – rather than 'on demand'. Thus,

in ordinary conditions, a 1000 mg dose four times daily for three to four days is sufficient for postoperative pain control in dental implant surgeries.

Opiates and morphinomimetics

These drugs are rarely used to control pain and discomfort after dental implant therapy.

Non-steroidal anti-inflammatory drugs (NSAIDs)

Aspirin and other NSAIDs are not indicated after surgery, because they have more side-effects than paracetamol and increase the risk of haemorrhage.

Steroids

There is no reason for the use of corticosteroids when dental implants are placed in ordinary conditions. They may cause a range of side-effects, including the risk of bleeding and infection. However, corticosteroids may also relieve inflammation, pain and discomfort after advanced dental implant surgeries, such as alveolar ridge augmentation or sinus procedures. These drugs should be reserved for these specific indications in combination with the use of antibiotics.

Key points

Provided that a possible allergy is proven by the medical questionnaire, in ordinary conditions the prescription should include the following:
- amoxicillin 1000 mg: 2 tablets 1 hour before the surgery
- paracetamol 1000 mg: 1 tablet every 6 hours for 4 days
- chlorhexidine 0.2% mouth rinse: rinse twice daily for 2 weeks.

57 Postoperative management

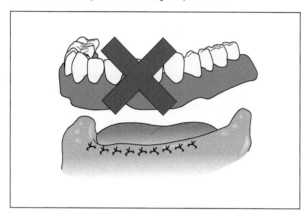

Figure 57.1 Patients are not allowed to wear a removable denture for 10 days after the surgical procedure

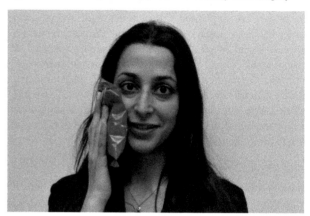

Figure 57.2 An ice pack is applied immediately after surgery

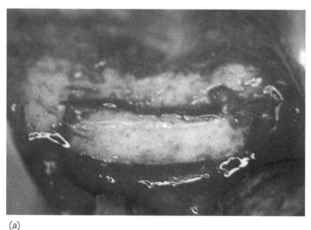

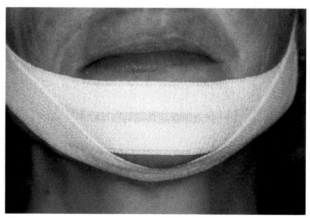

Figure 57.3 Advanced surgical procedures: specific postoperative management. (a) Chin bone harvesting. (b) Elastic tapes are used to provide pressure to the chin

(a)

(b)

Patients are instructed to contact the doctor's office immediately if they are concerned about any abnormalities. If a postoperative complication occurs, it must be managed as soon as possible (see Chapters 58–60). Postoperative instructions must be provided to the patient *before* the surgical procedure, with the informed consent form. Written forms are convenient and can be customised by the surgeon (see Appendices E and H).

Whatever the procedure, patients are asked not to wear a removable denture for 10 days postoperatively if there is a risk of hard pressure on the wound (Figure 57.1). Provisional fixed partial dentures (FPDs) can be inserted immediately. Care is taken to avoid pressure from the provisional restoration on the wound.

Standard procedure

The postoperative considerations are similar to those applied for most oral surgeries; that is, the postoperative course is often minimal. Recuperation normally takes one to five days after implant placement, depending on patient condition and patient compliance with prescription. Sutures are optimally removed ten days after the surgical procedure. Standard hygiene procedures can be reintroduced. The denture is carefully relined with a soft material after primary healing of the wound (at least ten days).

Cold therapy is beneficial to reduce bleeding, swelling and muscle spasm, and to decrease metabolic rate (Figure 57.2).

Implant Dentistry at a Glance, Second Edition. Jacques Malet, Francis Mora and Philippe Bouchard.
© 2018 John Wiley & Sons Ltd. Published 2018 by John Wiley & Sons Ltd.
Companion website: www.wiley.com/go/malet/implant

Instant ice packs, activated by squeezing the pack with both hands, are convenient.

Pressure at the surgical site, elevation of the head and rest are recommended. The patient is advised to stop smoking and to discontinue any physical activity that may lead to bleeding or suture disruption, or interfere with wound healing.

Tooth brushing should be continued, except on the surgical site. Chlorhexidine mouth rinses should be used (twice daily for two weeks) to reduce the risk of infection at the surgical site. Chlorhexidine gel applications (three per day) may also be helpful.

Advanced procedures

The postoperative management of advanced procedures is similar to the standard procedure. However, in advanced procedures prescriptions differ from those of standard implant placement procedures. Antibiotics are prescribed for a minimum of seven days. Non-steroidal anti-inflammatory drugs (NSAIDs) or corticosteroids may be used to reduce the inflammatory process. Pain is controlled with appropriate analgesics, including opiates and morphinomimetics if necessary. Depending on the surgical procedure employed, specific advice can be given.

Chin bone harvesting

A pressure dressing should be applied to the chin for five days to minimise swelling and haematoma formation, and to ensure close adaptation of the mentalis muscles (Figure 57.3). Elastic tapes are normally used to provide pressure to the chin region. Postoperative pain at the donor site is usually minimal to moderate and can be controlled by regular analgesics.

Ramus harvesting

The postoperative course is reduced, compared to chin bone harvesting, and complications are less frequent.

Sinus procedures

Postoperative considerations for the maxillary sinus grafting procedure are similar to those for most oral surgery and sinus manipulation procedures. Swelling and bruising are the chief postoperative sequelae. Occasionally, minor bleeding may arise from the nose. Recuperation normally takes one to two weeks.

Blowing the nose and sucking liquid through a straw create negative pressure and should be avoided for at least two weeks after a sinus grafting procedure. Coughing or sneezing should be done with an open mouth to relieve pressure. Decongestants can be prescribed to minimise sneezing. A nasal spray may be used on an as-needed basis for nasal congestion. Air travel and sports such as scuba diving must be absolutely avoided during the first two weeks after sinus procedures.

Key points

- Postoperative instructions must be provided to the patient *before* the surgical procedure.
- The postoperative considerations are similar to those applied for most oral surgeries.
- Cold therapy is efficient.
- Advanced surgical procedures require special attention.

58 Surgical complications: Local complications

Figure 58.1 Bone dehiscence management. (a) Bone dehiscence (white arrow) and bone fenestration (black arrow) at the end of implant drilling. (b) A graft material (BioOss®) is placed after the implants. (c) A guided bone regeneration membrane (Osseoguard®) is stabilised with resorbable sutures. (d) Tension-free flap closure

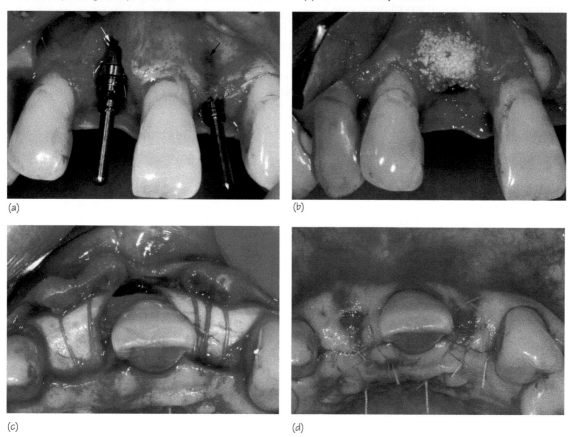

(a)

(b)

(c)

(d)

Figure 58.2 Implant placed a few millimetres into the sinus cavity (red arrow). Radiography at five years. In this case, no clinical signs were reported

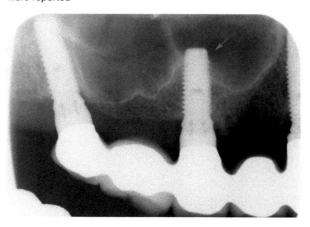

Implant Dentistry at a Glance, Second Edition. Jacques Malet, Francis Mora and Philippe Bouchard.
© 2018 John Wiley & Sons Ltd. Published 2018 by John Wiley & Sons Ltd.
Companion website: www.wiley.com/go/malet/implant

Figure 58.3 Wound dehiscence. (a) Clinical view one week after surgery. Note the wound opening with exposure of underlying tissues. (b) Clinical view three weeks after surgery and after two weeks of topical application of chlorhexidine. Note second-intention healing

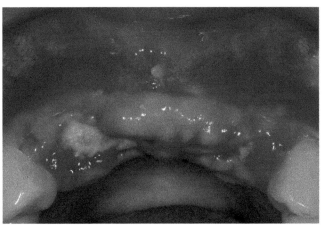

(a)

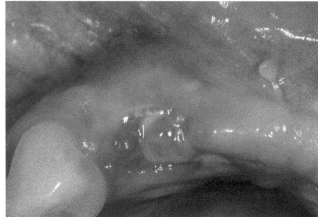

(b)

Box 58.1 General factors that may prevent surgical complications

Thorough medical and oral examination
Preoperative imaging
• CT scan
Thorough presurgical planning
• Knowledge of the anatomy
• Adequate dental implant size, shape and dimensions
Training of surgical staff
• Knowledge of standards of behaviour and aseptic techniques
• Knowledge of the surgical procedure
• Experience in rare surgical procedures and emergency situations
Environment
• Aseptic environment
• Working knowledge of the use and function of all operating theatre equipment
Surgical procedure
• Atraumatic and planned surgical procedures
  • Incisions in keratinised tissues
  • Limited extent of flap reflection
  • No high vertical releasing incisions
  • Deep sutures and flap adaptation
  • Safety margin of 2 mm between the implant body and any nerve canal
• Duration of intervention: no more than 2.5 hours (local anaesthesia)
• Strict postsurgical follow-up

Box 58.2 Factors that may negatively influence primary stability

Overworking of the implant bed
Prevention
• Sequential and controlled drilling
• Use of osteotomes in conjunction with drilling

Poor bone quality (class IV)
Prevention
• Use of imaging (CT scan) to determine regional bone quality
• Use of self-tapping implants dedicated to poor bone quality
• Undersized bed preparation

Implant placement in fresh extraction sockets
Prevention – see Chapter 41

Surgical complications can occur perioperatively (during the surgical procedure) and/or postoperatively (following the surgical procedure). They are uncommon and can be minimised or prevented in most cases (Box 58.1).

Perioperative complications
Dental implant mobility

When primary stability is lacking i.e. when there is a horizontal mobility (Box 58.2), the dental implant must be removed and the surgical placement postponed by at least two months. When the hard and soft tissue environment is optimal, the compromised implant may be replaced by a wider and/or longer self-tapping implant. When primary stability is questionable (ongoing rotation after final tightening), dental implants with rough surfaces can be kept. In this case, the *healing period must be extended.*

Bone dehiscence and fenestration

This may occur during surgery when the implant axis is tilted and inadequately positioned between the cortical plates (facial malposition). Small defects do not jeopardise implant prognosis. However, when combined with a thin soft tissue biotype, there is a risk of *postoperative recession* of the facial mucosal margin (Chen *et al.*, 2009). A conventional grafting approach may be used to fill the bone defect (Figure 58.1).

Maxillary sinus or nasal fossa penetration

Violation of the maxillary or nasal floor while drilling warrants antibiotic therapy. Dental implants inadvertently placed a few millimetres into the sinus or nasal cavities are normally well tolerated (Branemark *et al.*, 1984; Figure 58.2).

Postoperative complications
Wound dehiscence

This is the most common postoperative complication for submerged implants (Giglio *et al.*, 1998; Figure 58.3). It can be prevented during surgery by tension-free coaptation of the flaps.

After surgery, the best prevention is to avoid any trauma to the wound, in particular with dentures that must be carefully relined after primary wound healing (at least 10 days). Such dehiscence is often managed by topical application or rinsing with chlorhexidine. If the follow-up indicates a risk of infection, an antibiotic regimen and/or resuturing may be considered.

Key points

- Surgical complications are infrequent.
- Most local complications can be managed and do not jeopardise dental implant prognosis.
- Most surgical complications can be prevented.

59

Surgical complications: Rare and regional complications

Figure 59.1 Haematoma with skin discoloration

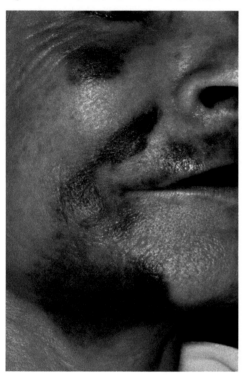

Figure 59.3 Displacement of an implant into the posterior region of the maxillary sinus cavity (red arrow)

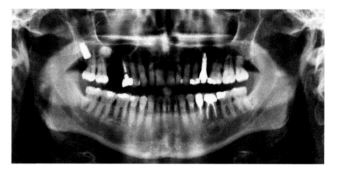

Ecchymosis and haematoma

These complications are not infrequent and affect approximately 24% of surgical sites (Goodacre *et al.*, 2003). They can be reduced with careful soft tissue management and by avoiding high vertical-releasing incisions. Skin discoloration usually appears after one to two days and disappears in two to three weeks (Figure 59.1).

Neurosensory dysfunctions

Anaesthesia, hypoaesthesia, hyperaesthesia, paraesthesia or dysaesthesia may occur after placement of dental implants (Figure 59.2). These changes in sensation following implant surgery considerably lower patient satisfaction and must be managed (Box 59.1). These dysfunctions are the consequences of transient or permanent injury to the branches of the mandibular nerve, which include the following.

Lingual nerve

This can be damaged by careless elevation of lingual flaps, excessive flap reflection or the use of lingual vertical-releasing incisions.

Inferior alveolar nerve

This may be permanently damaged if the mandibular canal is violated. If the apical part of the dental implant is too close to the mandibular canal, subsequent pressure caused by the apical haematoma may induce reversible neurosensory dysfunction (Figure 59.2). Meta-analyses have highlighted a short-term incidence of 13% in altered sensations (ten days after implant placement; Lin *et al.*, 2016). However, an incidence of only 3% is evident one year after surgery. Candidates for mandibular implant surgery must be informed of the risk of transient altered sensation.

The high prevalence of neurosensory disturbance following inferior alveolar nerve repositioning for dental implant placement should be noted (Vetromilla *et al.*, 2014).

Mental nerve

Damage may induce neurosensory alterations in the chin and lower lip. The best way to prevent injury of the mental nerve is to display the mental foramen and visualise the nerve.

Implant Dentistry at a Glance, Second Edition. Jacques Malet, Francis Mora and Philippe Bouchard.
© 2018 John Wiley & Sons Ltd. Published 2018 by John Wiley & Sons Ltd.
Companion website: www.wiley.com/go/malet/implant

Figure 59.2 Clinical management of inferior alveolar nerve injury. (a) Implant 34 is too close to the mental foramen, leading to paraesthesia. (b) The implant is removed. (c) A shorter implant is placed three months later. At this stage, paraesthesia has decreased but persists. (d) Five years later, the paraesthesia persists (area outlined in blue on the skin)

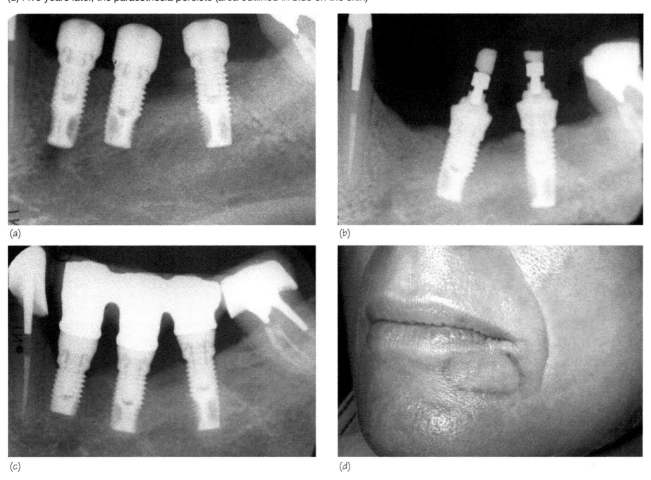

(a) (b) (c) (d)

Rare complications

Nowadays, most of these can be easily avoided.

Mandibular fractures

This infrequent perioperative or postoperative complication has been described. Dental implant placement in an atrophic mandible must be atraumatic and requires a minimum bone volume at least 7 mm high by 6 mm wide (Park and Wang, 2005).

Damage to the adjacent teeth

This surgical error can be easily avoided by respecting the parallelism of the dental implant with the neighbouring tooth.

Drill fracture within the implant bed

Disposable drills must be used to avoid this problem. In such cases, the broken instrument must be removed using a surgical trepan with a wider diameter.

Displacement of the implant into the maxillary sinus cavity

This can happen accidentally during surgery or in the postoperative period. In either case, the implant must be removed by creating a window into the sinus. The major problem is localisation of the dental implant within the sinus cavity. An endoscope can be used to pinpoint the dental implant. However, such a device is rarely available in a dentist's operating room. We recommend placing the patient in a seated position to prevent the implant from passing into the posterior section of the sinus (Figure 59.3). The surgical suction tip should then be used to explore the sinus in order to grasp the end of the dental implant and extract it from the sinus cavity.

Chronic postsurgical pain

Persistent orofacial pain has very occasionally been reported after dental implant placement (Devine *et al.*, 2016). It may occur with no apparent organic cause and without any neurosensory deficits, particularly in patients with a significant medical history.

Key points

- Ecchymosis and haematoma are the most frequent regional complications.
- Some surgical complications are rare and can be easily prevented.

60 Life-threatening surgical complications

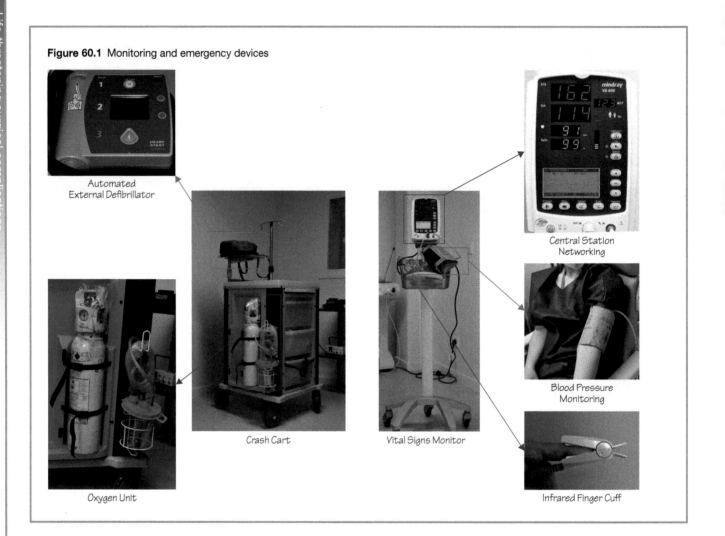

Figure 60.1 Monitoring and emergency devices

Automated External Defibrillator

Crash Cart

Vital Signs Monitor

Oxygen Unit

Central Station Networking

Blood Pressure Monitoring

Infrared Finger Cuff

Life-threatening complications are, fortunately, extremely rare. In any case, the surgeon must have the phone number of the closest emergency medical centre. The operating room (OR) should be equipped with monitoring and emergency devices (Figure 60.1). An automated external defibrillator (AED) and an oxygen unit should be located in the dental setting or in the operating room.

A vital signs monitor that can measure blood pressure, pulse rate and blood oxygen saturation is recommended in the OR. A crash cart containing the tools and drugs needed to treat a person in or near cardiac arrest should be located close to the OR. However, the emergency training of the operator may not be sufficient for adequate use of the drugs included in the crash cart.

The most serious complications occur during surgery and may be life-threatening (Box 60.1).

Haemorrhages

Haemorrhages during dental implant surgery are normally limited to class I; that is, blood loss does not involve more than 15% of the blood volume and does not require fluid resuscitation (Manning, 2004). Thus, bleeding is usually controlled locally (Box 60.2). Haemorrhages occur most frequently at the mandible in the interforaminal region (Hofschneider *et al.*, 1999).

Excessive bleeding of the implant bed is usually stopped by inserting the implant.

Blood supply to the mandibular lingual surface is provided by two arteries, with anastomoses between them (see Chapter 4). These arteries give off branches that penetrate into the bone and can be damaged during drilling.

• The *sublingual artery* is responsible for bleeding in the anterior, lingual region. It can be severed and may then retract into

Implant Dentistry at a Glance, Second Edition. Jacques Malet, Francis Mora and Philippe Bouchard.
© 2018 John Wiley & Sons Ltd. Published 2018 by John Wiley & Sons Ltd.
Companion website: www.wiley.com/go/malet/implant

Box 60.1 Life-threatening complications

Airway obstruction by haemorrhage

Damage to the mandibular lingual cortical plate is usually described in association with haemorrhagic accidents during dental implant placement. There is much anatomical variation in this area, making identification of a bleeding artery difficult.

Floor-of-the-mouth bleeding can lead to respiratory obstruction (a life-threatening complication). Massive internal haemorrhage of the floor of the mouth results in a dramatic swelling that produces protrusion and displacement of the tongue, obstructing the airways. This dramatic complication may occur several hours after the surgical procedure (ten Bruggenkate *et al.*, 1993)

If the symptoms persist, call for emergency help.

Airway obstruction by foreign body aspiration

Aspiration of an instrument or a dental implant may be a life-threatening complication. An acute episode of coughing is the most common but inconstant sign. Acute choking, with respiratory failure associated with tracheal or laryngeal foreign body obstruction, may be successfully treated at the scene with the Heimlich manoeuvre.

Figure 60.2 The Heimlich manoeuvre

Heimlich Maneuver

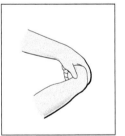

1. Lean the person forward slightly and stand behind him or her.

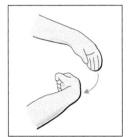

2. Make a fist with one hand.

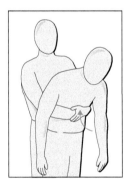

3. Put your arms around the person and grasp your fist with your other hand near the top of the stomach, just below the center of the rib cage.

4. Make a quick, hard movement inward and upward.

Box 60.2 Management of vascular complications

1 Compression
2 Infiltration of vasoconstrictor
Local anaesthetic injection directly in the bleeding site (soft tissues and/or bone canal)
3 Local haemostatic agents
Glue, sponge, powder, dressing, mesh
4 Bone wax
Intraosseous bleeding
5 Electrocoagulation
6 Vessel ligation

If bleeding persists, call for emergency help.

In fact, the arteries themselves are not often damaged during implant placement, but the intraosseous branches are more liable to be damaged.

Foreign body ingestion/aspiration

Ingestion of a direction indicator or a dental implant is normally not a major complication. The object can pass through naturally. In contrast, aspiration of an instrument can be a life-threatening complication. Staff should be familiar with the Heimlich manoeuvre (Figure 60.2).

Even without any symptoms, a patient who has swallowed a foreign body must be referred for evaluation to a physician specialist.

When using a screwdriver or a direction indicator, a suture can be tied to the instrument to prevent accidents. Intraoral gauze can also be used like a net during surgery to more easily retrieve an object accidentally dropped in the mouth.

the sublingual space. Even though the sublingual artery may be small, the anastomoses may create a copious blood flow.

• The *submental artery* is responsible for bleeding in the medial, lingual region. Usually larger than the sublingual artery, this artery can produce much more blood flow than the sublingual artery. It may be controlled by strong finger pressure in the inferior medial mandibular border.

Key points

• Some surgical complications can be life-threatening.
• An emergency medical centre near the operating room is mandatory.

61 Peri-implant diseases: Diagnosis

Figure 61.1 Radiographic interpretation of bone loss around dental implants

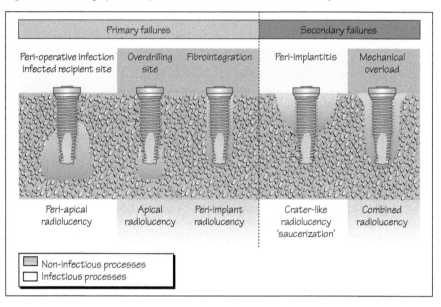

Figure 61.2 Peri-implant mucositis. (a) Clinical view (implant no. 12). Note the redness of the marginal mucosa, which reflects the inflammatory process. (b) Radiographic control. Note the absence of marginal bone loss

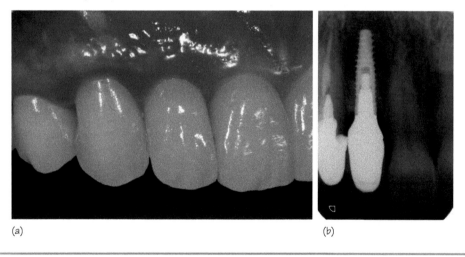

(a)　　　　　　　　　　(b)

Peri-implant diseases are inflammatory processes of the tissues surrounding a dental implant (Albrektsson and Isidor, 1994). Animal studies have shown that excessive mechanical load does not result per se in marginal bone loss in the presence of healthy peri-implant mucosal tissues (Heitz-Mayfield *et al.*, 2004), but can rather lead to loss of osseointegration (Isidor, 1996, 1997). In contrast, in the absence of mechanical stress, dental plaque accumulation may lead to marginal peri-implant bone loss and ultimately to dental implant loss. The pathological process may also be initiated by various factors (Box 61.1). Thus, plaque-induced peri-implant diseases can develop and should be prevented.

Diagnostic parameters

Systematic monitoring of peri-implant tissues is recommended over time (Lang *et al.*, 2004). Clinical parameters recommended in expert consensus reports (Meyle, 2008; Lang and Berglundh,

Implant Dentistry at a Glance, Second Edition. Jacques Malet, Francis Mora and Philippe Bouchard.
© 2018 John Wiley & Sons Ltd. Published 2018 by John Wiley & Sons Ltd.
Companion website: www.wiley.com/go/malet/implant

Figure 61.3 Peri-implantitis on a dental implant replacing tooth #46. (a) Postoperative radiograph 12 months after loading. Note the lack of marginal bone loss. (b) Clinical view after two years. Peri-implantitis has occurred, which is diagnosed by a thorough clinical examination. This examination includes peri-implant probing and radiographic control. Note the suppuration after probing (arrow). (c) Corresponding radiograph showing a typical saucerisation of the bone surrounding the dental implant neck

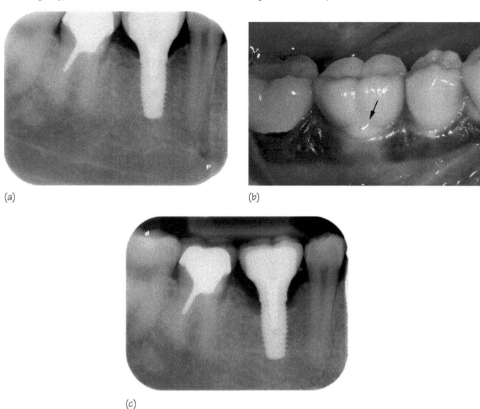

(a)

(b)

(c)

Box 61.1 Factors associated with dental implant failure (ranking according to the level of evidence)

- Plaque accumulation
- History of periodontitis
- Smoking
- Excess cement
- Lack of maintenance
- Genetic polymorphisms (IL-1RN, OPG, IL-6, RANKL, CD14, TNFα)
- Diabetes
- History of dental implant failure
- Lack of keratinised tissue

Box 61.2 Clinical parameters recorded at baseline evaluation and routinely used to longitudinally assess peri-implant conditions

- Plaque assessment
- Soft tissue conditions
  - Bleeding on probing (dichotomic measurement)
  - Suppuration
- Probing depth
  - Light forces (0.2–0.25 N)
- Radiographic evaluation
  - Long-cone paralleling technique
  - At one-year follow-up, then adapted to individual clinical assessment
- Implant mobility

2011; Academy Report, 2013) can be easily used to assess peri-implant conditions (Box 61.2). Follow-up measurements must be compared to baseline values at the time of prosthesis placement (end-of-treatment appraisal).

Bleeding on probing has been suggested as an indicator of soft tissue inflammation. It is considered a key clinical parameter for distinguishing between peri-implant health and disease (Jepsen *et al.*, 2015). Based on a narrative review, authors indicate that there is limited clinical evidence to support this hypothesis (Coli *et al.*, 2017). Indeed, from a histological perspective, the tip of the probe can easily penetrate the connective tissue due to the parallel direction of the fibres, leading to false positive values. However, it may be assumed that the absence of bleeding has a positive predictive value associated with the absence of soft tissue inflammation. Consequently, this clinical parameter must be recorded over time and compared against baseline values.

Peri-implant probing depth, under healthy conditions, should be less than 4 mm. However, deeper baseline values may be found, specifically in areas where soft tissue augmentations have been required for aesthetic reasons. Thus, the absolute value of the peri-implant probing depth appears to be of little importance in identifying dental implants at risk of failure. This is in contrast with the periodontal probing depth, which is a reliable indicator of periodontal conditions. The relative value of the peri-implant probing depth – that is, changes in probing depth over time – seems more relevant when detecting continuous bone loss, even if the level of evidence is low. This assertion is mostly based on animal studies (Lang *et al.*, 1993; Schou *et al.*, 1993a, b) and on the principal assumption that the tip of the probe for constant pressure (0.2–0.25 N) is always located at the same distance from the peri-implant bone crest, regardless of the inflammatory status.

The major problem associated with the monitoring of peri-implant probing depth over time is the lack of fixed reference point, like the cemento-enamel junction when probing around teeth. Regardless of the authors' opinions that challenge the use of the peri-implant probing depth to assess the peri-implant condition (Coli *et al.*, 2017), it makes sense to follow expert consensus recommendations that advocate peri-implant probing for dental implant monitoring. Further studies are required in order to establish the predictive value of peri-implant probing in assessing the progression of peri-implant diseases.

X-rays are essential (i) to verify the lack of complications during the bone healing process; (ii) to gain a better understanding of the reasons for the pathological condition; and (iii) for follow-up of the peri-implant bone level. Radiographic interpretation of the failures may be convenient in clinical practice (Figure 61.1). There is no evidence of specific scheduling for radiographic monitoring. However, the link between bleeding on probing (BOP) and increased pocket depth (PD) at a probing site, over time, indicates that X-rays are mandatory.

Dental implant mobility indicates the loss of osseointegration and consequently has no predictive value. There is no treatment for implant mobility except explantation.

Other parameters, such as analysis of peri-implant sulcus fluid, microbiological evaluation of the peri-implant pocket or evaluation of implant stability by resonance frequency analysis, are currently of limited assistance in routine practice.

Peri-implant mucositis

Peri-implant mucositis is a reversible inflammatory process in the soft tissues surrounding a functioning dental implant (Berglundh *et al.*, 2008). The clinical characteristics are similar to those of gingivitis (Figure 61.2). If left untreated, this may lead to peri-implantitis (Mombelli, 1999). BOP, as a surrogate variable for peri-implant mucositis, seems highly prevalent around dental implants (73–90%). Limited evidence indicates that mucositis is a reversible process.

Peri-implantitis

Peri-implantitis is an inflammatory process in the soft tissues surrounding a functioning dental implant additionally characterised by peri-implant bone loss (Berglundh *et al.*, 2008). The clinical characteristics are similar to peri-implant mucositis, but pus and/or increased probing depth are commonly found at peri-implantitis sites (Figure 61.3). The differential diagnosis is based on radiograph examination aiming to detect peri-implant bone loss. The occurrence of peri-implantitis is not rare, with prevalence ranging from 25% to 45% (Berglundh *et al.*, 2008). A recent study in a Swedish population indicated a 14.5% prevalence of moderate/severe peri-implantitis (Derks *et al.*, 2016).

Patients at risk of implant failure may constitute a specific group. Failures seem to affect a small number of patients (Ellegaard *et al.*, 1997; Roos-Jansåker *et al.*, 2006). An increasing risk of implant loss has been highlighted in patients with a history of implant failure (Weyant and Burt, 1993).

Key points

- Good oral hygiene is a prerequisite for long-term survival of dental implants.
- Systematic monitoring of peri-implant tissues is recommended to prevent peri-implant pathologies. Annual monitoring seems reasonable.
- A follow-up regime with more frequent controls than usual is recommended for patients at risk of developing peri-implant diseases.
- A combination of bleeding on probing and increased probing depth are adequate parameters to trigger dental X-rays.
- There is no evidence that peri-implant treatment is mandatory when the decision-making process is based on bleeding on probing and/or increased peri-implant probing depth alone.

62 Peri-implant diseases: Treatment

Figure 62.1 Localised peri-implantitis: surgical procedure. (a) Preoperative view. (b) Preoperative radiography. (c) Perioperative view. Note the bone defect morphology, which is characteristic of peri-implant defects. (d) One-year postoperative view. (e) One-year postoperative radiography

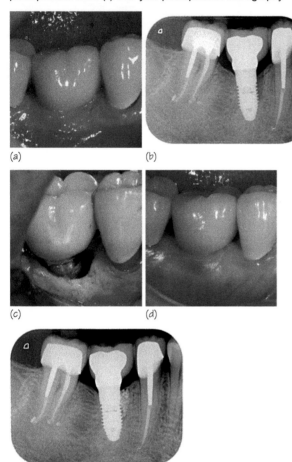

(a) (b)

(c) (d)

(e)

Box 62.1 Guidelines for the treatment of peri-implant diseases

Peri-implant mucositis
Non-surgical therapy
- Mechanical debridement
- Polishing
- Antiseptics

Peri-implantitis
- Surgical therapy + systemic antibiotics
- Explantation

Box 62.2 Explantation techniques

Unscrewing technique
After removal of the cover screw (or the abutment), an implant holder, transfer piece or screw is positioned in the implant body. A ratchet wrench is then set in an anticlockwise direction to unscrew the dental implant. This technique is the most conservative, but is limited to loose implants or when residual bone anchorage is low.

Trephine technique
A trephine with a diameter and length corresponding to the dimensions of the dental implant is sunk over the implant to the apex at low speed. A stem guide into the implant body, giving the implant direction, is recommended for trephine use. This non-conservative technique increases the diameter of the implant bed. It cannot be used when the diameter of the implant neck is larger than the diameter of the implant body.

Extraction-like technique
Osteotomy around the dental implant using a small round burr with a long shaft (copious running saline is mandatory), followed by the use of dental forceps turned clockwise and anticlockwise. A periotome can be extremely useful for trained operators. This approach is traumatic and therefore not recommended.

Explantation kits
Special explantation kits are commercially available. They are based on the insertion of a stem guide screwed into the implant body to indicate the correct direction for a trephine. A ratchet wrench is then inserted onto the trephine and used in an anticlockwise direction. The use of these devices is recommended due to the atraumatic approach.

The microflora associated with peri-implant diseases closely resembles that found in chronic periodontitis. Consequently, it is hardly surprising that peri-implant therapies are based on the available evidence for the treatment of periodontal diseases.

Treatment procedures must be aimed at eliminating the infection to resolve inflammatory lesions in peri-implant tissues.

Thus, the initial phase of therapy must always include plaque-control procedures. However, the differences between peri-implant mucositis and peri-implantitis must be considered when selecting treatment strategies for this disease (Box 62.1).

The following main treatments, either alone or combined, have been proposed to treat peri-implant diseases in humans.

Implant Dentistry at a Glance, Second Edition. Jacques Malet, Francis Mora and Philippe Bouchard.
© 2018 John Wiley & Sons Ltd. Published 2018 by John Wiley & Sons Ltd.
Companion website: www.wiley.com/go/malet/implant

Box 62.3 Standard surgical protocols based on the personal opinion and clinical experience of the authors

Open-flap debridement
Granulation tissue removal
- Titanium curettes in contact with the bone surface as opposed to the implant surface[1]
- Ultrasonic with non-metal tip
Implant surface smoothing (optional)
- Elimination of threads and roughness with carbide burrs
- Thorough rinsing with saline for 1 minute
Decontamination of the implant surface
- Tetracycline hydrochloride (50 mg/ml) burnished into the implant surface with small pieces of gauze for minutes
- Thorough rinsing with saline for 3 minutes
- Air-polishing[2] (optional) + rinsing with saline for 3 minutes
Treatment of the bone surface
- Perforation of the cortical bone
- Osteoplasty

Additional regenerative surgery[3]
- Bone-derived xenograft (Bio-Oss® 0.25–1 mm particles) moistened with saline[4]

Antimicrobial regimen[5]
- Amoxicillin per os (by mouth) 1000 mg twice a day for 8 days
- Chlorhexidine rinses three times a day (TID) for 10 days

Notes
1 Manual plastic scalers are not effective for removing granulation tissue.
2 Care must be taken with soft tissues by protecting them with pieces of gauze to prevent the risk of emphysema due to air-blasting.
3 Animal studies indicate that re-osseointegration is partly possible, but unpredictable on a previously contaminated implant surface (Renvert *et al.*, 2009). This may justify a regenerative surgical approach. However, the decision is based on the surgeon's personal experience.
4 Resorbable membranes (Bio-Gide®) can be used to cover the bone substitute. However, membranes must be submerged beneath the flap. This allows removal of the prosthesis.
5 Prescribed after open-flap debridement and regenerative surgery.

Non-surgical procedures
Mechanical debridement and polishing
- Manual with plastic scalers
- Ultrasonic with non-metal tip (carbon fibres, nylon or plastic sheaths or tips)
- Cleaning with saline-saturated surgical gauzes
- Polishing:
  - Rubber cup with toothpaste or polishing paste
  - Rotating titanium brush
  - Air-polishing with sodium bicarbonate or hydroxyapatite particles.

Plaque removal can be performed on SLA (sandblasted, large grit, acid-etched) surfaces using air-polishing, titanium brushes or ultrasonic scalers with non-metal tips (Louropoulou *et al.*, 2014). Air-abrasive systems also seem effective in removing plaque on machined and TPS (titanium plasma-sprayed) surfaces.

Laser beam: Er:YAG laser
Systematic reviews fail to demonstrate the superiority of laser treatment compared to conventional treatment of peri-implantitis (Kotsakis *et al.*, 2014). In addition, conventional treatment strategies offer comparably better value for money than Er:YAG laser monotherapy (Listl *et al.*, 2015).

Pharmaceutical therapy
Non-surgical therapy
Local antiseptics:
- Mouth rinses
- Subgingival irrigation with 0.2% chlorhexidine irrigation/gel
- Chlorhexidine chips.

Local antibiotics:
- Subgingival injection of 25% metronidazole gel
- Subgingival injection of 8.5% doxycycline gel.

Surgical therapy
Decontamination of the implant surface:
- Rinsing/cleaning for 1–3 minutes with a 2% chlorhexidine solution or with 0.12% chlorhexidine + 0.05% cetylpyridinium chloride
- Rubbing a tetracycline hydrochloride solution onto the implant surface.

For both non-surgical or surgical therapy;
- Systemic antibiotics: amoxicillin per os (by mouth), 2 x 1g amoxicillin/day (based on 50 mg/kg/day depending on the patient's weight) for 8 to 13 days, initiated 1 hour to 3 days before surgery, respectively.

A recent study indicates that (i) the local use of chlorhexidine during surgery does not seem to affect treatment outcomes; and (ii) adjunctive systemic antibiotics (amoxicillin 2 g/day for 13 days) has a positive but minimal effect on treatment success using implants with a modified surface only (Carcuac *et al.*, 2016).

Surgical procedures
All surgical procedures are based on the open-flap debridement technique (Figure 62.1).
- Granulation tissue removal
- Implant surface smoothing
- Decontamination of the implant surface using antibacterial agents or laser beam
- Correction of anatomical conditions by osteoplasty
- Regeneration of the surrounding bone using different materials:
  - Nanocrystalline hydroxyapatite
  - Bovine-derived xenograft
  - Resorbable membrane.

The decision-making process must balance the benefit of surgical intervention with the inconvenience of implant removal (Box 62.2). Indeed, the surgeon must carefully evaluate the percentage success rate of repeat surgical intervention, because the risk of recurrence of peri-implantitis appears to be high after one year (Esposito *et al.*, 2010).

Conclusion
It has not been established which therapeutic approach is the best. Long-term outcomes of mucositis therapy have not been sufficiently documented (Salvi and Ramseier, 2015). Regarding the treatment of peri-implantitis, a systematic review indicates that successful 12-month treatment outcomes have been recorded in most patients (Heitz-Mayfield and Mombelli, 2014). Decision-making approaches using relevant pre-determined protocols and decision trees have been proposed but

strong, evidence-based, programmed therapies are still lacking. Consequently, peri-implant treatment protocols are mostly based on expert opinions.

Our personal experience indicates that the non-surgical approach may prevent and possibly treat mucositis at a peri-implant probing depth less than or equal to 4 mm, but cannot treat peri-implantitis. In the light of the current literature, clear evidence-based recommendations should be proposed for the treatment of peri-implant diseases. In the absence of these data, Box 62.3 indicates the standard surgical protocols we use in our department.

Key points

- Non-surgical therapy is reserved solely for mucositis.
- Peri-implantitis must be treated using a surgical approach.
- Manual scalers and ultrasonic tips must be non-metal.
- The additional use of chlorhexidine during surgical peri-implantitis treatment does not seem to enhance clinical treatment outcomes.
- The use of adjunctive systemic antibiotics should be limited to dental implants with a modified surface.
- Most of the clinical proposals aimed at treating peri-implant diseases are expert based. Further studies are required to specify universally accepted guidelines.

63 Dental implant maintenance

Figure 63.1 Materials for individual plaque control around dental implants. (a) Powered toothbrush; (b) soft sulcular toothbrush; (c) interproximal brush; (d) special floss

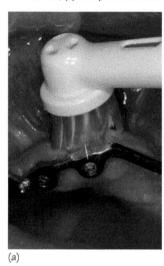

(a)

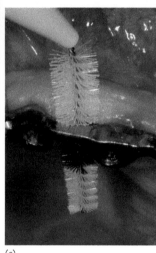

(c)

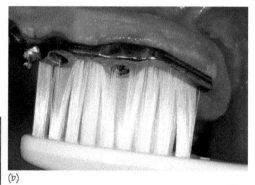

(b)

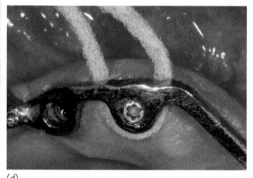

(d)

One of the key factors in the long-term success of oral implants is the maintenance of healthy tissues around them. The lack of regular maintenance in patients with peri-implant mucositis appears to be associated with an increased risk for onset of peri-implantitis (Jepsen *et al.*, 2015). Besides the maintenance of the prosthesis, patients who have experienced the benefits of implant dentistry must be enrolled in a systematic, individualized supportive care programme, alternating visitations between the surgeon and the restorative dentist, to maintain the health of the peri-implant tissues. They must be informed of this before implant placement (see Appendix E).

Rationale for plaque elimination around dental implants

Experimental and human studies have shown that long-standing plaque accumulation around dental implants induces inflammatory changes in the soft tissues that increase the risk of peri-implant diseases (Schou *et al.*, 1993; Pontoriero *et al.*, 1994). Consequently, one of the key factors for the long-term success of dental implants is the maintenance of healthy tissues around them

(Esposito *et al.*, 2010). However, there is no reliable evidence as to which regimens are most effective for long-term maintenance. Systematic appraisals of regular peri-implant maintenance on the occurrence of biological implant complications and implant loss indicate a clear influence of plaque-control protocols on dental implant survival (Salvi and Zitzmann, 2014). For implant survival, implants with regular maintenance have 0.958 the incident event compared to those with no maintenance (Monje *et al.*, 2016). There is a limited improvement in peri-implant tissue health with regular maintenance, and patients can still develop soft and hard tissue complications. In other words, despite good maintenance complications can occur, and it is unclear that the prevention of peri-implant mucositis prevents the onset of peri-implantitis. Consequently, further well-crafted prospective studies exploring other criteria than peri-implant tissue health, such as patient-, clinical- and implant-related factors, are needed to better understand peri-implant complications.

The development of peri-implant diseases is associated with an increase of bacterial species, such as *P. gingivalis*, *T. forsythia* and *A. actinomycetemcomitans*, which are involved in the pathogenesis of

Implant Dentistry at a Glance, Second Edition. Jacques Malet, Francis Mora and Philippe Bouchard.
© 2018 John Wiley & Sons Ltd. Published 2018 by John Wiley & Sons Ltd.
Companion website: www.wiley.com/go/malet/implant

Figure 63.2 Materials for professional plaque control around dental implants. (a) Plastic periodontal probe for peri-implant probing; (b) graphite tip scaler for sonic scalers; (c) graphite implant scalers; (d) plastic tip scaler for sonic scalers

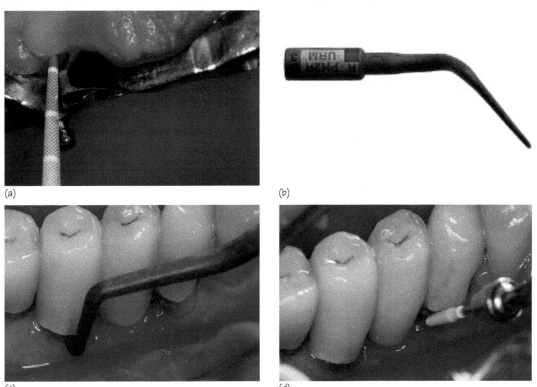

(a)

(b)

(c)

(d)

periodontal diseases (Heitz-Mayfield and Lang, 2010). However, more recent studies indicate that the implant surface may be colonised with opportunistic pathogens different from periodontal bacteria such as *P. aeruginosa*, *S. aureus* and *C. albicans*, which may be associated with implant failure (Albertini *et al.*, 2015). Therefore, it is not surprising that the prevention of peri-implant diseases is similar to the prevention of periodontal diseases, and may include daily implant cleaning by patients and regular cleaning by dental professionals.

Individual plaque control

At baseline, at the time of prosthesis insertion, the patient must be informed about how to carry out individual plaque-control procedures (Figure 63.1). Powered toothbrushes and soft sulcular toothbrushes are primary plaque-control devices; they are both effective in reducing plaque and marginal bleeding around implant-supported reconstructions. There is no evidence that powered toothbrushes perform better than manual toothbrushes.

The design of the implant-supported prosthesis must allow access for individual and professional plaque control to prevent inflammation in the peri-implant tissues. Depending on the design of the prosthetic reconstruction, different types of toothbrushes and/or floss should be used. Gauze strips, yarn, thicker dental floss or dental tape can also assist with plaque control. An interproximal brush is indicated when embrasure space permits (wire centre coated with plastic or nylon). For smaller spaces, an end-tuft brush may be a convenient device.

Daily use of triclosan or stannous fluoride dentifrices is safe after dental implant placement. There is no evidence of superiority for a toothpaste composition (Salvi and Ramseier, 2015).

The efficacy of adjunctive patient-administered antiseptic rinse, irrigation or gel remains to be established. Antibacterial mouth rinses, such as chlorhexidine or fluoride/stannous fluoride mouthwash, may help reduce plaque around dental implants.

Professional plaque control

The recall frequency for follow-up of implant-treated patients should be adapted to individual risk factors. A maintenance appointment once a year may be sufficient when patients are free of risk and compliant with dental hygiene procedures. Following the surgical treatment of peri-implantitis, patients with a high standard of oral hygiene, and enrolled in a recall system every six months, have been shown to be stable during a five-year period (Serino *et al.*, 2015).

During the maintenance appointment, the dentist or dental hygienist should remove calculus, bacterial plaque and staining (Figure 63.2). Cleaning is accomplished with implant-safe instruments: plastic (not very efficient), graphite (fragile and brittle), titanium and gold-tipped curettes. An ultrasonic tip may only be used with a plastic covering that prevents damages to the implant surface. The visible portion of the implant, if any, can be polished with rubber cups and non-abrasive polishing paste.

Numerous local antibacterial agents that can be professionally administered have been proposed to maintain soft tissue health. There is no reliable evidence to recommend their use for long-term maintenance in the absence of peri-implant pathology.

Key points

- The maintenance of peri-implant soft tissue health is mandatory to establish the conditions for long-term success, but does not guarantee the absence of complications over time.
- Nowadays, the prevention of peri-implant diseases is similar to the prevention of periodontal diseases.
- Despite regular maintenance, some patients can still develop soft and hard tissue complications.

Appendix A: Glossary

Allograft (adjective, allogeneic): living tissue transferred between two genetically different individuals of the same species (Stevenson, 1999).

Autograft (adjective, autogenous or autogeneic): a graft moved from one site to another within the same individual.

Bioactive: refers to a material that induces specific biological activity, as opposed to bioinert (Williams, 1987).

Combined tooth/implant-supported prosthesis: non-removable (fixed) prosthetic device, which is tooth and implant supported.

Conventional loading: implants are functional 2 months or more following implantation.

Delayed implantation: *Syn.: early implantation with partial bone healing:* Implant placement at least 2 months after tooth extraction.

Dental implant: in a general sense, a biomedical device usually composed of an inert metal or metallic alloy that is surgically placed (implanted) on or within the osseous tissues. Nowadays, the biomedical device refers to a titanium threaded root-form osseointegrated implant that is placed within the bone. *Syn.: oral implant, fixture, implant, osseointegrated implants.*

Denture: removable prosthetic device, which is supported by soft tissue only, or by soft tissue and roots remaining in the jaw bone if present.

Early loading: implants are functional between 1 week and 2 months following implantation.

End-of-treatment appraisal: critical appraisal of the outcome at the time of prosthesis placement. The recording measurements include BOP, PD, radiographic, and esthetic evaluation. *Syn.: baseline evaluation.*

Immediate-delayed implantation: any implant placed in an extraction socket within 8 weeks after tooth extraction. *Syn.: early implantation with soft tissue healing.*

Immediate implantation: implant placement within the extraction socket at the time of the extraction.

Immediate loading: implants are functional within 1 week following implantation.

Implant: non-viable material, such as bone that has been frozen, freeze-dried, or sterilized by irradiation (Urist, 1980; Burwell, 1994).

Implant failure: the dental implant and the prosthetic reconstruction, if any, cannot be used or are no longer present in the mouth of the patient. *Syn.: implant loss.*

Implant restoration: dental prosthesis attached to the implant by means of components (American Academy of Periodontology, 2000) *Syn.: implant reconstruction.*

Implant-supported prosthesis: removable or non-removable (fixed) prosthetic device, which is implant supported.

Late implantation: implant placement after complete bone healing of the extraction site.

Osseointegration: a process whereby clinically asymptomatic rigid fixation of alloplastic materials is achieved, and maintained, in bone during functional loading (Albrektsson & Johansson, 2001). The stable anchorage of a dental implant is achieved by direct bone-to-implant contact (Brånemark *et al.*, 1977).

Osteoconduction: the process by which bone grows to a surface (Albrektsson & Johansson, 2001). This phenomenon is regularly seen in the case of bone implants. In the case of dental implants, bone conduction is not only dependent on conditions for bone repair, but also on the biomaterial used and its reactions.

Osteogenesis: in a general sense, osteogenesis refers to bone formation with no indication of cellular origin; new bone may originate from live cells in the graft or cells of host origin (Stevenson, 1999). In a stricter and more commonly used definition, osteogenesis refers to bone formation by transplanted living cells (Mulliken *et al.*, 1984; Fitch *et al.*, 1997).

Osteoinduction: the process by which osteogenesis is induced (Albrektsson & Johansson, 2001). It implies the recruitment of primitive, undifferentiated and pluripotent cells, and the stimulation of these cells to develop into preosteoblasts. It involves the participation of tissue factors.

Osteoproduction: bone proliferation resulting from the combined properties (i.e. osteoinductive, osteoconductive, and/or osteogenic properties) of a grafting material.

Overdenture: removable or non-removable prosthetic device with a denture design, which is supported by dental implants only, or by soft tissues and dental implants.

Peri-implant diseases: inflammatory processes that involve the soft tissues and/or the bone surrounding a functioning dental implant.

Peri-implant mucositis: reversible plaque-induced inflammatory process of the peri-implant soft tissues without appreciable bone loss (Salvi & Lang, 2004; Grusovin *et al.*, 2010).

Peri-implantitis: plaque-induced inflammatory process of the peri-implant tissues characterized by localized marginal bone loss with or without soft tissue complications (Salvi & Lang, 2004; Esposito *et al.*, 2010).

Primary stability: absence of implant mobility immediately after the final tightening of the implant at the time of surgery. It can be evaluated by subjective hand-felt perception and/or by insertion torque.

Prosthetic failure: the reconstruction cannot be used or is no longer present in the mouth of the patient.

Removable prosthesis: prosthetic device that can be removed by the patient without the aid of a professional.

Secondary stability: absence of implant mobility after the healing phase. It can be evaluated by subjective hand-felt perception and/or by resonance frequency analysis.

Teeth-retained prosthesis: removable or non-removable (fixed) prosthetic device, which is tooth supported.

Xenograft (adjective, xenogeneic): transfer of viable tissue from a donor of a different species.

Implant Dentistry at a Glance, Second Edition. Jacques Malet, Francis Mora and Philippe Bouchard.
© 2018 John Wiley & Sons Ltd. Published 2018 by John Wiley & Sons Ltd.
Companion website: www.wiley.com/go/malet/implant

Appendix B: Basic surgical table and instrumentation

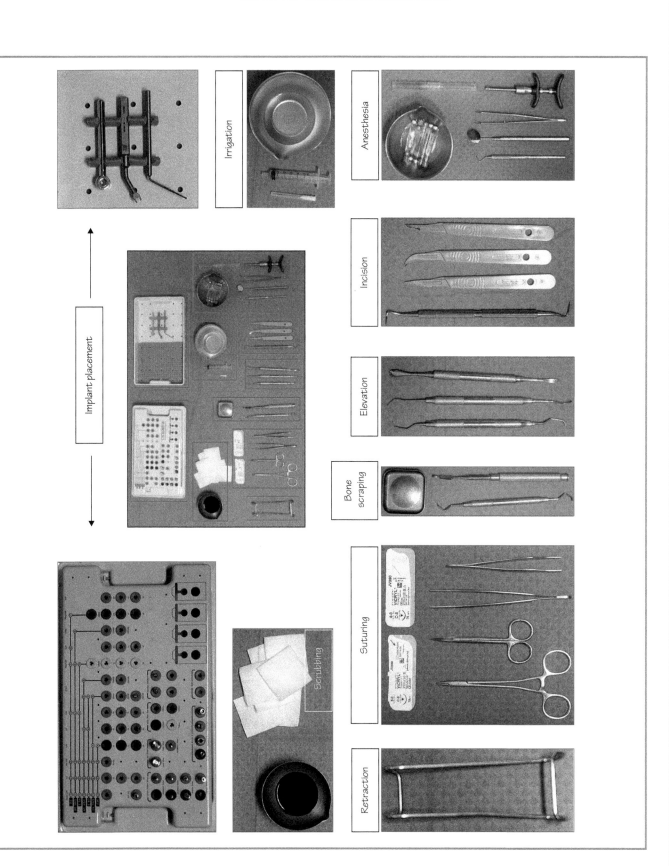

Implant Dentistry at a Glance, Second Edition. Jacques Malet, Francis Mora and Philippe Bouchard.
© 2018 John Wiley & Sons Ltd. Published 2018 by John Wiley & Sons Ltd.
Companion website: www.wiley.com/go/malet/implant

Appendix C: Preparation of the members of the sterile team

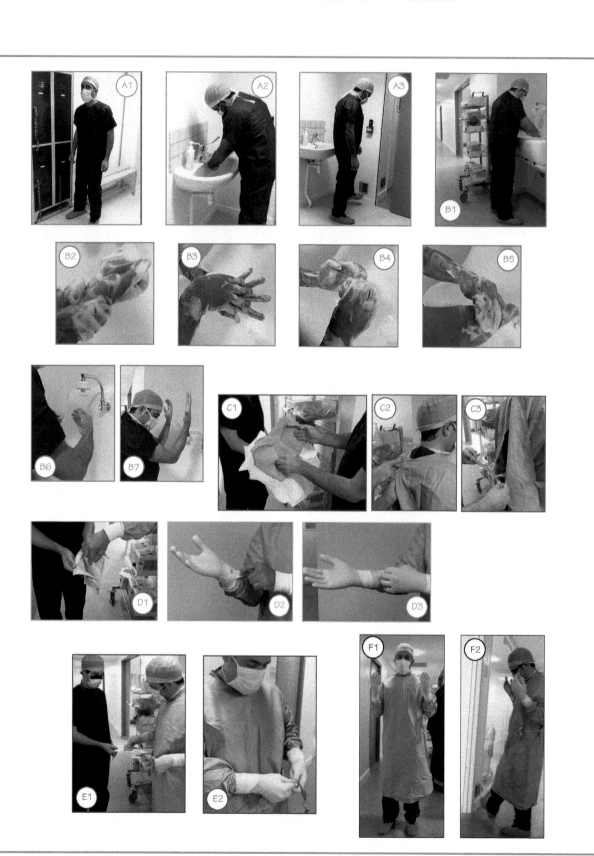

Implant Dentistry at a Glance, Second Edition. Jacques Malet, Francis Mora and Philippe Bouchard.
© 2018 John Wiley & Sons Ltd. Published 2018 by John Wiley & Sons Ltd.
Companion website: www.wiley.com/go/malet/implant

Appendix D: Medical history form

Patient's copy

Your answers on this form will help your surgeon understand your medical concerns and conditions better. If you are uncomfortable with any question, do not answer it. If you cannot remember specific details, please provide your best guess.

Name:_____ **Date:** □ Day □ Month □ Year

Occupation: _____ Retired □

Live with: □ Parents □ Children □ Friends □ Spouse/Partner □ Alone

Person to notify in case of emergency:_____Phone_____

How would you rate your general health?

□ Excellent □ Good □ Fair □ Poor □ Don't know

Main reason for your visit?

_____

Other concerns: _____

Last medical **check-up**: □ Month □ Year □ Don't Know

Last **blood tests**: □ Month □ Year □ Don't Know

Are you or have you been treated for a cancer? □ Yes □ No □ Don't know

Have you had an organ transplant? □ Yes □ No □ Don't know

Do you have prosthetic material in your body? □ Yes □ No □ Don't know

If yes, what type of prosthetic material do you have?

□ Artificial heart valves □ Pacemaker □ Artificial joints □ Other

---

Are you **nervous or anxious about implant surgery**? □ Yes □ No □ Don't know

If yes, would you say that your anxiety is: □ Very high □ High □ Mild

If yes, could you say why? _____

_____

_____

Medical status

For women:

□ Pregnant □ Planning pregnancy □ Nursing □ Birth control pills □ IUD □ Menopause

Do you have hormonal therapy? □ Yes □ No □ Don't know

Implant Dentistry at a Glance, Second Edition. Jacques Malet, Francis Mora and Philippe Bouchard.
© 2018 John Wiley & Sons Ltd. Published 2018 by John Wiley & Sons Ltd.
Companion website: www.wiley.com/go/malet/implant

I am not aware of any current or past medical condition or any disease that could be applicable to me. I am healthy and having read the contents of the box below, I am able to answer "no" to each item.

Name: **Signature:**

Please check the following in the box below, and indicate if it is a current or a past condition (if applicable).

Genetic Disease   ☐ Yes   ☐ No   ☐ Don't know

If yes, what type of genetic disease do you have?…….…….…….…….…….…….…….…….…….…….…….…….…….…….…….…….…..

Heart and Vascular Diseases   ☐ Yes   ☐ No   ☐ Don't know   ☐ Current   ☐ Past

If yes, what type of heart and vascular diseases do you have?

          ☐ Rheumatic fever   ☐ Heart murmur   ☐ Mitral valve prolapse

          ☐ Chest pain/angina   ☐ Heart attack(s)   ☐ Stroke   ☐ Other   ☐ Don't know

If other, what type of cardiovascular disease do you have?…….…….…….…….…….…….…….…….…….…….…….…….…….…….

Bleeding Disorder   ☐ Yes   ☐ No   ☐ Don't know   ☐ Current   ☐ Past

If yes, what type of bleeding disorder do you have?

          ☐ Hemophilia   ☐ Anemia   ☐ Leukemia   ☐ Other   ☐ Don't know

If other, what type of bleeding disorder do you have?…….…….…….…….…….…….…….…….…….…….…….…….…….…….……

High Blood Pressure   ☐ Yes   ☐ No   ☐ Don't know   ☐ Current   ☐ Past

If yes, are you treated for this high blood pressure?   ☐ Yes   ☐ No   ☐ Don't know

Cancer   ☐ Yes   ☐ No   ☐ Don't know   ☐ Current   ☐ Past

If yes, what type of cancer do you have?…….…….…….…….…….…….…….…….…….…….…….…….…….…….…….…….…..

What type of treatment do you have? ☐ Chemotherapy   ☐ Radiation treatment   ☐ Other   ☐ Don't know

If you have radiation treatment, is it to head/neck?   ☐ Yes   ☐ No   ☐ Don't know

If other, what type of treatment do you have?…….…….…….…….…….…….…….…….…….…….…….…….…….…….…….

Kidney Disease   ☐ Yes   ☐ No   ☐ don't know   ☐ Current   ☐ Past

If yes, what type of disease do you have?…….…….…….…….…….…….…….…….…….…….…….…….…….…….

Are you on dialysis?   ☐ Yes   ☐ No   ☐ Don't know

Liver Disease   ☐ Yes   ☐ No   ☐ Don't know   ☐ Current   ☐ Past

If yes, what type of liver disease do you have?   ☐ Hepatitis   ☐ Cirrhosis| ☐ Other   ☐ Don't know

If other, what type of liver disease do you have?…….…….…….…….…….…….…….…….…….…….…….…….…….…….

Diabetes   ☐ Yes   ☐ No   ☐ Don't know   ☐ Current   ☐ Past

If yes, what type of diabetes do you have?…….…….…….…….…….…….…….…….…….…….…….…….…….…….

If yes, how is your diabetes controlled?

          ☐ Well controlled   ☐ Poorly controlled   ☐ Not controlled   ☐ Don't know

If yes, do you have complications?   ☐ Yes   ☐ No   ☐ Don't know   ☐ Current   ☐ Past

If yes, what type of complication?…….…….…….…….…….…….…….…….…….…….…….…….…….…….

Bone Disease   ☐ Yes   ☐ No   ☐ Don't know   ☐ Current   ☐ Past

If yes, what type of bone disease do you have?

          ☐ Osteoporosis   ☐ Rheumatoid arthritis   ☐ Paget's disease   ☐ Arthritis   ☐ Other   ☐ Don't know

If other, what type of bone disease do you have?…….…….…….…….…….…….…….…….…….…….…….…….…….

Transmissible Disease   ☐ Yes   ☐ No   ☐ Don't know   ☐ Current   ☐ Past

If yes, what type of transmissible disease do you have?

          ☐ AIDS/HIV positive   ☐ Tuberculosis   ☐ Venereal disease   ☐ Other   ☐ Don't know

If other, what type of transmissible disease do you have?…….…….…….…….…….…….…….…….…….…….…….…….……

Respiratory Disease   □ Yes   □ No   □ Don't know   □ Current   □ Past

If yes, what type of respiratory disease do you have?

□ Lung disease   □ Emphysema   □ Shortness of breath   □ Asthma   □ Sleep apnea   □ Other   □ Don't know

If other, what type of respiratory disease do you have?…………………………………………………………………………

Sinus Trouble   □ Yes   □ No   □ Don't know   □ Current   □ Past

If yes, what type of sinus trouble do you have?…………………………………………………………………………… ……

Have you been operated for sinus trouble?   □ Yes   □ No   □

If yes, what type of operation have you had?…………………………………………………………………… …

Stomach Disease   □ Yes   □ No   □ Don't know   □ Current   □ Past

If yes, what type of stomach disease do you have?

        □ Reflux   □ Ulcer   □ Crohn's disease   □ Other   □ Don't know

If other, what type of stomach disease do you have?………………………………………………………………… ………

Skin Disease   □ Yes   □ No   □ Don't know   □ Current   □ Past

If yes, what type of skin disease do you have?

    □ Scleroderma   □ Lichen planus   □ Ectodermal dysplasia   □ Arthritis   □ Other   □ Don't know

If other, what type of skin disease do you have?…………………………………………………………………………

Psychiatric/Neurological Disorders   □ Yes   □ No   □ Don't know   □ Current   □ Past

If yes, what type of disorder do you have?

    □ Depression   □ Epilepsy/seizures   □ Convulsions   □ Parkinson's disease   □ Other   □ Don't know

If other, what type of disorder do you have?………………………………………………………………………………

Miscellaneous   □ Yes   □ No   □ Don't know   □ Current   □ Past

Do you have the following condition?

□ Eating disorder   □ Sjögren's disease   □ Lupus   □ Thyroid disease   □ Glaucoma   □ Other   □ Don't know

Do you have any disease or condition that has not been listed so far?

        □ Yes   □ No   □ Don't know   □ Current   □ Past

If yes, please detail:

………

………

………………………………………………………………………………………

………

…………………………………………………………………………………………

Medication intake

Do you take the following medications?

Bisphosphonates   □ Yes   □ No | Don't know   □ Current   □ Past

If past, when did you stop the bisphosphonates?…………………………………………………………………………..

If yes, why do you take bisphosphonates?………………………………………………………………………………

If yes, do you take the bisphosphonates by   □ Pills   □ Injections   □ Don't know

Anticoagulants   □ Yes   □ No   □ Don't know   □ Current   □ Past

If yes, why do you take anticoagulants?………………………………………………………………………………

Aspirin   □ Yes   □ No   □ Don't know   □ Current   □ Past

If yes, why do you take aspirin?……………………………………………………………………………

Steroids of any type   □ Yes   □ No   □ Don't know   □ Current   □ Past

If yes, why do you take steroids?………………………………………………………………………………

Please **list all the current medications you take** (including appetite suppressants, vitamins, herbal supplements, or any homeopathic medication):

MEDICATION	DOSAGE	FREQUENCY	MEDICATION	DOSAGE	FREQUENCY

Allergies

Please check the following in the box below, and indicate if it is a current or a past condition (if applicable).

Do you have or have you had in the past any **allergies and/or sensitivities** to the following substances?

Antibiotics   ☐ Yes   ☐ No   ☐ Don't know   ☐ Current   ☐ Past

If yes, indicate if possible the type of antibiotic:…………………………………………………………………

Local anesthetics   ☐ Yes   ☐ No   ☐ Don't know   ☐ Current   ☐ Past

If yes, indicate if you can the type of anesthetics:………………………………………………………………

Latex   ☐ Yes   ☐ No   ☐ Don't know   ☐ Current   ☐ Past

Other   ☐ Yes   ☐ No   ☐ Don't know   ☐ Current   ☐ Past

If yes, indicate if you can the type of substance:………………………………………………………………

Personal behavior

Please check the following in the box below, and indicate if it is a current or a past condition (if applicable).

Cigarette Smoking   ☐ Never smoker   ☐ Current smoker   ☐ Former smoker   ☐ Passive smoker

Current smoker: number of cigarettes per day? ☐ Number of years   ☐

Former smoker: number of cigarettes per day? ☐ Number of years   ☐ Quit date

Passive smoker: Number of years ☐

Other Tobacco Use   ☐ Cigar   ☐ Pipe   ☐ Snuff   ☐ Chew

Consumption (number per day): ………………………………………………………………………………

Are you interested in quitting? ☐ Yes   ☐ No   ☐ Don't know

Alcohol Use   ☐ Yes   ☐ No   ☐ Former drinker

If yes, indicate the number of glasses per week: ☐ Wine   ☐ Beer   ☐ Aperitif   ☐ Other

If yes, is your alcohol use a concern for you and/or others? ☐ Yes   ☐ No   ☐ Don't know

Drug Use   ☐ Yes   ☐ No   ☐ Former drug user

Any other habit or behavior that you consider as an addiction (please detail)?

……

Surgical history

Previous dental treatment

Have you had any previous local anesthesia for a dental treatment?

☐ Yes ☐ No ☐ Don't know ☐ Current ☐ Past

If yes, have you had any abnormal reaction following this anesthesia? ☐ Yes ☐ No

If yes, indicate the type of reaction:...

Indicate when you experienced this reaction: ☐ Year

Please list all **previous hospitalization/operations**, including cosmetic, in the **last 5 years** (details)

YEAR	DESCRIPTION	COMPLICATION (if any)

In your opinion, is there any additional information on your health state that would be of interest to the surgeon? ☐ Yes ☐ No ☐ Don't know

If yes, please detail:

....
....
....
....
....

I hereby state that I have answered all of the questions accurately to the best of my knowledge. This form will reveal my complete medical history and assist my surgeon in providing the best care possible. I will not hold the surgeon or the clinic responsible for any errors or omissions that I have made in completing this form.

Signature of patient/parent or guardian if minor   Date ☐ ☐ ☐

Reviewed by: ☐ ☐
Doctor's initials

The information in this document is intended only for the person/persons directly involved with the patients' care and may contain confidential and/or privileged material. Any review, retransmission, dissemination or other use of or taking of any action in reliance upon this information by persons or entities other than the intended care provider is prohibited by law.

Appendix E: Consent form for dental implant surgery

Please read this form carefully before signing it and ask about anything that you do not understand.

You have the right to be given information about your proposed implant placement so that you are able to make the decision as to whether to proceed with the surgery. What you are being asked to sign is a confirmation that we have discussed the nature and purpose of the treatment, the known risks associated with the treatment, and the feasible treatment alternatives; that you have been given an opportunity to ask questions; that all your questions have been answered in a satisfactory manner.

After a study of my oral condition, the dentist has advised me that my missing tooth/teeth may be replaced with artificial teeth supported by one or more dental implants. The procedure involves placing dental implant into the jawbone. This procedure has two phases: a surgical phase (*placing the dental implants to serve as anchors to replace a missing tooth or teeth*), followed, after a healing phase from 2 to 6 months, by a prosthetic phase (*getting a crown, cap, bridge or denture attached to the dental implant*). This office only does the surgical phase. I understand that my general dentist or prosthodontist will do the prosthetic phase and that the cost for that work is not included in the charge for the surgical procedure.[1]

Surgical options

We will utilize the options that are best suited for your condition. The decision is made in agreement with the general dentist or prosthodontist who will do the prosthetic phase.

One-stage/two-stage

I understand that dental implants may be placed by either a one-stage technique or two-stage technique. One-stage technique requires only one surgery to place the implant and the healing cap. Two-stage surgery requires two surgeries: (1) to place the implant; (2) to uncover the implant and place a healing cap.

Your procedure is intended to be: □ One-stage □ Two-stage

Immediate loading

In certain unusual circumstances, and with very specific criteria, we may elect to restore some or all of the implants immediately or shortly after the placement procedure. This technique carries some increased concerns about bone and implant healing.

Your dental implants are intended to be:
□ Normally loaded □ Immediately loaded

[1]The phrases in blue are optional, according to whether the practitioner performs all the procedures or not.

Temporary dental implants

In certain unusual circumstances, additional special implants may be placed to temporarily anchor a provisional dental restoration while the other dental implants heal. These special implants are usually surgically removed in the final treatment phase.

Your treatment is intended to include temporary implants:
□ Yes □ No

Additional materials and procedures

In certain cases, the surgery may involve gum and/or bone augmentation using bone grafts, artificial bone substitute, and/or healing membranes associated with fixation devices. When planned, these additional procedures are subject to a separate consent form. However, the need for those procedures may not be apparent until after the surgery has begun. Consequently, complete information is given to you before the surgery on the nature of these materials, whether or not they are planned to be used during the surgical procedure.

Your procedure intends to use:
□ Gingival grafting □ Bone grafting □ Bone substitute
□ Healing membrane □ Fixation screws □ Sinus lift procedures

Anesthesia

I have been informed on a separate consent form of the anesthetic risks.

_____
Initials

The anesthetic I have chosen for my surgery is:
□ Local □ Local with Nitrous Oxide/Oxygen Analgesia
□ Local with Oral Premedication
□ Local with Intravenous Sedation □ General Anesthesia

Surgical procedure

The gum will be incised (cut) and pulled away to expose the jawbone; a hole or holes will be drilled into the jawbone, and the titanium dental implant screw(s) will be placed within the hole.

One-stage technique

The gum will be closed by sutures around the dental implant neck. Thus, a portion of the dental implant will protrude through the gum at the completion of the surgery, and will remain uncovered during the 2–6-month healing phase.

Two-stage technique

The gum will be closed by sutures over the dental implant, which will probably remain covered by the gum during the 2–6-month healing phase. A second surgical procedure will be required to uncover the top of the dental implant to prepare for the prosthetic phase, which may start 4–5 weeks after.

Implant Dentistry at a Glance, Second Edition. Jacques Malet, Francis Mora and Philippe Bouchard.
© 2018 John Wiley & Sons Ltd. Published 2018 by John Wiley & Sons Ltd.
Companion website: www.wiley.com/go/malet/implant

Whatever the technique, if non-resorbable sutures are used, they will be removed 8–14 days after the surgical procedure.

It has been explained to me that during the course of surgery unforeseen conditions may be revealed that will necessitate extension of the original procedure or a different procedure from that which was planned (for example, changing from a one-stage to a two-stage process, use of bone grafting techniques involving substitute material or locally available particles, etc.). I give my permission for such unforeseen additional procedures, and I authorize the surgeon to do whatever he/she deems necessary and advisable under the circumstances according to his/her professional judgment.

_____
Initials

Principal risks and complications of the surgery

These include, but are not limited to, the following.

• Postoperative discomfort and swelling that may require several days of at-home recuperation. Prolonged or heavy bleeding that may require additional treatment.

• Skin discoloration may rarely occur after 1–2 days. Discoloration is usually gone in 2–3 weeks.

• Damage to adjacent teeth or roots of adjacent teeth.

• Postoperative infection that may require additional treatment, and possible loss of the implant(s).

• Stretching of the corners of the mouth that may cause cracking and bruising and may heal slowly.

• Restricted mouth opening for several days. Sometimes related to swelling and muscle soreness and sometimes related to stress on the jaw joints.

• Injury to sensory nerve branches in the jaw or soft tissue resulting in tingling, numbness, or pain in the chin, lips, cheek, gums, tongue (including possible loss of taste sensation) or teeth on the operated side(s). These symptoms usually persist for several weeks or months, and in some cases may be permanent.

• Opening into the sinus (a normal hollow chamber in the bone above the roots of back upper teeth) requiring additional treatment. If the sinus is entered there may be symptoms of sinusitis for several weeks that may require certain medications and additional recovery time.

• Fracture of the jaw or of thin bony plates.

• Bone loss around the implants.

• Certain other fixation devices may be used (screws, plates, membranes, etc.) that may either stay in place permanently or require later removal by another surgery. There may be unexpected exposure of these devices through the gum, causing their premature loss or removal, and possible loss of the implant.

• Implant or prosthesis failure. Rarely, the implant or parts of the structure holding the replacement tooth, or the replacement tooth itself, may fail due to chewing stresses.

No warranty or guarantee

Some patients do not respond successfully to dental implant surgery and in such cases, the implant may be lost. If the implant is lost during the healing phase, it is usually possible to replace it in a later surgery after the bony defect has healed or been bone grafted to achieve adequate bone volume for another implant placement procedure. Should it happen, I understand that a charge will be made for this procedure. It is also always possible to have a successful, solid dental implant and the connection between the implant and the gum and/or bone may fail months or years later, necessitating the removal of the implant.

Therefore, I hereby acknowledge that no guarantee, warranty or assurance has been given to me that the proposed surgery will be completely successful in eliminating all pretreatment symptoms or complaints. I acknowledge that there is the risk of failure, relapse, selective retreatment, or worsening of my present condition, despite efforts at optimal care. In the event of implant failure, there will be no refund of fees.

I understand that once the implant is inserted, the entire treatment plan must be followed and completed on schedule. If the planned schedule is not carried out, the implant(s) may fail.

I understand that my doctor is not a seller of the implant device itself and makes no warranty or guarantee regarding success or failure of the implant or its attachments used in this procedure.

_____
Initials

Alternatives to dental implant(s)

The advantages and disadvantages of possible alternative methods of replacing my missing teeth have been explained to me, including:

• no treatment at all

• keeping, or attempting to improve, my present denture or bridge

• restoring missing teeth with a new standard dental prosthesis such as removable dentures and/or dental bridges.

Finally, after reviewing the pros and cons of the non-implant-based restorations and of the dental implant therapies, I choose to proceed with insertion of the dental implant(s).

_____
Initials

Patient co-operation

I agree and understand that the degree of success of any dental treatment is related to my co-operation. I have read and understood the postsurgical instruction form, and I will be compliant with it. Specifically, I agree, if applicable, not to wear my denture for 1–2 weeks after the surgical procedure according to my surgeon's advice.

I understand that tobacco use is extremely detrimental to the success of dental implant therapy. I agree to make efforts to cease all use of tobacco in view of the surgical procedure and during the healing phase. I also understand that any abuse, including alcohol, drug, and dietary practices, may jeopardize the dental implant success.

I understand that the success of dental implants depends to a great extent on my maintenance and hygiene throughout my mouth and especially around the implant posts where they come through the gum tissue.

I agree to return at regular intervals as specified by the doctor for inspection of my mouth and implant cleansings by the doctor or the hygienist and to have performed such dental services as may be needed to maintain my oral health.

I agree to report immediately any evidence of pain, swelling, or inflammation around my implant(s) and agree to attend the office/hospital if necessary.

_____
Initials

Authorization of use of dental records

I authorize that photographs, X-rays, or other viewing of my care and treatment during its progress may be used for educational purposes and research.

I authorize sending any documents and other information pertaining to my treatment before, during, and after its completion with my insurance carriers, the doctor's billing agency, my general dentist, and any other healthcare provider I may have who may have a need to know about my dental treatment.

_____
Initials

I certify that I have read and fully understand the above informed consent form and that all my questions have been fully answered. I have had the opportunity to take this form and to review it before signing it. I understand and agree that my initial on each page along with my signature below will be considered conclusive proof that I have read and understand the content of this document. I have been informed on the nature of the different materials that can be used during the surgical procedure. I acknowledge that the procedure has been explained to my full understanding, including the number and location of incisions and the type of implant(s) that will be used. Consequently I hereby give my consent to proceed with dental implant treatment and related surgery, including any ancillary grafting procedures.

_____

Signature of Patient or Guardian   Guardian's Relationship to Patient

_____

Surgeon Signature

_____

Witness Signature

Date: _____

Appendix F: Postoperative patient records: stage 1

POSTOPERATIVE RECORD (Stage 1) Contact Clinic											
LAST NAME				First Name				Date of Birth			
Home Address											
Phone		Business				Home			Mobile		
Referred by											
STAGE 1						Date of the Surgery					
Surgeon							Nurse				
Premedication											
Anesthesia		Local		EMONO*			I.V.		General		
Tooth # (implant location)											
Dental Implant	**Brand**										
	Type										
	Length										
	Diameter										
	Angulation										
	Head										
	Neck										
	Reference										
Immediate Implant	YES										
Loading	Immediate										
	Early										
Submerged	YES										
	NO										
Healing Abutment	Height										
	Diameter										
Bone Resorption	A (Low)										
	B (Moderate)										
	C (Advanced)										
Bone Density	1 (Extreme)										
	2 (High)										
	3 (Moderate)										
	4 (Poor)										
Primary Stability	Good										
	Questionable										
Comments											
Prescription											

POSTOPERATIVE CONTROLS		
Date	Radiographs	Comments

TRACEABILITY

Implant Dentistry at a Glance, Second Edition. Jacques Malet, Francis Mora and Philippe Bouchard.
© 2018 John Wiley & Sons Ltd. Published 2018 by John Wiley & Sons Ltd.
Companion website: www.wiley.com/go/malet/implant

Appendix G: Postoperative patient records: stage 2

POSTOPERATIVE RECORD (Stage 2)								
Contact Clinic								

LAST NAME		First name				Date of Birth		
Home Address								
Phone	Business			Home		Mobile		
Referred by								

STAGE 2				Date of the Surgery				
Surgeon					**Nurse**			
Premedication								
Anesthesia	Local		EMONO*		I.V.		General	
Tooth # (implant location)								
Healing Abutment	Height							
	Diameter							
Secondary Stability	Good							
	Questionable							
Comments								
Prescription								

POSTOPERATIVE CONTROLS		
Date	Radiographs	Comments

CONTROLS AFTER LOADING		
Date	Radiographs	Comments

Implant Dentistry at a Glance, Second Edition. Jacques Malet, Francis Mora and Philippe Bouchard.
© 2018 John Wiley & Sons Ltd. Published 2018 by John Wiley & Sons Ltd.
Companion website: www.wiley.com/go/malet/implant

Appendix H: Postoperative instructions

Do not drive on the day of surgery or while taking narcotic pain medication.

Medications

• <u>Do not stop your regular medications</u> prescribed by your physician (for diabetes, high blood pressure, etc.) unless advised to do otherwise.

• <u>Take the medications that have been prescribed</u> by the surgeon (painkillers, antibiotics, etc.), and respect the drug dosage.

Pain

• <u>Pain will be most severe within the first 6–8 hours after the operation.</u> Moderate pain usually does not last longer than 48 hours, and mild discomfort usually diminishes after the third day.

• If the pain seems beyond your tolerance, please call the office.

Healing

• DO NOT DISTURB THE AREA OF SURGERY.
• <u>Do not chew on the surgical area for 10 days.</u>
• <u>Do not brush on the surgical area until the day after surgery.</u>
• Avoid checking the implant with your tongue.
• Smokers must refrain from smoking during healing. <u>Try to avoid smoking completely,</u> for at least 4 days after surgery.

Bleeding

• Minor bleeding or oozing from the operative site is expected. Thus, during the few hours after the surgery, your saliva may be red.

• The best thing for bleeding control is pressure. You can wrap a moistened tea bag (a good blood-clotting agent) in a <u>gauze sponge and gently bite on it</u>. This minor bleeding may continue throughout the first day. Renew the gauze every 30–45 minutes until cessation of bleeding.

• <u>Do not rinse your mouth on the day of the surgery.</u>
• <u>Do not spit.</u> Wipe your mouth with a tissue.

Swelling and bruising

• Mild swelling usually develops, if it does occur, during the first 24–48 hours following surgery. It should begin to subside by the third day.

• Some blue/yellow marks (bruising) may rarely appear on the skin of the face during the first few days after surgery. They will slowly disappear within a week. It is unesthetic but does not jeopardize the outcome of the surgery.

• <u>Swelling and bruising can be minimized a great deal by using an ice pack</u> on the sides of your face, 10 minutes on and 10 minutes off, as often as possible during the first day following the surgery.

Rest

• <u>Limit physical activity</u> during the first 24–48 hours after surgery and avoid strenuous exercise for 1 week. Overexertion may lead to postoperative bleeding and discomfort.

• When you lie down, keep your head elevated on a pillow. You may wish to place a towel on your pillowcase to avoid staining from any blood-tainted saliva.

Diet

• <u>Drink plenty of fluids:</u> cold water, soda, tea or juices are suitable.
• Avoid hot liquids.
• Do not use a straw for 1 week.
• Do not drink alcoholic beverages while taking prescription medication.
• <u>Eat soft, cool foods.</u> They are most easily tolerated. Eating prevents nausea.
• Yogurt with active cultures or acidophilus should be taken while on antibiotics, if applicable, to prevent diarrhea.

Oral hygiene

• <u>You need to brush the area after the first 24 hours</u> with a very soft toothbrush. Be gentle on the stitches. The tooth brushing on the surgical area must be painless. If this is not the case, delay the brushing 1 day more.
• Do not use a syringe or Water Pik®.
• Do not rinse forcefully.

Denture or nightguard

• If you wear a denture or a nightguard, follow the instruction of your surgeon to set the right time for its reinsertion. Insertion of removable dentures too early may jeopardize a successful healing process.
• You can wear your denture or nightguard from . . . .

Special Procedures

Special procedures may imply a longer postoperative period, and require special attention in addition to the above recommendations.

Bone grafting

You may find some small granules in your mouth for the first several days. This will not jeopardize the outcome of the surgery.

Sinus grafting

ANYTHING THAT CAUSES PRESSURE IN YOUR NASAL CAVITY MUST BE AVOIDED.
• Do not blow your nose.
• If you must sneeze, do so with your mouth open.
• Scuba diving, flying in pressurized aircraft, playing a wind instrument, blowing up balloons should be avoided.
• You may have some bleeding from the nose. This is not uncommon and should pass quickly. Lie down with your head back, and place cotton in the nostril that is bleeding.

Implant Dentistry at a Glance, Second Edition. Jacques Malet, Francis Mora and Philippe Bouchard.
© 2018 John Wiley & Sons Ltd. Published 2018 by John Wiley & Sons Ltd.
Companion website: www.wiley.com/go/malet/implant

Next appointment

Your next appointment is scheduled on . . . .
for suture removal (if applicable) and postoperative evaluation.

Emergency Calls

If bleeding persists or is active; if swelling and/or bruising are excessive or do not decrease; if you have any postoperative problem or additional question, call the following phone number . . . .

Appendix I: Treatment planning: fully edentulous patient

Table I.1 Prosthetic options according the number of implant, placed in the mandible

Number of implants	Removable option			
	Prosthetic design	Attachment system	Retention	Number of replaced teeth
2	Overdenture	Ball/bar/magnet	Friction/clip/magnetism	All
4	Overdenture	Bar	Clip	All
5	Overdenture	Bar	Clip	All
6	NA	NA	NA	NA
8	NA	NA	NA	NA

Number of implants	Fixed option			
	Prosthetic design	Attachment system	Retention	Number of replaced teeth
2	NA	NA	NA	NA
4	Denture design (tilted implants)	Metal framework	Screw	10
5	Denture design (parallel implants)	Metal framework	Screw	10 to 12
6	Denture/bridge design	Metal framework/ porcelain-fused-to-metal	Screw/screw or cement	10 to 14
8	Bridge design	Porcelain-fused-to-metal	Screw or cement	14

Table I.2 Prosthetic options according the number of implants placed in the maxilla

Number of implants	Removable option			
	Prosthetic design	Attachment system	Retention	Number of replaced teeth
4	Overdenture	Bar	Clips/spring pins/ others	All
6	Overdenture	Bar	Clips/spring pins/ others	All
8 to 10	NA	NA	NA	NA

Number of implants	Fixed option			
	Prosthetic design	Attachment system	Retention	Number of replaced teeth
4	Denture design (tilted implants)	Metal framework	Screw	10
6	Denture/bridge design	Metal framework/ porcelain-fused-to-metal	Screw/screw or cement	10 to 12
8 to 10	Bridge design	Porcelain-fused-to-metal	Screw or cement	12 to 14

Implant Dentistry at a Glance, Second Edition. Jacques Malet, Francis Mora and Philippe Bouchard.
© 2018 John Wiley & Sons Ltd. Published 2018 by John Wiley & Sons Ltd.
Companion website: www.wiley.com/go/malet/implant

Table I.3 Advantages/disadvantages of removable overdentures over fixed prosthesis

- **Advantages**
  - Fewer implants
  - Fewer surgical augmentation procedures
  - Easier management of esthetics
  - Easier provisional phase
  - Easier oral hygiene maintenance
  - Easier repair
  - Allow for easier changes to other types of reconstruction
  - Immediate lower costs

- **Disadvantages**
  - Removability
    - May not correspond to patient's expectation
  - Higher space for prosthetic components
    - Specially with bars at the maxilla
  - Demanding professional maintenance requirement
    - Attachments replacement
    - Relines
    - Overdenture replacement due to the wear
  - Long-term costs

Table I.4 Advantages and disadvantages of fixed denture design restorations versus fixed bridge design restorations

	Denture design	Bridge design	
	Screw-retained	Screw-retained	Cement-retained
Advantages	Can compensate the volume of bone resorption	Allow porcelain-fused-to-metal restoration	Allow porcelain-fused-to-metal restoration
	Can be removed for professional maintenance	Can be removed for professional maintenance	Allow the replacement of all teeth with a minimum of 8 implants
	Lower cost	Allow the replacement of all teeth with a minimum of 8 implants	Possible psychological advantage
Disadvantages	Possible psychological disadvantage	Cannot compensate the volume of bone resorption	Cannot compensate the volume of bone resorption
		High cost	Cannot be removed for professional maintenance
			High cost

Appendix J: Overdenture supported by two implants: surgical procedure

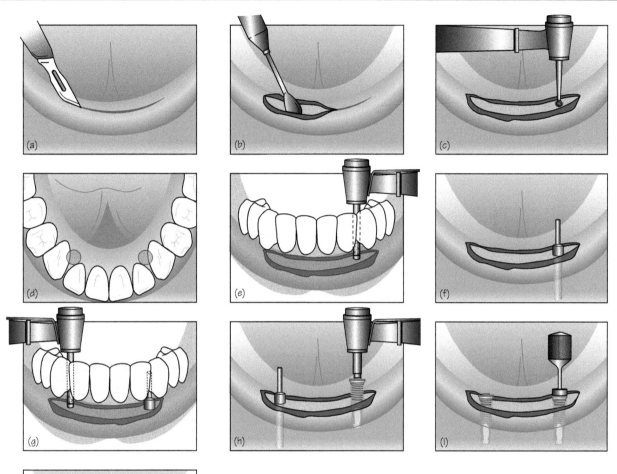

Figure J.1 Standard one step procedure. (a) Midcrestal incision, ending distally to the implant position, with or without 2 small releasing incisions. (b) Buccal and lingual full-thickness flap. (c) Osseous recontouring, if applicable, to obtain a wide and flat ridge. (d) The surgical guide is placed. Implants need to be placed slightly lingual. (e) Implant bed is drilled through the surgical guide. (f) A guide pin is inserted to ensure the parallelism of the second implant. (G) The second implant bed is drilled through the surgical guide. (h) The first implant is placed, leaving the guide pin inserted in the other implant bed. (i) Healing abutments are placed 1 mm to 2 mm above the final flap position. (j) The flap is secured using a vertical mattress or interrupted suturing technique

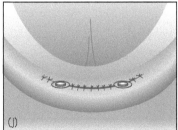

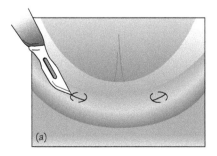

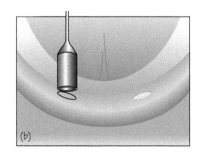

Figure J.2 Two stage procedure: uncovering techniques. Minimally invasive approaches: (a) Flapless technique. (b) Punch technique

Implant Dentistry at a Glance, Second Edition. Jacques Malet, Francis Mora and Philippe Bouchard.
© 2018 John Wiley & Sons Ltd. Published 2018 by John Wiley & Sons Ltd.
Companion website: www.wiley.com/go/malet/implant

Appendix K: Overdenture supported by two implants: prosthetic procedure

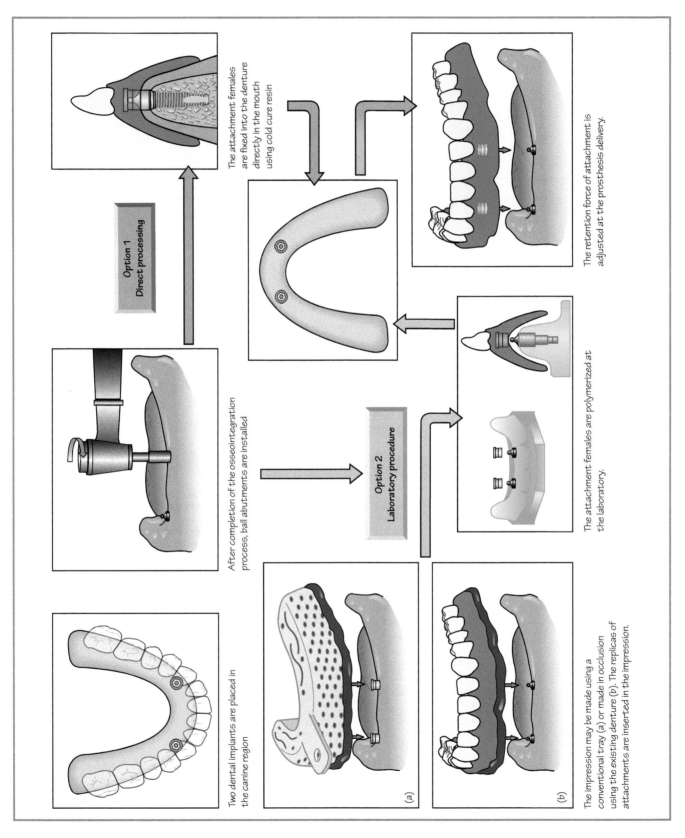

The attachment females are fixed into the denture directly in the mouth using cold cure resin

Option 1
Direct processing

The retention force of attachment is adjusted at the prosthesis delivery.

After completion of the osseointegration process, ball abutments are installed

The attachment females are polymerized at the laboratory.

Option 2
Laboratory procedure

Two dental implants are placed in the canine region

The impression may be made using a conventional tray (a) or made in occlusion using the existing denture (b). The replicas of attachments are inserted in the impression.

(a)

(b)

Implant Dentistry at a Glance, Second Edition. Jacques Malet, Francis Mora and Philippe Bouchard.
© 2018 John Wiley & Sons Ltd. Published 2018 by John Wiley & Sons Ltd.
Companion website: www.wiley.com/go/malet/implant

Appendix L: Fixed prosthesis (mandible) supported by four implants

Surgical procedure

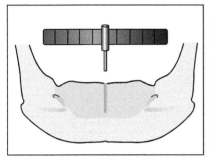

(a) after mucoperiosteal flap elevation, an osteotomy is drilled (10x2mm) in the midline and a pliant guide is placed.

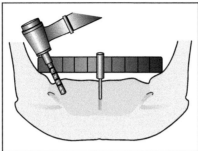

(b) after indentification of the mental foraminae, 2 posterior implant beds are prepared (15x2mm; 50 Ncm) and tilted to a maximum angle of 45°. Angulated abutments (30°) are tightened (15 Ncm).

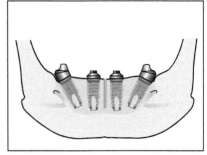

(c) after placement of the 2 posterior implants (15x4mm), 2 parallel anterior implants (10x4mm) are placed. Straight abutments are tightened (15 Ncm).

Prosthetic procedure
Immediate loading

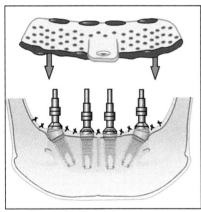

(d) An impression is taken using silicone soft putty material.

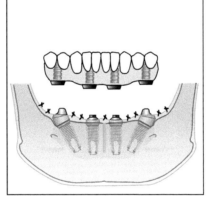

(e) After the laboratory procedure, the all-acrylic provisional restoration is placed in the patient's mouth.

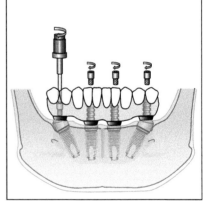

(f) The provisional restoration is connected to the abutments and the occlusion is checked.

Implant Dentistry at a Glance, Second Edition. Jacques Malet, Francis Mora and Philippe Bouchard.
© 2018 John Wiley & Sons Ltd. Published 2018 by John Wiley & Sons Ltd.
Companion website: www.wiley.com/go/malet/implant

Appendix M: Fixed prosthesis (maxilla) supported by four implants

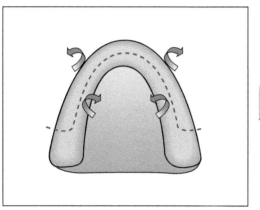

(a) One horizonal incision is made on the crest and two releasing incisions are made distally. Buccal and palatal mucoperiosteal flaps are elevated.

Surgical procedure

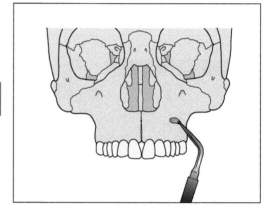

(b) The anterior wall of the maxillary sinus is explored with a periodontal probe through a small opening drilled on the lateral wall of the maxilla.

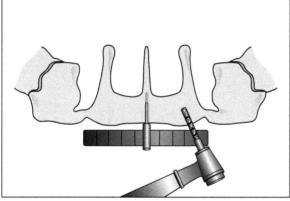

(c) The guide is placed in the midline and 2 posterior implant beds are prepared (15x2mm; 50 Ncm) 4 to 5 mm along the sinus wall and tilted to a maximum angle of 45˚. Angulated abutments (30˚) are tightened (15 Ncm).

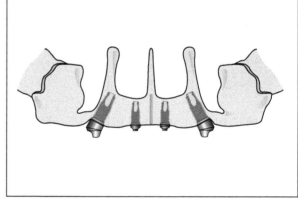

(d) After placement of the 2 posterior implants (15x4mm), 2 parallel anterior implants (10x4mm) are placed at the central/lateral incisor sites. Straight abutments are tightened (15 Ncm).

Implant Dentistry at a Glance, Second Edition. Jacques Malet, Francis Mora and Philippe Bouchard.
© 2018 John Wiley & Sons Ltd. Published 2018 by John Wiley & Sons Ltd.
Companion website: www.wiley.com/go/malet/implant

Appendix N: Overview of the digital implant dentistry

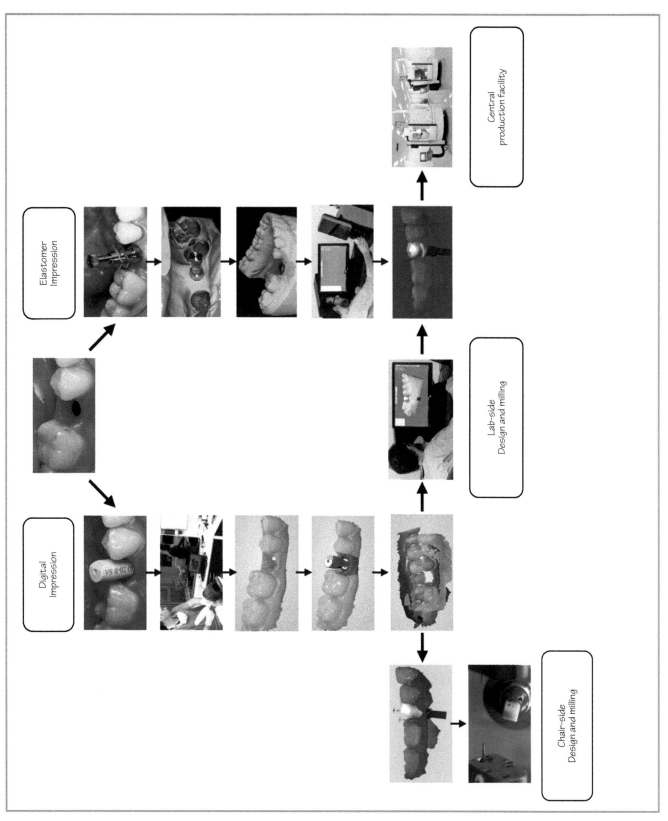

Implant Dentistry at a Glance, Second Edition. Jacques Malet, Francis Mora and Philippe Bouchard.
© 2018 John Wiley & Sons Ltd. Published 2018 by John Wiley & Sons Ltd.
Companion website: www.wiley.com/go/malet/implant

Appendix O: The double scanning method

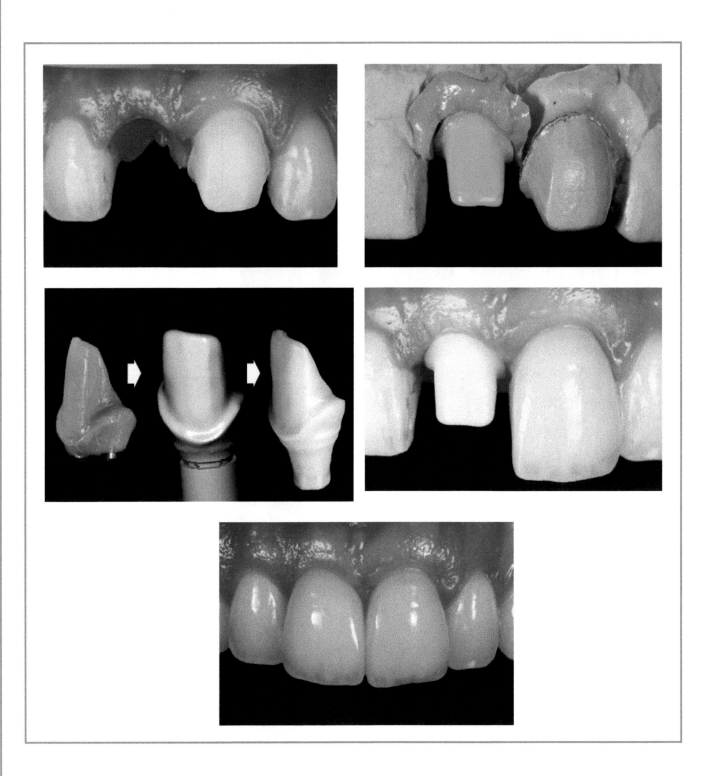

Implant Dentistry at a Glance, Second Edition. Jacques Malet, Francis Mora and Philippe Bouchard.
© 2018 John Wiley & Sons Ltd. Published 2018 by John Wiley & Sons Ltd.
Companion website: www.wiley.com/go/malet/implant

Appendix P: The virtual modelling method

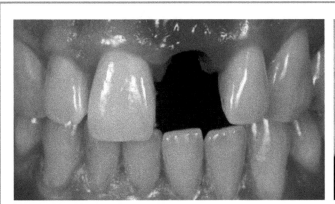
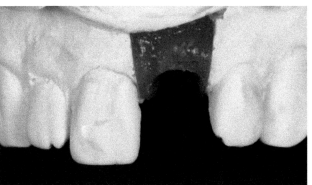

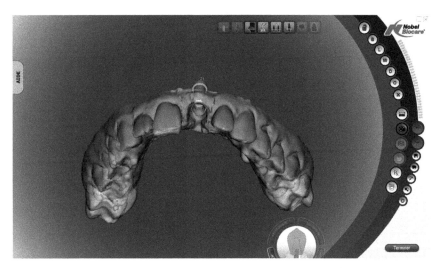

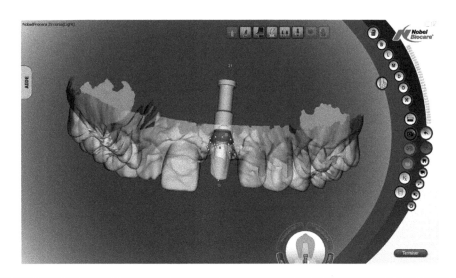

Implant Dentistry at a Glance, Second Edition. Jacques Malet, Francis Mora and Philippe Bouchard.
© 2018 John Wiley & Sons Ltd. Published 2018 by John Wiley & Sons Ltd.
Companion website: www.wiley.com/go/malet/implant

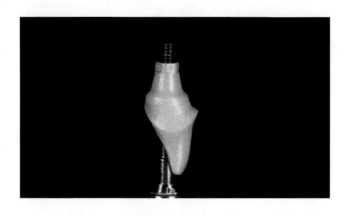

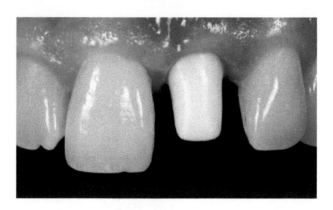

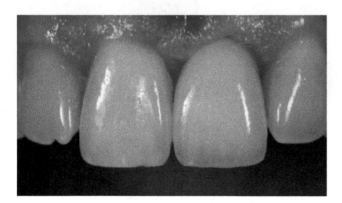

Appendix Q: Guided bone regeneration

Box Q.1 Clinical recommendations for the GBR technique

- Prerequisites
  - Low plaque index (<20%)
  - No infection at the defect site
- Strict observance of the basic principles of open flap debridement (OFD)
- Perforations in the bony surface of the defect
- Space between the inner portion of the membrane and the defect
  - May be filled by the blood clot alone
    - Use non-resorbable space-maintaining membranes only
  - May be filled by bone substitute (large or non-naturally space-making defects)
    - Resorbable non-space-maintaining membranes can be used
- Complete coverage of the defect area with the membrane
- Lack of contamination of the membrane
  - Avoid contact with the saliva
  - Minimise handling
- Complete coverage of the defect area with the membrane
  - The membrane must extend by at least 3 mm beyond the defect margins
- Stabilisation of the membrane
  - Fixation screws or pins may be used (large defects)
- Complete soft tissue coverage
  - Membrane completely submerged beneath the flap
  - Tension-free primary wound closure
- Strict oral hygiene maintenance plan

Box Q.2 Postoperative management of membrane exposure

DO NOT CLOSE THE OPENING SURGICALLY
- Exposure without infection
  - Topical application of an antiseptic gel (chlorhexidine) at least three times daily using a cotton swab or an applicator
  - Increase antibacterial rinsing protocol
  - Patient recall weekly
  - Membrane removal after at least four weeks[1] if the exposure is getting larger over time
- Exposure with infection (pus)
  - Immediate removal of the membrane
  - Antibiotic regimen

Note: 1. Membrane barriers should remain in place for at least four weeks to avoid compromising the regenerative process.

Figure Q.1 Time difference between the staged and the combined approach

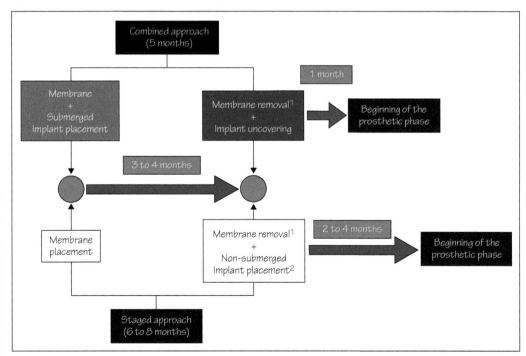

[1] Only for non-resorbable membranes; [2] a submerged implant requires an additional month.

Implant Dentistry at a Glance, Second Edition. Jacques Malet, Francis Mora and Philippe Bouchard.
© 2018 John Wiley & Sons Ltd. Published 2018 by John Wiley & Sons Ltd.
Companion website: www.wiley.com/go/malet/implant

References and further reading

Preface

Lang, N.P., Lindhe, J. and Karring, T (eds) (2008) *Clinical Periodontology and Implant Dentistry*, 5th edn, Blackwell, Oxford.

Chapter 1

Abuzar, M.A., Humplik, A.J. and Shahim N. (2015) The shortened dental arch concept: Awareness and opinion of dentists in Victoria, Australia. *Aust. Dent. J.*, **60** (3), 294–300.

Adolph, M., Darnaud, C., Thomas, F. *et al.* (2017) Oral health in relation to all-cause mortality: The IPC cohort study. *Sci. Rep.*, **7**, 44604.

Angkaew, C., Serichetaphongse, P., Krisdapong, S. *et al.* (2016) Oral health-related quality of life and esthetic outcome in single anterior maxillary implants. *Clin. Oral. Implants Res.*, **28** (9), 1089–1096.

Antunes, J.L., Tan, H., Peres, K.G. and Peres, M.A. (2016) Impact of shortened dental arches on oral health-related quality of life. *J. Oral. Rehabil.*, **43** (3), 190–197.

Becker, W., Hujoel, P., Becker, B.E. and Wohrle, P. (2016) Dental implants in an aged population: Evaluation of periodontal health, bone loss, implant survival, and quality of life. *Clin. Implant. Dent. Relat. Res.*, **18** (3), 473–479.

Bouchard, P., Renouard, F., Bourgeois, D. *et al.* (2009) Cost-effectiveness modeling of dental implant vs. bridge. *Clin. Oral Implants Res.*, **20** (6), 583–587.

Boven, G.C., Raghoebar, G.M., Vissink, A. and Meijer, H.J. (2015) Improving masticatory performance, bite force, nutritional state and patient's satisfaction with implant overdentures: A systematic review of the literature. *J. Oral Rehabil.*, **42** (3), 220–233.

Brennan, M., Houston, F., O'Sullivan, M. and O'Connell, B. (2010) Patient satisfaction and oral health-related quality of life outcomes of implant overdentures and fixed complete dentures. *Int. J. Oral Maxillofac. Implants*, **25** (4), 791–800.

Broder, H.L. and Wilson-Genderson, M. (2007) Reliability and convergent and discriminant validity of the Child Oral Health Impact Profile (COHIP Child's version). *Community Dent. Oral Epidemiol.*, **35** (Suppl. 1), 20–31.

CDC (2000) Measuring Healthy Days: Population Assessment of Health-Related Quality of Life. November. Centers for Disease Control and Prevention, Atlanta, GA.

Darnaud, C., Thomas, F., Pannier, B. *et al.* (2015) Oral health and blood pressure: The IPC cohort. *Am. J. Hypertens.*, **28** (10), 1257–1261.

El Osta, N., Hennequin, M., Tubert-Jeannin, S. *et al.* (2014) The pertinence of oral health indicators in nutritional studies in the elderly. *Clin. Nutr.*, **33** (2), 316–321.

Esfandiari, S., Lund, J.P., Penrod, J.R. *et al.* (2009) Implant overdentures for edentulous elders: Study of patient preference. *Gerodontology* **26** (1), 3–10.

Feine, J.S., Carlsson, G.E., Awad, M.A. *et al.* (2002) The McGill consensus statement on overdentures. Mandibular two-implant overdentures as first choice standard of care for edentulous patients. Montreal, Quebec, May 24–25, 2002. *Int. J. Oral Maxillofac. Implants*, **17** (4), 601–602.

Godlewski, A.E., Veyrune, J.L., Nicolas, E. *et al.* (2011) Effect of dental status on changes in mastication in patients with obesity following bariatric surgery. *PLoS One*, **6** (7), e22324.

Hennequin, M., Allison, P.J., Veyrune, J.L. *et al.* (2005) Clinical evaluation of mastication: Validation of video versus electromyography. *Clin. Nutr.*, **24** (2), 314–320.

Jensen, P.M., Saunders, R.L., Thierer, T. and Friedman, B. (2008) Factors associated with oral health-related quality of life in community-dwelling elderly persons with disabilities. *J. Am. Geriatr. Soc.*, **56** (4), 711–717.

Klages, U., Bruckner, A. and Zentner, A. (2004) Dental aesthetics, self-awareness, and oral health-related quality of life in young adults. *Eur. J. Orthod.*, **26** (5), 507–514.

Leung, K.C. and McGrath, C.P. (2010) Willingness to pay for implant therapy: A study of patient preference. *Clin. Oral Implants Res.*, **21** (8), 789–793.

Moreira, N.C., Krausch-Hofmann, S., Matthys, C. *et al.* (2016) Risk factors for malnutrition in older adults: A systematic review of the literature based on longitudinal data. *Adv. Nutr.*, **7** (3), 507–522.

Nickenig, H.J., Wichmann, M., Andreas, S.K. and Eitner, S. (2008) Oral health-related quality of life in partially edentulous patients: Assessments before and after implant therapy. *J. Craniomaxillofac. Surg.*, **36** (8), 477–480.

Pavel, K., Seydlova, M., Dostalova, T. *et al.* (2012) Dental implants and improvement of oral health-related quality of life. *Community Dent. Oral Epidemiol.*, **40** (Suppl. 1), 65–70.

Petersen, P.E. and Yamamoto, T. (2005) Improving the oral health of older people: The approach of the WHO Global Oral Health Programme. *Community Dent. Oral Epidemiol.*, **33** (2), 81–92.

Pisetkul, C., Chanchairujira, K., Chotipanvittayakul, N. *et al.* (2010) Malnutrition-inflammation score associated with atherosclerosis, inflammation and short-term outcome in hemodialysis patients. *J. Med. Assoc. Thai.*, **93** (Suppl. 1), S147–S156.

Tan, H., Peres, K.G. and Peres, M.A. (2015) Do people with shortened dental arches have worse oral health-related quality of life than those with more natural teeth? A population-based study. *Community Dent. Oral Epidemiol.*, **43** (1), 33–46.

Tan, H., Peres, K.G. and Peres, M.A. (2016) Retention of teeth and oral health-related quality of life. *J. Dent. Res.*, **95** (12), 1350–1357.

Thomason, J.M., Feine, J., Exley, C. *et al.* (2009) Mandibular two implant-supported overdentures as the first choice standard of care for edentulous patients – the York Consensus Statement. *Br. Dent. J.*, **207** (4), 185–186.

Vogel, R., Smith-Palmer, J. and Valentine, W. (2013) Evaluating the health economic implications and cost-effectiveness of dental implants: A literature review. *Int. J. Oral Maxillofac. Implants*, **28** (2), 343–356.

von der Gracht, I., Derks, A., Haselhuhn, K. and Wolfart, S. (2016) EMG correlations of edentulous patients with implant overdentures and fixed dental prostheses compared to conventional complete dentures and dentates: A systematic review and meta-analysis. *Clin. Oral Implants Res.*, **28** (7), 765–773.

WHO (1946) Constitution of the World Health Organization. *Official Records of the World Health Organization*, **2**, 100–122.

WHO (1997) WHOQOL Measuring Quality of Life. WHO (MNH/PSF/97.4). World Health Organization, Geneva.

WHO (2017) Health topics: Nutrition. http://www.who.int/topics/nutrition/en/ (accessed 10 November 2017).

Implant Dentistry at a Glance, Second Edition. Jacques Malet, Francis Mora and Philippe Bouchard.
© 2018 John Wiley & Sons Ltd. Published 2018 by John Wiley & Sons Ltd.
Companion website: www.wiley.com/go/malet/implant

Witter, D.J., van Palenstein Helderman, W.H., Creugers, N.H. and Kayser, A.F. (1999) The shortened dental arch concept and its implications for oral health care. *Community Dent. Oral Epidemiol.*, **27** (4), 249–258.

Woda, A., Nicolas, E., Mishellany-Dutour, A. *et al.* (2010) The masticatory normative indicator. *J. Dent. Res.*, **89** (3), 281–285.

Wood, A.D., Strachan, A.A., Thies, F. *et al.* (2014) Patterns of dietary intake and serum carotenoid and tocopherol status are associated with biomarkers of chronic low-grade systemic inflammation and cardiovascular risk. *Br. J. Nutr.*, **112** (8), 1341–1352.

Chapter 2

Abrahamsson, I., Berglundh, T., Linder, E. et al. (2004) Early bone formation adjacent to rough and turned endosseous implant surfaces: An experimental study in the dog. *Clin. Oral Implants Res.*, **15** (4), 381–392.

Berglundh, T., Abrahamson, I., Lang, N.P. and Lindhe, J. (2003) De novo alveolar bone formation adjacent to endosseous implants: A model study in the dog. *Clin. Oral Implants Res.*, **14** (3), 251–262.

Berglundh, T., Abrahamsson, I. and Lindhe, J. (2005) Bone reactions to longstanding functional load at implants: An experimental study in dogs. *J. Clin. Periodontol.*, **32** (9), 925–932.

Further reading

Lindhe, J., Berglundh, T. and Lang, N.P. (2008) Osseointegration, in *Clinical Periodontology and Implant Dentistry*, 5th edn (eds N.P. Lang, J. Lindhe and T. Karring), Blackwell, Oxford, pp. 99–107.

Chapter 3
Further reading

Berglundh, T. (1999) Soft tissue interface and response to microbial challenge, in *Implant Dentistry: Proceedings of the Third European Workshop on Periodontology* (eds N.P. Lang, J. Lindhe and T. Karring), Quintessence, Berlin, pp. 153–174.

Lindhe, J., Wennström, J.L. and Berglundh, T. (2008) The mucosa at teeth and implants, in *Clinical Periodontology and Implant Dentistry*, 5th edn (eds N.P. Lang, J. Lindhe and T. Karring), Blackwell, Oxford, pp. 69–85.

Chapter 4
Further reading

Greenstein, G. and D. Tarnow (2006) The mental foramen and nerve: Clinical and anatomical factors related to dental implant placement: A literature review. *J. Periodontol.*, **77** (12), 1933–1943.

Chapter 5
Further reading

Greenstein, G., Cavallaro, J., Romanos, G. and Tarnow, D. (2008) Clinical recommendations for avoiding and managing surgical complications associated with implant dentistry: A review. *J. Periodontol.*, **79** (8), 1317–1329.

Chapter 6

Lekholm, U. and Zarb, G.A. (1985) Patient selection, in *Tissue Integrated Prostheses: Osseointegration in Clinical Dentistry* (eds P.I. Bränemark, G.A. Zarb and T. Albrektsson), Quintessence, Chicago, IL, pp. 199–209.

Wolff, J. (1986) *The Law of Bone Remodeling*, Springer, New York (translation of German 1892 edn).

Further reading

Ericsson, J., Randow, K., Glantz, P.O. *et al.* (1994) Some clinical and radiographic features of submerged and non-submerged titanium implants. *Clin. Oral Implants Res.*, **5** (3), 185–189.

Esposito, M., Hirsch, J.M., Lekholm, U. and Tomsen, P. (1998) Biological factors contributing to failures of osseointegrated oral implant (II): Etiopathogenesis. *Eur. J. Oral Sci.*, **106** (3), 721–764.

Quirynen, M. and Lekholm, U. (2008) The surgical site, in *Clinical Periodontology and Implant Dentistry*, 5th edn (eds N.P. Lang, J. Lindhe and T. Karring), Blackwell, Oxford, pp. 1068–1079.

Rangert, B., Jemt, T. and Jorneus, L. (1989) Forces and moments on Brånemark implants. *Int. J. Oral Maxillofac. Implants*, **4** (3), 241–247.

Chapter 7

Abuhussein, H., Pagni, G., Rebaudi, A. and Wang, H.L. (2010) The effect of thread pattern upon implant osseointegration. *Clin. Oral Implants Res.*, **21** (2), 129–136.

Esposito, M. (2007) Interventions for replacing missing teeth: Different types of dental implants (Review). *Cochrane Database Syst. Rev.*, **4**, CD003815.

Lang, N., Tonetti, M., Suvan, J. *et al.* (2007) Immediate implant placement with transmucosal healing in areas of aesthetic priority: A multicentre randomized-controlled clinical trial I. Surgical outcomes. *Clin. Oral Implants Res.*, **18** (2), 188–196.

Steigenga, J., Al-Shammari, K., Misch, C. *et al.* (2004) Effects of implant thread geometry on percentage of osseointegration and resistance to reverse torque in the tibia of rabbits. *J. Periodontol.*, **75** (9), 1233–1241.

Further reading

Renouard, F. and Nisand, D. (2006) Impact of implant length and diameter on survival rates. *Clin. Oral Implants Res.*, **17** (Suppl. 2), 35–51.

Chapter 8

Fan, T., Li, Y., Deng, W.W. *et al.* (2017) Short implants (5 to 8 mm) versus longer implants (>8 mm) with sinus lifting in atrophic posterior maxilla: A meta-analysis of RCTs. *Clin. Implant Dent. Relat. Res.* **19** (1), 207–215.

Garaicoa-Pazmino, C., Suarez-Lopez del Amo, F., Monje, A. *et al.* (2014) Influence of crown/implant ratio on marginal bone loss: A systematic review. *J. Periodontol.* **85** (9), 1214–1221.

Javed, F., Ahmed, H.B., Crespi, R. *et al.* (2013) Role of primary stability for successful osseointegration of dental implants: Factors of influence and evaluation. *Interv. Med. Appl. Sci.*, **5** (4), 162–167.

Monje, A., Suarez, F., Galindo-Moreno, P. *et al.* (2014) A systematic review on marginal bone loss around short dental implants (<10 mm) for implant-supported fixed prostheses. *Clin. Oral Implants Res.*, **25** (10), 1119–1124.

Nisand, D. and Renouard, F. (2014) Short implant in limited bone volume. *Periodontol. 2000*, **66** (1), 72–96.

Telleman, G., Raghoebar, G.M., Vissink, A. *et al.* (2011) A systematic review of the prognosis of short (<10 mm) dental implants placed in the partially edentulous patient. *J. Clin. Periodontol.*, **38** (7), 667–676.

Thoma, D.S., Zeltner, M., Husler, J. *et al.* (2015) EAO Supplement Working Group 4 – EAO CC 2015. Short implants versus sinus lifting with longer implants to restore the posterior maxilla: A systematic review. *Clin. Oral Implants Res.*, **26** (Suppl. 11), 154–169.

Chapter 9

Antoszewska-Smith, J., Sarul, M., Lyczek, J. *et al.* (2017) Effectiveness of orthodontic miniscrew implants in anchorage reinforcement during en-masse retraction: A systematic review and meta-analysis. *Am. J. Orthod. Dentofacial Orthop.*, **151** (3), 440–455.

Bidra, A.S. and Almas, K. (2013) Mini implants for definitive prosthodontic treatment: A systematic review. *J. Prosthet. Dent.*, **109** (3), 156–164.

Chen, Y.J., Chang, H.H., Huang, C.Y. *et al.* (2007) A retrospective analysis of the failure rate of three different orthodontic skeletal anchorage systems. *Clin. Oral Implants Res.*, **18** (6), 768–775.

Lambert, F., Botilde, G., Lecloux, G. *et al.* (2016) Effectiveness of temporary implants in teenage patients: A prospective clinical trial. *Clin. Oral Implants Res.*, **28** (9), 1152–1157.

Lemos, C.A., Verri, F.R., Batista, V.E. *et al.* (2017) Complete overdentures retained by mini implants: A systematic review. *J. Dent.*, **57**, 4–13.

Melsen, B. and Costa, A. (2000) Immediate loading of implants used for orthodontic anchorage. *Clin. Orthod. Res.*, **3** (1), 23–28.

Reynders, R., Ronchi, L. and Bipat, S. (2009) Mini-implants in orthodontics: A systematic review of the literature. *Am. J. Orthod. Dentofacial Orthop.*, **135** (5), 564.e1–19; discussion 564–565.

Watanabe, H., Deguchi, T., Hasegawa, M. *et al.* (2013) Orthodontic miniscrew failure rate and root proximity, insertion angle, bone contact length, and bone density. *Orthod. Craniofac. Res.*, **16** (1), 44–55.

Zygogiannis, K., Wismeijer, D. and Parsa, A. (2016) A pilot study on mandibular overdentures retained by mini dental implants: Marginal bone level changes and patient-based ratings of clinical outcome. *Int. J. Oral Maxillofac. Implants*, **31** (5), 1171–1178.

Chapter 10

Crespi, R., Cappare, P. and Gherlone, E. (2009) Radiographic evaluation of marginal bone levels around platform-switched and non-platform-switched implants used in an immediate loading protocol. *Int. J. Oral Maxillofac. Implants*, **24** (5), 920–926.

Hansson, S. (2003) A conical implant-abutment interface at the level of the marginal bone improves the distribution of stresses in the supporting bone: An axisymmetric finite element analysis. *Clin. Oral Implants Res.*, **14** (3), 286–293.

Piermatti, J., Yousef, H., Luke, A. *et al.* (2006) An in vitro analysis of implant screw torque loss with external hex and internal connection implant systems. *Implant Dent.*, **15** (4), 427–435.

Chapter 11

Jarmar, T., Palmquist, A., Brånemark, R. *et al.* (2008) Characterization of the surface properties of commercially available dental implants using scanning electron microscopy, focused ion beam and high resolution transmission electron microscopy. *Clin. Implant Dent. Relat. Res.*, **10** (1), 11–22.

Wennerberg, A. and Albrektsson, T. (2010) On implant surfaces: A review of current knowledge and opinions. *Int. J. Oral Maxillofac. Implants*, **25** (1), 63–74.

Further reading

Albrektsson, T. and Wennerberg, A. (2004) Oral implant surfaces. Part 1: Review focusing on topographic and chemical properties of different surfaces and in vivo responses to them. *Int. J. Prosth. Dent.*, **17** (5), 536–543.

Albrektsson, T. and Wennerberg, A. (2004) Oral implant surfaces. Part 2: Review focusing on clinical knowledge of different surfaces. *Int. J. Prosth. Dent.*, **17** (5), 544–564.

Albrektsson, T., Zarb, G., Woorthington, P. and Eriksson, R.A. (1986) The long-term efficacy of currently used dental implants: A review and proposed criteria of success. *Int. J. Oral Maxillofac. Implants*, **1** (1), 11–25.

Chapter 12

Cionca, N., Hashim, D. and Mombelli, A. (2017) Zirconia dental implants: Where are we now, and where are we heading? *Periodontol. 2000*, **73** (1), 241–258.

Sennerby, L., Rocci, A., Becker, W. *et al.* (2008) Short-term clinical results of Nobel Direct implants: A retrospective multicenter analysis. *Clin. Oral Implants Res.*, **19** (3), 219–226.

Chapter 13

Bornstein, M.M., Schmid, B., Belser, U.C. *et al.* (2005) Early loading of non-submerged titanium implants with a sandblasted and acid-etched surface: 5-year results of a prospective study in partially edentulous patients. *Clin. Oral Implants Res.*, **16** (6), 631–638.

Cionca, N., Hashim, D. and Mombelli, A. (2017) Zirconia dental implants: Where are we now, and where are we heading? *Periodontol. 2000*, **73** (1), 241–258.

De Bruyn, H., Raes, S., Ostman, P.O. and Cosyn, J. (2014) Immediate loading in partially and completely edentulous jaws: A review of the literature with clinical guidelines. *Periodontol. 2000*, **66** (1), 153–187.

Karl, M. and Taylor, T.D. (2016) Effect of cyclic loading on micromotion at the implant-abutment interface. *Int. J. Oral Maxillofac. Implants*, **31** (6), 1292–1297.

Klein, M.O., Schiegnitz, E. and Al-Nawas, B. (2014) Systematic review on success of narrow-diameter dental implants. *Int. J. Oral Maxillofac. Implants*, **29** (Suppl.), 43–54.

Koodaryan, R. and Hafezeqoran, A. (2016) Evaluation of implant collar surfaces for marginal bone loss: A systematic review and meta-analysis. *Biomed. Res. Int.*, **2016**, 4987526.

Lang, N.P., Salvi, G.E., Huynh-Ba, G. *et al.* (2011) Early osseointegration to hydrophilic and hydrophobic implant surfaces in humans. *Clin. Oral Implants Res.*, **22** (4), 349–356.

Saulacic, N., Bosshardt, D.D., Bornstein, M.M. *et al.* (2012) Bone apposition to a titanium-zirconium alloy implant, as compared to two other titanium-containing implants. *Eur. Cell Mater.*, **23**, 273–286; discussion 276–278.

Shah, F.A., Trobos, M., Thomsen, P. and Palmquist, A. (2016) Commercially pure titanium (cp-Ti) versus titanium alloy (Ti6Al4V) materials as bone anchored implants: Is one truly better than the other? *Mater. Sci. Eng. C. Mater. Biol. Appl.*, **62**, 960–966.

Smeets, R., Stadlinger, B., Schwarz, F. *et al.* (2016) Impact of dental implant surface modifications on osseointegration. *Biomed. Res. Int.*, **2016**, 6285620.

Stach, R.M. and Kohles, S.S. (2003) A meta-analysis examining the clinical survivability of machined-surfaced and osseotite implants in poor-quality bone. *Implant Dent.*, **12** (1), 87–96.

Sullivan, D., Vincenzi, G. and Feldman, S. (2005) Early loading of osseotite implants 2 months after placement in the maxilla and mandible: A 5-year report. *Int. J. Oral Maxillofac. Implants*, **20**, 905–912.

Chapter 14

Berglundh, T., Persson, L. and Klinge, B. (2002) A systematic review of the incidence of biological and technical complications in implant dentistry reported in prospective longitudinal studies of at least 5 years. *J. Clin. Periodontol.*, **29** (Suppl. 3), 197–212.

Blanes, R.J. (2009) To what extent does the crown-implant ratio affect the survival and complications of implant-supported reconstructions? A systematic review. *Clin. Oral Implants Res.*, **20** (Suppl. 4), 67–72.

Bouchard, P., Renouard, F., Bourgeois, D. *et al.* (2009) Cost-effectiveness modeling of dental implant vs. bridge. *Clin. Oral Implants Res.*, **20** (6), 583–587.

Derks, J. and Tomasi, C. (2015) Peri-implant health and disease: A systematic review of current epidemiology. *J. Clin. Periodontol.*, **42** (Suppl. 16), S158–S171.

Esposito, M., Grusovin, M.G., Achille, H. *et al.* (2009) Interventions for replacing missing teeth: Different times for loading dental implants. *Cochrane Database Syst. Rev.*, **1**, CD003878.

Lang, N.P., Berglundh, T., Heitz-Mayfield, L.J. *et al.* (2004) Consensus statements and recommended clinical procedures regarding implant survival and complications. *Int. J. Oral Maxillofac. Implants*, **19** (Suppl.), 150–154.

Lang, N.P. and Salvi, G.E. (2008) Implants in restorative dentistry, in *Clinical Periodontology and Implant Dentistry*, 5th edn (eds N.P. Lang, J. Lindhe and T. Karring), Blackwell, Oxford, pp. 1138–1145.

Moraschini, V., Poubel, L.A., Ferreira, V.F. and Barboza Edos, S. (2015) Evaluation of survival and success rates of dental implants reported in longitudinal studies with a follow-up period of at least 10 years: A systematic review. *Int. J. Oral Maxillofac. Surg.*, **44** (3), 377–388.

Papaspyridakos, P., Chen, C.J., Singh, M. *et al.* (2012) Success criteria in implant dentistry: A systematic review. *J. Dent. Res.*, **91** (3), 242–248.

Pjetursson, B.E. (2008) Systematic reviews of survival and complication rates of implant-supported fixed dental prostheses and single crowns, 14–26, in *Osseointegration and Dental Implants* (ed. A. Jokstad), Wiley-Blackwell, Oxford, p. 429.

Popelut, A., Rousval, B., Fromentin, O. *et al.* (2010a) Tooth extraction decision model in periodontitis patients. *Clin. Oral Implant Res.*, **21** (1), 80–89.

Popelut, A., Valet, F., Fromentin, O. *et al.* (2010b) Relationship between sponsorship and failure rate of dental implants: A systematic approach. *PLoS ONE*, **5** (4), e10274.

Further reading

Berglundh, T., Persson, L. and Klinge, B. (2002) A systematic review of the incidence of biological and technical complications in implant dentistry reported in prospective longitudinal studies of at least 5 years. *J. Clin. Periodontol.*, **29** (Suppl. 3), 197–212.

Karoussis, I.K., Bragger, U., Salvi, G.E. *et al.* (2004) Effect of implant design on survival and success rates of titanium oral implants: A 10-year prospective cohort study of the ITIs dental implant system. *Clin. Oral Implants Res.*, **15** (1), 8–17.

Lang, N.P., Pjetursson, B.E., Tan, K. *et al.* (2004) A systematic review of the survival and complication rates of fixed partial dentures (FPDs) after an observation period of at least 5 years. II. Combined tooth-implant-supported FPDs. *Clin. Oral Implants Res.*, **15** (6), 643–653.

Pjetursson, B.E., Tan, K., Lang, N.P. *et al.* (2004) A systematic review of the survival and complication rates of fixed partial dentures (FPDs) after an observation period of at least 5 years. *Clin. Oral Implants Res.*, **15** (6), 625–642.

Tan, K., Pjetursson, B.E., Lang, N.P. and Chan, E.S. (2004) A systematic review of the survival and complication rates of fixed partial dentures (FPDs) after an observation period of at least 5 years. *Clin. Oral Implants Res.*, **15** (6), 654–666.

Zurdo, J., Romão, C. and Wennström, J.L. (2009) Survival and complication rates of implant-supported fixed partial dentures with cantilevers: A systematic review. *Clin. Oral Implants Res.*, **20** (Suppl. 4), 59–66.

Chapter 17

Brasseur, M., Brogniez, V., Grégoire, V. *et al.* (2006) Effects of irradiation on bone remodelling around mandibular implants: An experimental study in dogs. *Int. J. Oral Maxillofac. Surg.*, **35** (9), 850–855.

Esposito, M., Grusovin, M.G., Patel, S. *et al.* (2008) Interventions for replacing missing teeth: Hyperbaric oxygen therapy for irradiated patients who require dental implants. *Cochrane Database Syst. Rev.*, **1**, CD003603.

Lazarovici, T.S., Yahalom, R., Taicher, S. *et al.* (2010) Bisphosphonate-related osteonecrosis of the jaw associated with dental implants. *J. Oral Maxillofac. Surg.*, **68** (4), 790–796.

Madrid, C. and Sanz, M. (2009) What influence do anticoagulants have on oral implant therapy? A systematic review. *Clin. Oral Implants Res.*, **20** (Suppl. 4), 96–106.

National Patient Safety Agency (2007) *Managing Patients Who Are Taking Warfarin and Undergoing Dental Treatment*. National Patient Safety Agency/British Dental Association/British Society for Haematology, London.

RPSGB/BMA (2006) *British National Formulary 52*. Royal Pharmaceutical Society of Great Britain/British Medical Association, London, pp. 24–25.

Sanz, M. and Naert, I. (2009) Biomechanics/risk management (Working Group 2). *Clin. Oral Implants Res.*, **20** (Suppl. 4), 107–111.

Further reading

Gomez-de Diego, R., Mang-de la Rosa Mdel, R., Romero-Perez, M.J. *et al.* (2014) Indications and contraindications of dental implants in medically compromised patients: Update. *Med. Oral Patol. Oral Cir. Bucal*, **19** (5), e483–e489.

Mucke, T., Krestan, C.R., Mitchell, D.A. *et al.* (2016) Bisphosphonate and medication-related osteonecrosis of the jaw: A review. *Semin. Musculoskelet. Radiol.*, **20** (3), 305–314.

Chapter 18

Bornstein, M.M., Cionca, N. and Mombelli, A. (2009) Systemic conditions and treatments as risks for implant therapy. *Int. J. Oral Maxillofac. Implants*, **24** (Suppl.), 12–27.

Chambrone, L., Preshaw, P.M., Ferreira, J.D. *et al.* (2014) Effects of tobacco smoking on the survival rate of dental implants placed in areas of maxillary sinus floor augmentation: A systematic review. *Clin. Oral Implants Res.*, **25** (4), 408–416.

Chrcanovic, B.R., Albrektsson, T. and Wennerberg, A. (2014a) Periodontally compromised vs. periodontally healthy patients and dental implants: A systematic review and meta-analysis. *J. Dent.*, **42** (12), 1509–1527.

Chrcanovic, B.R., Albrektsson, T. and Wennerberg, A. (2014b) Diabetes and oral implant failure: A systematic review. *J. Dent. Res.*, **93** (9), 859–867.

Cochran, D.L., Schou, S., Heitz-Mayfield, L.J. *et al.* (2009) Consensus statements and recommended clinical procedures regarding risk factors in implant therapy. *Int. J. Oral Maxillofac. Implants*, **24** (Suppl.), 86–89.

Ferreira, S.D., Silva, G.L., Cortelli, J.R. *et al.* (2006) Prevalence and risk variables for peri-implant disease in Brazilian subjects. *J. Clin. Periodontol.*, **33** (12), 929–935.

Heitz-Mayfield, L.J. and Huynh-Ba, G. (2009) History of treated periodontitis and smoking as risks for implant therapy. *Int. J. Oral Maxillofac. Implants*, **24** (Suppl.), 39–68.

Keenan, J.R. and Veitz-Keenan, A. (2016) The impact of smoking on failure rates, postoperative infection and marginal bone loss of dental implants. *Evid. Based Dent.*, **17** (1), 4–5.

Madrid, C. and Sanz, M. (2009) What impact do systemically administered bisphosphonates have on oral implant therapy? A systematic review. *Clin. Oral Implants Res.*, **20** (Suppl. 4), 87–95.

Monje, A., Alcoforado, G., Padial-Molina, M. *et al.* (2014) Generalized aggressive periodontitis as a risk factor for dental implant failure: A systematic review and meta-analysis. *J. Periodontol.*, **85** (10), 1398–1407.

Monje, A., Catena, A. and Borgnakke, W.S. (2017) Association between diabetes mellitus/hyperglycemia and peri-implant diseases: Systematic review and meta-analysis. *J. Clin. Periodontol.* **44** (6), 636–648.

Noda, K., Arakawa, H., Kimura-Ono, A. *et al.* (2015) A longitudinal retrospective study of the analysis of the risk factors of implant failure by the application of generalized estimating equations. *J. Prosthodont. Res.*, **59** (3), 178–184.

Renvert, S. and Polyzois, I. (2015) Risk indicators for peri-implant mucositis: A systematic literature review. *J. Clin. Periodontol.*, **42** (Suppl. 16), S172–S186.

Shi, Q., Xu, J., Huo, N. *et al.* (2016) Does a higher glycemic level lead to a higher rate of dental implant failure? A meta-analysis. *J. Am. Dent. Assoc.*, **147** (11), 875–881.

Sousa, V., Mardas, N., Farias, B. *et al.* (2016) A systematic review of implant outcomes in treated periodontitis patients. *Clin. Oral Implants Res.*, **27** (7), 787–844.

Srinivasan, M., Meyer, S., Mombelli, A. and Müller, F. (2017) Dental implants in the elderly population: A systematic review and meta-analysis. *Clin. Oral Implants Res.*, **28** (8), 920–930.

Yap, A.K. and Klineberg, I. (2009) Dental implants in patients with ectodermal dysplasia and tooth agenesis: A critical review of the literature. *Int. J. Prosthodont.*, **22** (3), 268–276.

Zangrando, M.S., Damante, C.A., Sant'Ana, A.C. *et al.* (2015) Long-term evaluation of periodontal parameters and implant outcomes in periodontally compromised patients: A systematic review. *J. Periodontol.* **86** (2), 201–221.

Further reading

Turri, A., Rossetti, P.H., Canullo, L. *et al.* (2016) Prevalence of peri-implantitis in medically compromised patients and smokers: A systematic review. *Int. J. Oral Maxillofac. Implants*, **31** (1), 111–118.

Chapter 19

Bengazi, F., Wennström, J.L. and Lekholm, U. (1996) Recession of the soft tissue margin at the oral implants: A 2 year longitudinal prospective study. *Clin. Oral Implants Res.*, **7** (4), 303–310.

Cochran, D.L., Schou, S., Heitz-Mayfield, L.J. *et al.* (2009) Consensus statements and recommended clinical procedures regarding risk factors in implant therapy. *Int. J. Oral Maxillofac. Implants*, **24** (Suppl.), 86–89.

Esposito, M., Maghaireh, H., Grusovin, M.G. *et al.* (2012) Interventions for replacing missing teeth: Management of soft tissues for dental implants. *Cochrane Database Syst. Rev.*, **2**, CD006697.

Martin, W., Lewis, E. and Nicol, A. (2009) Local risk factors for implant therapy. *Int. J. Oral Maxillofac. Implants*, **24** (Suppl.), 28–38.

Molly, L. (2006) Bone density and primary stability in implant therapy. *Clin. Oral Implants Res.*, **17** (Suppl 2), 124–135.

Chapter 20

Heitz-Mayfield, L.J. and Huynh-Ba, G. (2009) History of treated periodontitis and smoking as risks for implant therapy. *Int. J. Oral Maxillofac. Implants*, **24** (Suppl.), 39–68.

Salvi, G.E. and Bragger, U. (2009) Mechanical and technical risks in implant therapy. *Int. J. Oral Maxillofac. Implants*, **24** (Suppl.), 69–85.

Van Steenberghe, D., Lekholm, U., Bolender, C. *et al.* (1990) Applicability of osseointegrated oral implants in the rehabilitation of partial edentulism: A prospective multicenter study on 558 fixtures. *Int. J. Oral Maxillofac. Implants*, **5** (3), 272–281.

Chapter 21

Cochran, D.L., Schou, S., Heitz-Mayfield, L.J. *et al.* (2009) Consensus statements and recommended clinical procedures regarding risk factors in implant therapy. *Int. J. Oral Maxillofac. Implants*, **24** (Suppl.), 86–89.

Heitz-Mayfield, L.J. and Huynh-Ba, G. (2009) History of treated periodontitis and smoking as risks for implant therapy. *Int. J. Oral Maxillofac. Implants*, **24** (Suppl.), 39–68.

Ong, C.T.T., Ivanovski, S., Needleman, I.G. *et al.* (2008) Systematic review of implant outcomes in treated periodontitis subjects. *J. Clin. Periodontol.*, **35** (5), 438–462.

Popelut, A., Rousval, B., Fromentin, O. et al. (2010) Tooth extraction decision model in periodontitis patients. *Clin. Oral Implants Res.*, **21** (1), 80–89.

Wen, X., Liu, R., Li, G. *et al.* (2014) History of periodontitis as a risk factor for long-term survival of dental implants: A meta-analysis. *Int. J. Oral Maxillofac. Implants*, **29** (6), 1271–1280.

Chapter 22

Araújo, M. and Lindhe, J. (2005) Dimensional ridge alterations following tooth extraction: An experimental study in the dog. *J. Clin. Periodontol.*, **32** (2), 212–218.

Buser, D., Martin, W. and Belser, U.C. (2004) Optimizing esthetics for implant restorations in the anterior maxilla: Anatomic and surgical considerations. *Int. J. Oral Maxillofac. Implants*, **19** (Suppl.), 43–61.

Choquet, V., Hermans, M., Adriaenssens, P. *et al.* (2001) Clinical and radiographic evaluation of the papilla level adjacent to single-tooth dental implants: A retrospective study in the maxillary anterior region. *J. Periodontol.*, **72** (10), 1364–1371.

Olsson, M. and Lindhe, J. (1991) Periodontal characteristics in individuals with varying form of the upper central incisors. *J. Clin. Periodontol.*, **18** (1), 78–82.

Tarnow, D.P., Cho, S.C. and Wallace, S.S. (2000) The effect of inter-implant distance on the height of inter-implant bone crest. *J. Periodontol.*, **71** (4), 546–549.

Chapter 24

Vercruyssen, M., Laleman, I., Jacobs, R. and Quirynen, M. (2015) Computer-supported implant planning and guided surgery: A narrative review. *Clin. Oral Implants Res.*, **26** (Suppl. 11), 69–76.

Further reading

Pozzi, A., Polizzi, G. and Moy, P.K. (2016) Guided surgery with tooth-supported templates for single missing teeth: A critical review. *Eur. J. Oral Implantol.*, **9** (Suppl. 1), S135–S153.

Chapter 25

Further readingJacobs, R. (2003) Preoperative radiologic planning of implant surgery in compromised patients. *Periodontol. 2000*, **33** (1), 12–25.

Tyndall, D.A. and Brooks, S.L. (2000) Selection criteria for dental implant site imaging: A position paper of the American Academy of Oral and Maxillofacial Radiology. *Oral Surg. Oral Med. Oral Pathol. Oral Radiol. Endod.*, **89** (5), 630–637.

Zitzmann, N.U., Margolin, M.D., Filippi, A. *et al.* (2008) Patient assessment and diagnosis in implant treatment. *Aust. Dent. J.*, **53** (Suppl. 1), S3–S10.

Chapter 27

Belser, U., Buser, D. and Bernard, J.P. (2008a) Implants in the posterior dentition, in *Clinical Periodontology and Implant Dentistry*, 5th edn (eds N.P. Lang, J. Lindhe and T. Karring), Blackwell, Oxford, pp. 1175–1207.

Belser, U., Bernard, J.P. and Buser, D. (2008b) Implants in the esthetic zone, in *Clinical Periodontology and Implant Dentistry*, 5th edn (eds N.P. Lang, J. Lindhe and T. Karring), Blackwell, Oxford, pp. 1146–1174.

Renouard, F. and Rangert, B. (1999) *Risk Factors in Implant Dentistry*, Quintessence, Chicago, IL.

Further reading

Lang, N.P., Wilson, T. and Corbet, E.F. (2000) Biological complications with dental implants: Their prevention, diagnosis and treatment. *Clin. Oral Implants Res.*, **11** (Suppl. 1), 146–155.

Magne, P., Magne, M. and Belser, U.C. (1993) Natural and restorative oral esthetics. Part I: Rationale and basic strategies for successful esthetic rehabilitations. *J. Esthet. Dent.*, **5** (4), 161–173.

Quirynen, M., van Assche, N., Botticelli, D. and Berglundh, T. (2007) How does the timing of implant placement to extraction affect oucome? *Int. J. Oral Maxillofac. Implants*, **22** (Suppl.), 203–223.

Salvi, G.E. and Brägger, U. (2009) Mechanical and technical risks in implant therapy. *Int. J. Oral Maxillofac. Implants*, **24** (Suppl.), 69–85.

Weber, H.P., Morton, D., Gallucci, G.O. *et al.* (2009) Consensus statements and recommended clinical procedures regarding loading protocols. *Int. J. Oral Maxillofac. Implants*, **24** (Suppl.), 180–185.

Zistman, N.U. and Marinello, C.P. (1999) Treatment plan for restoring the edentulous maxilla with implant supported restorations: Removable overdenture versus fixed partial denture design. *J. Prosthet. Dent.*, **82** (2), 188–196.

Chapter 28

Ivanoff, C.J., Grondahl, K., Sennerby, L. *et al.* (1999) Influence of variations in implant diameters: A 3- to 5-year retrospective clinical report. *Int. J. Oral Maxillofac. Implants*, **14** (2), 173–180.

Further reading

Nisand, D. and Renouard, F. (2014) Short implant in limited bone volume. *Periodontol. 2000*, **66** (1), 72–96.

Telleman, G., Raghoebar, G.M., Vissink, A. *et al.* (2011) A systematic review of the prognosis of short (<10 mm) dental implants placed in the partially edentulous patient. *J. Clin. Periodontol.*, **38** (7), 667–676.

Chapter 29
Further reading

Siadat, H., Alikhasi, M. and Beyabanaki, E. (2017) Interim prosthesis options for dental implants, *J. Prosthodont.*, **26** (4), 331–338.

Chapter 30

Esposito, M., Grusovin, M.G., Achille, H. *et al.* (2009) Interventions for replacing missing teeth: Different times for loading dental implants. *Cochrane Database Syst. Rev.*, **1**, CD003878.

Gallucci, G.O., Morton, D. and Weber, H.P. (2009) Loading protocols for dental implants in edentulous patients. *Int. J. Oral Maxillofac. Implants*, **24** (Suppl.), 132–146.

Roccuzzo, M., Aglietta, M. and Cordaro, L. (2009) Implant loading protocols for partially edentulous maxillary posterior sites. *Int. J. Oral Maxillofac. Implants*, **24** (Suppl.), 147–157.

Chapter 31

Belser, U., Bernard, J.P. and Buser, D. (2008) Implants in the esthetic zone, in *Clinical Periodontology and Implant Dentistry*, 5th edn (eds N.P. Lang, J. Lindhe and T. Karring), Blackwell, Oxford, pp. 1146–1174.

Bouchard, P., Renouard, F., Bourgeois, D. *et al.* (2009) Cost-effectiveness modeling of dental implant vs. bridge. *Clin. Oral Implants Res.*, **20**, 583–587.

Chapter 32

Pjetursson, B. and Lang, N. (2008) Prosthetic treatment planning on the basis of scientific evidence. *J. Oral Rehabil.*, **35** (Suppl. 1), 72–79.

Chapter 33

Cehreli, M.C., Karasoy, D., Kökat, A.M. *et al.* (2010) A systematic review of marginal bone loss around implants retaining or supporting overdentures. *Int. J. Oral Maxillofac. Implants*, **25** (2), 266–277.

Cune, M., Burgers, M., van Kampen, F. *et al.* (2010) Mandibular overdentures retained by two implants: 10-year results from a crossover clinical trial comparing ball-socket and bar-clip attachments. *Int. J. Prosthodont.*, **23** (4), 310–317.

Cune, M., van Kampen, F., van der Bilt, A. and Bosman, F. (2005) Patient satisfaction and preference with magnet, bar-clip, and ball-socket retained mandibular implant overdentures: A cross-over clinical trial. *Int. J. Prosthodont.*, **18** (2), 99–105.

Esposito, M., Grusovin, M.G., Chew, Y.S. *et al.* (2009) One-stage versus two-stage implant placement: A Cochrane systematic review of randomised controlled clinical trials. *Eur. J. Oral Implantol.*, **2** (2), 91–99.

Gotfredsen, K., Carlsson, G.E., Jokstad, A. *et al.* (2008) Scandinavian Society for Prosthetic Dentistry, Danish Society of Oral Implantology. Implants and/or teeth: Consensus statements and recommendations. *J. Oral Rehabil.*, **35** (Suppl. 1), 2–8.

Preiskel, H.W. (ed.) (1996) *Overdentures Made Easy: A Guide to Implant and Root Supported Prostheses*, Quintessence, Chicago, IL, pp. 81–122.

Sadowsky, S. (2007) Treatment considerations for maxillary overdentures: A systematic review. *J. Prosthet. Dent.*, **97** (6), 340–348.

Semper, W., Heberer, S. and Nelson, K. (2010) Retrospective analysis of bar-retained dentures with cantilever extension: Marginal bone level changes around dental implants over time. *Int. J. Oral Maxillofac. Implants*, **25** (2), 385–393.

Chapter 34

Alsabeeha, N., Atieh, M. and Payne, A.G. (2010) Loading protocols for mandibular implant overdentures: A systematic review with meta-analysis. *Clin. Implant Dent. Relat. Res.*, **12** (Suppl. 1), e28–38.

Brånemark, P.I., Engstrand, P., Öhrnell, L.O. *et al.* (1999) Brånemark Novum: A new treatment concept for rehabilitation of the edentulous mandible. Preliminary results from a prospective clinical follow-up study. *Clin. Implant Dent. Relat. Res.*, **1** (1), 2–16.

Bryant, S.R., MacDonald-Jankowski, D. and Kim, K. (2007) Does the type of implant prosthesis affect outcomes for the completely edentulous arch? *Int. J. Oral Maxillofac. Implants*, **22** (Suppl.), 117–139.

Feine, J.S., Carlsson, G.E., Awad, M.A. *et al.* (2002) The McGill Consensus Statement on Overdentures. Montreal, Quebec, Canada. May 24–25, 2002. *Int. J. Prosthodont.*, **15** (4), 413–414.

Kawai, Y. and Taylor, J.A. (2007) Effect of loading time on the success of complete mandibular titanium implant retained overdentures: A systematic review. *Clin. Oral Implants Res.*, **18** (4), 399–408.

Maló, P., Rangert, B. and Nobre, M. (2003) 'All-on-Four' immediate-function concept with Brånemark System implants for completely edentulous mandibles: A retrospective clinical study. *Clin. Implant Dent. Relat. Res.*, **5** (Suppl. 1), 2–9.

Vercruyssen, M., Marcelis, K., Coucke, W. *et al.* (2010) Long-term, retrospective evaluation (implant and patient-centred outcome) of the two-implants-supported overdenture in the mandible. Part 1: survival rate. *Clin. Oral Implants Res.*, **21** (4), 357–365.

Chapter 35

Bueno-Samper, A., Hernández-Aliaga, M. and Calvo-Guirado, J.L. (2010) The implant-supported milled bar overdenture: A literature review. *Med. Oral Patol. Oral Cir. Bucal*, **15** (2), e375–e378.

Gallucci, G.O., Morton, D. and Weber, H.P. (2009) Loading protocols for dental implants in edentulous patients. *Int. J. Oral Maxillofac. Implants*, **24** (Suppl.), 132–146.

Lambert, F.E., Weber, H.P., Susarla, S.M. *et al.* (2009) Descriptive analysis of implant and prosthodontic survival rates with fixed implant-supported rehabilitations in the edentulous maxilla. *J. Periodontol.*, **80** (8), 1220–1230.

Maló, P., Rangert, B. and Nobre, M. (2003) 'All-on-Four' immediate-function concept with Brånemark System implants for completely edentulous mandibles: A retrospective clinical study. *Clin. Implant Dent. Relat. Res.*, **5** (Suppl. 1), 2–9.

Mericske-Stern, R. (2003) Prosthodontic management of maxillary and mandibular overdentures, in *Implant Overdentures: The Standard of Care for Edentulous Patients* (eds J.S. Feine and G.E. Carlsson), Quintessence, Chicago, IL, pp. 83–98.

Weber, H.P., Morton, D., Gallucci, G.O. *et al.* (2009) Consensus statements and recommended clinical procedures regarding loading protocols. *Int. J. Oral Maxillofac. Implants*, **24** (Suppl.), 180–183.

Chapter 36

Atieh, M.A., Duncan, W.J. and Faggion, C.M., Jr. (2016) Quality assessment of systematic reviews on oral implants placed immediately into fresh extraction sockets, *Int. J. Oral Maxillofac. Implants*, **31** (2), 338–351.

Buser, D., Martin, W. and Belser, U.C. (2004) Optimizing esthetics for implant restorations in the anterior maxilla: Anatomic and surgical considerations. *Int. J. Oral Maxillofac. Implants*, **19** (Suppl.), 43–61.

Cardaropoli, G., Lekholm, U. and Wennstrom, J.L. (2006) Tissue alterations at implant-supported single-tooth replacements: A 1-year prospective clinical study. *Clin. Oral Implants Res.*, **17** (2), 165–171.

Chen, S.T. and Buser, D. (2014) Esthetic outcomes following immediate and early implant placement in the anterior maxilla: A systematic review. *Int. J. Oral Maxillofac. Implants*, **29** (Suppl.), 186–215.

Chrcanovic, B.R., Albrektsson, T. and Wennerberg, A. (2015) Dental implants inserted in fresh extraction sockets versus healed sites: A systematic review and meta-analysis. *J. Dent.*, **43** (1), 16–41.

De Rouck, T., Collys, K., Wyn, I. and Cosyn, J. (2009) Instant provisionalization of immediate single-tooth implants is essential to optimize esthetic treatment outcome. *Clin. Oral Implants Res.*, **20** (6), 566–570.

Jemt, T. (1999) Restoring the gingival contour by means of provisional resin crowns after single-implant treatment. *Int. J. Periodontics Restorative Dent.*, **19** (1), 20–29.

Kan, J.Y., Rungcharassaeng, K., Lozada, J.L. *et al.* (2011) Facial gingival tissue stability following immediate placement and provisionalization of maxillary anterior single implants: A 2- to

8-year follow-up. *Int. J. Oral Maxillofac. Implants*, **26** (1), 179–187.

Lutz, R., Neukam, F.W., Simion, M. *et al.* (2015) Long-term outcomes of bone augmentation on soft and hard-tissue stability: A systematic review. *Clin. Oral Implants Res.*, **26** (Suppl. 11), 103–122.

Mello, C.C., Lemos, C.A.A., Verri, F.R. *et al.* (2017) Immediate implant placement into fresh extraction sockets versus delayed implants into healed sockets: A systematic review and meta-analysis. *Int. J. Oral Maxillofac. Surg.*, **46** (9), 1162–1177.

Schropp, L., Wenzel, A., Kostopoulos, L. *et al.* (2003) Bone healing and soft tissue contour changes following single-tooth extraction: A clinical and radiographic 12-month prospective study. *Int. J. Periodontics Restorative Dent.*, **23** (4), 313–323.

Chapter 37

Heij, D.G., Opdebeeck, H., van Steenberghe, D. *et al.* (2006) Facial development, continuous tooth eruption, and mesial drift as compromising factors for implant placement. *Int. J. Oral Maxillofac. Implants*, **21** (6), 867–878.

Karl, M. (2016) Outcome of bonded vs all-ceramic and metal-ceramic fixed prostheses for single tooth replacement. *Eur. J. Oral Implantol.*, **9** (Suppl. 1), S25–S44.

Kiliaridis, S., Sidira, M., Kirmanidou, Y. and Michalakis, K. (2016) Treatment options for congenitally missing lateral incisors. *Eur. J. Oral Implantol.*, **9** (Suppl. 1), S5–S24.

Lambert, F., Botilde, G., Lecloux, G. and Rompen, E. (2016) Effectiveness of temporary implants in teenage patients: A prospective clinical trial. *Clin. Oral Implants Res.*, **28** (9), 1152–1157.

Melsen, B. and Lang, N.P. (2001) Biological reactions of alveolar bone to orthodontic loading of oral implants. *Clin. Oral Implants Res.*, **12** (2), 144–152.

Terheyden, H. and Wusthoff, F. (2015) Occlusal rehabilitation in patients with congenitally missing teeth-dental implants, conventional prosthetics, tooth autotransplants, and preservation of deciduous teeth: A systematic review. *Int. J. Implant Dent.*, **1** (1), 30.

Chapter 38

Haanaes, H.R. (1990) Implants and infections with special reference to oral bacteria. *J. Clin. Periodontol.*, **17** (7), 516–524.

Parienti, J.J., Thibon, P., Heller, R. *et al.* (2002) Hand-rubbing with an aqueous alcoholic solution vs traditional surgical hand-scrubbing and 30-day surgical site infection rates: A randomized equivalence study. *JAMA*, **288** (6), 722–727.

Van Steenberghe, D., Yoshida, K., Papaioannou, W. *et al.* (1997) Complete nose coverage to prevent airborne contamination via nostrils is unnecessary. *Clin. Oral Implants Res.*, **8** (6), 512–516.

Chapter 39

Araujo, M.G. and Lindhe, J. (2005) Dimensional ridge alterations following tooth extraction: An experimental study in the dog. *J. Clin. Periodontol.*, **32** (2), 212–218.

Araújo, M.G. and Lindhe, J. (2009a) Ridge alterations following tooth extraction with and without flap elevation: An experimental study in the dog. *Clin. Oral Implants Res.*, **20** (6), 545–549.

Araújo, M.G. and Lindhe, J. (2009b) Ridge preservation with the use of Bio-Oss collagen: A 6-month study in the dog. *Clin. Oral Implants Res.*, **20** (5), 433–440.

Araújo, M.G. and Lindhe, J. (2011) Socket grafting with the use of autologous bone: An experimental study in the dog. *Clin. Oral Implants Res.*, **22** (1), 9–13.

Araujo, M.G., Wennström, J.L. and Lindhe, J. (2006) Modeling of the buccal and lingual bone walls of fresh extraction sites following implant installation. *Clin. Oral Implants Res.*, **17** (6), 600–614.

Atieh, M.A., Alsabeeha, N.H., Payne, A.G. *et al.* (2015) Interventions for replacing missing teeth: Alveolar ridge preservation techniques for dental implant site development. *Cochrane Database Syst. Rev.*, **5**, CD010176.

Carmagnola, D., Adriaens, P. and Berglundh, T. (2003) Healing of human extraction sockets filled with Bio-Oss. *Clin. Oral Implants Res.*, **14** (2), 137–143.

Darby, I., Chen, S.T. and Buser, D. (2009) Ridge preservation techniques for implant therapy. *Int. J. Oral Maxillofac. Implants*, **24** (Suppl.), 260–271.

Esposito, M., Worthington, H.V., Loli, V. *et al.* (2010) Interventions for replacing missing teeth: Antibiotics at dental implant placement to prevent complications. *Cochrane Database Syst. Rev.*, **7**, CD004152.

Iasella, J.M., Greenwell, H., Miller, R.H. *et al.* (2003) Ridge preservation with freeze-dried bone allograft and a collagen membrane compared to extraction alone for implant site development: A clinical and histologic study in humans. *J. Periodontol.*, **74** (7), 990–999.

Kim, J.J., Ben Amara, H., Schwarz, F. *et al.* (2017) Is ridge preservation/augmentation at periodontally compromised extraction sockets safe? A retrospective study. *J. Clin. Periodontol.*, **44** (10), 1051–1058.

Further reading

Fickl, S., Zuhr, O., Wachtel, H. *et al.* (2008) Tissue alterations after tooth extraction with and without surgical trauma: A volumetric study in the beagle dog. *J. Clin. Periodontol.*, **35** (4), 356–363.

Fiorellini, J., Howell, T., Cochran, D. *et al.* (2005) Randomized study evaluating recombinant human bone morphogenetic protein-2 for extraction socket augmentation. *J. Periodontol.*, **76** (4), 605–613.

Grunder, U. (2000) Stability of the mucosal topography around single-tooth implants and adjacent teeth: 1 year results. *Int. J. Periodont. Restorat. Dent.*, **20**, 11–17.

Quirynen, M., van Assche, N., Botticelli, D. and Berglundh, T. (2008) How does the timing of implant placement to extraction affect outcome? *Int. J. Oral Maxillofac. Implants*, **23** (1), 203–223.

Serino, G., Rao, W., Iezzi, G. and Piattelli, A. (2008) Polylactide and polyglycolide sponge used in human extraction socket: Bone formation following 3 months after its application. *Clin. Oral Implants Res.*, **19** (1), 26–31.

Chapter 40

Quirynen, M. and Lekholm, U. (2008) The surgical site, in *Clinical Periodontology and Implant Dentistry*, 5th edn (eds N.P. Lang, J. Lindhe and T. Karring), Blackwell, Oxford, pp. 1068–1079.

Further reading

Hämmerle, C.H.F., Araújo, M. and Lindhe, J. (2008) Timing of implant placement, in *Clinical Periodontology and Implant Dentistry*, 5th edn (eds N.P. Lang, J. Lindhe and T. Karring), Blackwell, Oxford, pp. 1053–1067.

Chapter 41

Araújo, M.G., Sukekava, F., Wennström, J.L. and Lindhe, J. (2006) Tissue modeling following implant placement in fresh extraction sockets. *Clin. Oral Implants Res.*, **17** (6), 615–624.

Botticelli, D., Berglundh, T. and Lindhe, J. (2004) Hard tissue alterations following immediate implant placement in extraction sites. *J. Clin. Periodontol.*, **31** (10), 820–828.

Chen, S.T. and Buser, D. (2008) Implants in post-extraction sites: A literature update, in *ITI Treatment Guide, Vol. 3. Implant Placement in Post-Extraction Sites: Treatment Options* (eds S. Chen and D. Buser). Quintessence, Chicago, IL, pp. 9–16.

Chen, S.T. and Buser, D. (2009) Clinical and esthetic outcomes of implants placed in the postextraction sites. *Int. J. Oral Maxillofac. Implants*, **24** (Suppl.), 186–217.

Esposito, M., Grusovin, M.G., Polyzos, I.P. *et al.* (2010) Interventions for replacing missing teeth: Dental implant in fresh extraction socket (immediate, immediate-delayed, delayed implants). *Cochrane Database Syst. Rev.*, **9**, CD005968.

Sanz, M., Cecchinato, D., Ferrus, J. *et al.* (2010) A prospective, randomized-controlled clinical trial to evaluate bone preservation using implants with different geometry placed into extraction sockets in the maxilla. *Clin. Oral Implants Res.*, **21** (1), 13–21.

Further reading

Hammerle, C.H., Chen, S.T. and Wilson, T.G., Jr. (2004) Consensus statements and recommended clinical procedures regarding the placement of implants in extraction sockets. *Int. J. Oral Maxillofac. Implants*, **19** (Suppl.), 26–28.

Lindeboom, J.A., Tjiook, Y. and Kroon, F.H. (2006) Immediate placement of implants in periapical infected sites: A prospective randomized study in 50 patients. *Oral Surg. Oral Med. Oral Pathol. Oral Radiol. Endod.*, **101** (6), 705–710.

Paolantonio, M., Dolci, M., Scarano, A. et al. (2001) Immediate implantation in fresh extraction sockets: A controlled clinical and histological study in man. *J. Periodontol.*, **72** (11), 1560–1571.

Chapter 42

Hammerle, C.H., Stone, P., Jung, R.E. *et al.* (2009) Consensus statements and recommended clinical procedures regarding computer-assisted implant dentistry. *Int. J. Oral Maxillofac. Implants*, **24** (Suppl.), 126–131.

Jung, R.E., Schneider, D., Ganeles, J. *et al.* (2009) Computer technology applications in surgical implant dentistry: A systematic review. *Int. J. Oral Maxillofac. Implants*, **24** (Suppl.), 92–109.

Vercruyssen, M., Laleman, I., Jacobs, R. *et al.* (2015) Computer-supported implant planning and guided surgery: A narrative review. *Clin. Oral Implants Res.*, **26** (Suppl. 11), 69–76.

Further reading

D'Haese, J., Ackhurst, J., Wismeijer, D. *et al.* (2017) Current state of the art of computer-guided implant surgery. *Periodontol. 2000*, **73** (1), 121–133.

Chapter 43

Abduo, J. and Lyons, K. (2013) Rationale for the use of CAD/CAM technology in implant prosthodontics. *Int. J. Dent.*, **2013**, 768121.

Abduo, J., Lyons, K., Waddell, N. *et al.* (2012) A comparison of fit of CNC-milled titanium and zirconia frameworks to implants. *Clin. Implant Dent. Relat. Res.*, **14** (Suppl. 1), e20–e29.

Glauser, R., Sailer, I., Wohlwend, A. *et al.* (2004) Experimental zirconia abutments for implant-supported single-tooth restorations in esthetically demanding regions: 4-year results of a prospective clinical study. *Int. J. Prosthodont.*, **17** (3), 285–290.

Joda, T., Ferrari, M., Gallucci, G.O. *et al.* (2017) Digital technology in fixed implant prosthodontics. *Periodontol. 2000*, **73** (1), 178–192.

Kapos, T., Ashy, L.M., Gallucci, G.O. *et al.* (2009) Computer-aided design and computer-assisted manufacturing in prosthetic implant dentistry. *Int. J. Oral Maxillofac. Implants*, **24** (Suppl.), 110–117.

Ortorp, A., Jemt, T., Back, T. *et al.* (2003) Comparisons of precision of fit between cast and CNC-milled titanium implant frameworks for the edentulous mandible. *Int. J. Prosthodont.*, **16** (2), 194–200.

Takahashi, T. and Gunne, J. (2003) Fit of implant frameworks: An in vitro comparison between two fabrication techniques. *J. Prosthet. Dent.*, **89** (3), 256–260.

van Noort, R. (2012) The future of dental devices is digital. *Dent. Mater.*, **28** (1), 3–12.

Yuzugullu, B. and Avci, M. (2008) The implant-abutment interface of alumina and zirconia abutments. *Clin. Implant Dent. Relat. Res.*, **10** (2), 113–121.

Chapter 44

Amin, S., Weber, H.P., Finkelman, M. *et al.* (2017) Digital vs. conventional full-arch implant impressions: A comparative study. *Clin. Oral Implants Res.*, **28** (11), 1360–1367.

Brown, S.D. and Payne, A.G. (2011) Immediately restored single implants in the aesthetic zone of the maxilla using a novel design: 1-year report. *Clin. Oral Implants Res.*, **22**, 445–454.

Ekfeldt, A., Furst, B. and Carlsson, G.E. (2011) Zirconia abutments for single-tooth implant restorations: A retrospective and clinical follow-up study. *Clin. Oral Implants Res.*, **22**, 1308–1314.

Flugge, T.V., Att, W., Metzger, M.C. *et al.* (2016) Precision of dental implant digitization using intraoral scanners. *Int. J. Prosthodont.*, **29** (3), 277–283.

Guess, P.C., Att, W. and Strub, J.R. (2012) Zirconia in fixed implant prosthodontics. *Clin. Implant Dent. Relat. Res.*, **14** (5), 633–645.

Guess, P.C., Bonfante, E.A., Silva, N.R. *et al.* (2013) Effect of core design and veneering technique on damage and reliability of Y-TZP-supported crowns. *Dent. Mater.*, **29** (3), 307–316.

Kohal, R.J., Wolkewitz, M. and Mueller, C. (2010) Alumina-reinforced zirconia implants: Survival rate and fracture strength in a masticatory simulation trial. *Clin. Oral Implants Res.*, **21** (12), 1345–1352.

Kokubo, Y., Tsumita, M., Kano, T. *et al.* (2011) The influence of zirconia coping designs on the fracture load of all-ceramic molar crowns. *Dent. Mater.*, **30** (3), 281–285.

Larsson, C. and Vult von Steyern, P. (2010) Five-year follow-up of implant-supported Y-TZP and ZTA fixed dental prostheses: A randomized, prospective clinical trial comparing two different material systems. *Int. J. Prosthodont.*, **23** (6), 555–561.

Larsson, C., Vult von Steyern, P. and Nilner, K. (2010) A prospective study of implant-supported full-arch yttria-stabilized tetragonal zirconia polycrystal mandibular fixed dental prostheses: Three-year results. *Int. J. Prosthodont.*, **23** (4), 364–369.

Papaspyridakos, P., Chen, C.J., Gallucci, G.O. *et al.* (2014) Accuracy of implant impressions for partially and completely edentulous patients: A systematic review. *Int. J. Oral Maxillofac. Implants*, **29** (4), 836–845.

Parpaiola, A., Norton, M.R., Cecchinato, D. *et al.* (2013) Virtual abutment design: A concept for delivery of CAD/CAM customized abutments – report of a retrospective cohort. *Int. J. Periodontics Restorative Dent.*, **33**, 51–58.

Rauscher, O. (2011) Impression-free implant restorations with Cerec InLab. *Int. J. Comput. Dent.*, **14** (2), 139–146.

Sailer, I., Philipp, A., Zembic, A. *et al.* (2009) A systematic review of the performance of ceramic and metal implant abutments supporting fixed implant reconstructions. *Clin. Oral Implants Res.*, **20** (Suppl. 4), 4–31.

Selz, C.F., Bogler, J., Vach, K. *et al.* (2015) Veneered anatomically designed zirconia FDPs resulting from digital intraoral scans: Preliminary results of a prospective clinical study. *J. Dent.*, **43** (12), 1428–1435.

Silva, N.R., Bonfante, E.A., Rafferty, B.T. *et al.* (2011) Modified Y-TZP core design improves all-ceramic crown reliability. *J. Dent. Res.*, **90** (1), 104–108.

Vandeweghe, S., Vervack, V., Dierens, M. *et al.* (2017) Accuracy of digital impressions of multiple dental implants: An in vitro study. *Clin. Oral Implants Res.*, **28** (6), 648–653.

Chapter 45

Chiapasco, M., Casentini, P. and Zaniboni, M. (2009) Bone augmentation procedures in implant dentistry. *Int. J. Oral Maxillofac. Implants*, **24** (Suppl.), 237–259.

Hammerle, C.H. and Lang, N. (2001) Single stage surgery combining transmucosal implant placement with guided bone regeneration and bioresorbable materials. *Clin. Oral Implants Res.*, **12** (1), 9–18.

Chapter 46

Wang, J., Wang, L., Zhou, Z. *et al.* (2016) Biodegradable polymer membranes applied in guided bone/tissue regeneration: A review, *Polymers*, **8** (4), 115.

Chapter 47

Antoun, H., Sitbon, J.M., Martinez, H. *et al.* (2001) A prospective randomized study comparing two techniques of bone augmentation: Onlay graft alone or associated with a membrane. *Clin. Oral Implants Res.*, **12** (6), 632–639.

Benic, G.I. and Hammerle, C.H. (2014) Horizontal bone augmentation by means of guided bone regeneration. *Periodontol. 2000*, **66** (1), 13–40.

Chiapasco, M. and Zaniboni, M. (2009) Clinical outcomes of GBR procedures to correct peri-implant dehiscences and fenestrations: A systematic review. *Clin. Oral Implants Res.*, **20** (Suppl. 4), 113–123.

Dahlin, C., Sennerby, L., Lekholm, U. *et al.* (1989) Generation of new bone around titanium implants using a membrane technique: An experimental study in rabbits. *Int. J. Oral Maxillofac. Implants*, **4** (1), 19–25.

Esposito, M., Grusovin, M.G., Felice, P. *et al.* (2009) Interventions for replacing missing teeth: Horizontal and vertical bone augmentation techniques for dental implant treatment. *Cochrane Database Syst. Rev.*, **4**, CD003607.

Esposito, M., Grusovin, M.G., Tzanetea, E. *et al.* (2010) Interventions for replacing missing teeth: Treatment of perimplantitis. *Cochrane Database Syst. Rev.*, **6**, CD004970.

Gottlow, J., Nyman, S., Karring, T. *et al.* (1984) New attachment formation as the result of controlled tissue regeneration. *J. Clin. Periodontol.*, **11** (8), 494–503.

Hurley, L.A., Stinchfield, F.E., Bassett, A.L. *et al.* (1959) The role of soft tissues in osteogenesis: An experimental study of canine spine fusions. *J. Bone Joint Surg. Am.*, **41-A**, 1243–1254.

Klinge, B. and Flemmig, T.F. (2009) Tissue augmentation and esthetics (Working Group 3). *Clin. Oral Implants Res.*, **20** (Suppl. 4), 166–170.

Tonetti, M.S. and Hammerle, C.H. (2008) Advances in bone augmentation to enable dental implant placement: Consensus Report of the Sixth European Workshop on Periodontology. *J. Clin. Periodontol.*, **35** (8 Suppl.), 168–172.

von Arx, T., Cochran, D.L., Hermann, J.S. *et al.* (2001) Lateral ridge augmentation using different bone fillers and barrier membrane application: A histologic and histomorphometric pilot study in the canine mandible. *Clin. Oral Implants Res.*, **12** (3), 260–269.

Chapter 48

Anitua, E. (1999) Plasma rich in growth factors: Preliminary results of use in the preparation of future sites of implants. *Int. J. Oral Maxillofac. Implants*, **14** (4), 529–535.

Berglundh, T. and Lindhe, J. (1997) Healing around implants placed in bone defects treated with Bio-Oss: An experimental study in the dog. *Clin. Oral Implants Res.*, **8** (2), 117–124.

Boyne, P. and James, R.A. (1980) Grafting of the maxillary sinus floor with autogenous marrow and bone. *J. Oral. Surg.*, **38** (8), 613–616.

Carmagnola, D., Berglundh, T., Araujo, M. *et al.* (2000) Bone healing around implants placed in a jaw defect augmented with Bio-Oss: An experimental study in dogs. *J. Clin. Periodontol.*, **27** (11), 799–805.

Daculsi, G. (1998) Biphasic calcium phosphate concept applied to artificial bone, implant coating and injectable bone substitute. *Biomaterials*, **19** (16), 1473–1478.

Davies, J.E. and Hosseini, M.M. (2000) Histodynamics of endosseus wound healing, in *Bone Engineering* (ed. J.E. Davies), Em Squared, Toronto, pp. 1–14.

Esposito, M., Grusovin, M.G., Felice, P. *et al.* (2009) Interventions for replacing missing teeth: Horizontal and vertical bone augmentation techniques for dental implant treatment. *Cochrane Database Syst. Rev.*, **4**, CD003607.

Hallman, M. and Thor, A. (2008) Bone substitutes and growth factors as an alternative/complement to autogenous bone for grafting in implant dentistry. *Periodontol. 2000*, **47** (1), 172–192.

Merkx, M.A., Fennis, J.P., Verhagen, C.M. and Stoelinga, P.J. (2004) Reconstruction of the mandible using preshaped 2, 3 mm titanium plates, autogenous particulate cortico-cancellous bone grafts and platelet rich plasma: A report on eight patients. *Int. J. Oral Maxillofac. Surg.*, **33**, 2029–2035.

Piatelli, M., Favero, G., Scarano, A. *et al.* (1999) Bone reactions to anorganic bovine (Bio-Oss) used in sinus augmentation procedures: A histologic long-term report of 20 cases in humans. *Int. J. Oral Maxillofac. Implants*, **14** (6), 835–840.

Terheyden, H., Jepsen, S., Möller, B. *et al.* (1999) Sinus floor augmentation with simultaneous placement of dental implants using a combination of deproteinized bone xenograft and recombinant human osteogenic protein-1: A histometric study in miniature pigs. *Clin. Oral Implants Res.*, **10** (6), 510–521.

Thor, A., Wannfors, K., Sennerby, L. and Rasmusson, L. (2005) Reconstruction of the severely resorbed maxilla with autogenous bone, platelet-rich plasma, and implants: 1-year results of a controlled prospective 5-year study. *Clin. Implant Dent. Relat. Res.*, **7** (4), 209–220.

Tonetti, M.S. and Hâmmerle, C.H.F. (2008) Advances in bone augmentation to enable dental implant placement: Consensus Report of the Sixth European Workshop on Periodontology. *J. Clin. Periodontol.*, **35** (Suppl. 8), 168–172.

Turunen, T., Peltola, J., YLI-Urpo, A. and Happonen, R. (2004) Bioactive glass granules as a bone adjunctive material in maxillary sinus floor augmentation. *Clin. Oral Implants Res.*, **15** (2), 135–141.

Valentini, P., Abensur, D., Densari, D. *et al.* (1998) Histological evaluation of Bio-Oss in a 2-stage sinus floor elevation and implantation procedure: A human case report, *Clin. Oral Implants Res.*, **9** (1), 59–64.

Wiltfang, J., Schlegel, K.A., Schultze-Mosgau, S. *et al.* (2003) Sinus floor augmentation with beta-tricalciumphosphate (beta-TCP): Does platelet-rich plasma promote its osseous integration and degradation? *Clin. Oral Implants Res.*, **14** (2), 213–218.

Yildirim, M., Spiekermann, H., Handt, S. and Edelhoff, D. (2001) Maxillary sinus augmentation with the xenograft Bio-Oss and autogenous intraoral bone for qualitative improvement of the implant site: A histologic and histomorphometric clinical study in humans. *Int. J. Oral Maxillofac. Implants*, **16** (1), 23–33.

Chapter 49

Chen, S.T., Beagle, J., Jensen, S.S. *et al.* (2009) Consensus statements and recommended clinical procedures regarding surgical techniques. *Int. J. Oral Maxillofac. Implants*, **24** (Suppl.), 272–278.

Chiapasco, M., Casentini, P. and Zaniboni, M. (2009) Bone augmentation procedures in implant dentistry. *Int. J. Oral Maxillofac. Implants*, **24** (Suppl.), 237–259.

Esposito, M., Grusovin, M.G., Felice, P. *et al.* (2009) Interventions for replacing missing teeth: Horizontal and vertical bone augmentation techniques for dental implant treatment. *Cochrane Database Syst. Rev.*, **4**, CD003607.

Chapter 50

Chen, S.T., Beagle, J., Jensen, S.S. *et al.* (2009) Consensus statements and recommended clinical procedures regarding surgical techniques. *Int. J. Oral Maxillofac. Implants*, **24** (Suppl.), 272–278.

Donos, N., Mardas, N. and Chadha, V. (2008) Clinical outcomes of implants following lateral bone augmentation: Systematic assessment of available options (barrier membranes, bone grafts, split osteotomy). *J. Clin. Periodontol.*, **35** (Suppl. 8), 173–202.

Chapter 51

Chiapasco, M., Casentini, P. and Zaniboni, M. (2009) Bone augmentation procedures in implant dentistry. *Int. J. Oral Maxillofac. Implants*, **24** (Suppl.), 237–259.

Del Fabbro, M., Testori, T., Francetti, L. and Weinstein, R. (2004) Systematic review of survival rates for implants placed in the grafted maxillary sinus. *Int. J. Periodontics Restorative Dent.*, **24** (6), 565–577.

Esposito, M., Felice, P. and Worthington, H.V. (2014) Interventions for replacing missing teeth: Augmentation procedures of the maxillary sinus. *Cochrane Database Syst. Rev.*, **5**, CD008397.

Graziani, F., Donos, N., Needleman, I. *et al.* (2004) Comparison of implant survival following sinus floor augmentation procedures with implants placed in pristine posterior maxillary bone: A systematic review. *Clin. Oral Implants Res.*, **15** (6), 677–682.

Lutz, R., Berger-Fink, S., Stockmann, P. *et al.* (2015) Sinus floor augmentation with autogenous bone vs. a bovine-derived xenograft: A 5-year retrospective study. *Clin. Oral Implants Res.*, **26**, 644–648.

Nkenke, E. and Stelzle, F. (2009) Clinical outcomes of sinus floor augmentation for implant placement using autogenous bone or bone substitutes: A systematic review. *Clin. Oral Implants Res.*, **20** (Suppl. 4), 124–133.

Pjetursson, B.E., Tan, W.C., Zwahlen, M. and Lang, N.P. (2008) A systematic review of the success of sinus floor elevation and survival of implants inserted in combination with sinus floor elevation. *J. Clin. Periodontol.*, **35** (8 Suppl.), 216–240.

Schmitt, C.M., Doering, H., Schmidt, T. *et al.* (2013) Histological results after maxillary sinus augmentation with Straumann® BoneCeramic, Bio-Oss®, Puros®, and autologous bone: A randomized controlled clinical trial. *Clin. Oral Implants Res.*, **24** (5), 576–585.

Tonetti, M.S. and Hammerle, C.H. (2008) Advances in bone augmentation to enable dental implant placement: Consensus Report of the Sixth European Workshop on Periodontology. *J. Clin. Periodontol.*, **35** (8 Suppl.), 168–172.

Wallace, S.S. and Froum, S.J. (2003) Effect of maxillary sinus augmentation on the survival of endosseous dental implants: A systematic review. *Ann. Periodontol.*, **8** (1), 328–343.

Chapter 52

Engelke, W. and Deckwer, I. (1997) Endoscopically controlled sinus floor augmentation: A preliminary report. *Clin. Oral Implants Res.*, **8** (6), 527–531.

Esposito, M., Felice, P. and Worthington, H.V. (2014) Interventions for replacing missing teeth: Augmentation procedures of the maxillary sinus. *Cochrane Database Syst. Rev.*, **5**, CD008397.

Franceschetti, G., Rizzi, A., Minenna, L. *et al.* (2017) Patient-reported outcomes of implant placement performed concomitantly with transcrestal sinus floor elevation or entirely in native bone. *Clin. Oral Implants Res.*, **28**, 156–162.

Franceschetti, G., Trombelli, L., Minenna, L. *et al.* (2015) Learning curve of a minimally invasive technique for transcrestal sinus floor elevation: A split-group analysis in a prospective case series with multiple clinicians. *Implant Dent.*, **24** (5), 517–526.

Fugazzotto, P.A. and De, P.S. (2002) Sinus floor augmentation at the time of maxillary molar extraction: Success and failure rates of 137 implants in function for up to 3 years. *J. Periodontol.*, **73** (1), 39–44.

Sohn, D.S., Lee, J.S., Ahn, M.R. *et al.* (2008) New bone formation in the maxillary sinus without bone grafts. *Implant Dent.*, **17** (3), 321–331.

Summers, R.B. (1994) The osteotome technique: Part 3 – Less invasive methods of elevating the sinus floor. *Compendium*, **15**, 698, 700, 702–704 passim; quiz 710.

Tan, W.C., Lang, N.P., Zwahlen, M. *et al.* (2008) A systematic review of the success of sinus floor elevation and survival of implants inserted in combination with sinus floor elevation. Part II: Transalveolar technique. *J. Clin. Periodontol.*, **35** (8 Suppl.), 241–254.

Trombelli, L., Minenna, P., Franceschetti, G. *et al.* (2010) Transcrestal sinus floor elevation with a minimally invasive technique. *J. Periodontol.*, **81** (1), 158–166.

Chapter 53

Allais, M., Maurette, P.E., Mazzonetto, R. and Filho, J.R.L. (2007) Patient's perception of the events during and after osteogenic alveolar distraction. *Med. Oral Patol. Oral Cir. Bucal*, **12**, E225–E228.

Chen, S.T., Beagle, J., Jensen, S.S. *et al.* (2009) Consensus statements and recommended clinical procedures regarding surgical techniques. *Int. J. Oral Maxillofac. Implants*, **24** (Suppl.), 272–278.

Chiapasco, M., Casentini, P. and Zaniboni, M. (2009) Bone augmentation procedures in implant dentistry. *Int. J. Oral Maxillofac. Implants*, **24** (Suppl.), 237–259.

Chiapasco, M., Zaniboni, M. and Rimondini, L. (2007) Autogenous onlay bone grafts vs. alveolar distraction osteogenesis for the correction of vertically deficient edentulous ridges: A 2–4-year prospective study on humans. *Clin. Oral Implants Res.*, **18** (4), 432–440.

Chin, M. (1999) Distraction osteogenesis for dental implants. *Oral Maxillofac. Surg. Clin. North Am.*, **7** (1), 41–63.

Esposito, M., Grusovin, M.G., Felice, P. *et al.* (2009) Interventions for replacing missing teeth: Horizontal and vertical bone augmentation techniques for dental implant treatment. *Cochrane Database Syst. Rev.*, **4**, CD003607.

Tonetti, M.S. and Hammerle, C.H.F. (2008) Advances in bone augmentation to enable dental implant placement: Consensus Report of the Sixth European Workshop on Periodontology. *J. Clin. Periodontol.*, **35** (8 Suppl), 168–172.

Chapter 54

Abrahamsson, I., Berglundh, T., Glantz, P.O. and Lindhe, J. (1998) The mucosal attachment at different abutments: An experimental study in dogs. *J. Clin. Periodontol.*, **25** (9), 721–727.

Abrahamsson, I., Zitzmann, N.U., Berglundh, T. *et al.* (2001) Bone and soft tissue integration to titanium implants with different surface topography: An experimental study in the dog. *Int. J. Oral Maxillofac. Implants*, **16** (3), 323–332.

Berglundh, T., Abrahamsson, I., Welander, M. *et al.* (2007) Morphogenesis of the peri-implant mucosa: An experimental study in dogs. *Clin. Oral Implants Res.*, **18** (1), 1–8.

Berglundh, T., Lindhe, J., Ericsson, I. *et al.* (1991) The soft tissue barrier at implants and teeth. *Clin. Oral Implants Res.*, **2** (2), 81–90.

Blanco, J., Carral, C., Linares, A. *et al.* (2012) Soft tissue dimensions in flapless immediate implants with and without immediate loading: An experimental study in the beagle dog. *Clin. Oral Implants Res.*, **23** (1), 70–75.

Canullo, L., Tallarico, M., Penarrocha-Oltra, D. *et al.* (2016) Implant abutment cleaning by plasma of argon: 5-year follow-up of a randomized controlled trial. *J. Periodontol.*, **87** (4), 434–442.

de Sanctis, M., Vignoletti, F., Discepoli, N. *et al.* (2009) Immediate implants at fresh extraction sockets: Bone healing in four different implant systems. *J. Clin. Periodontol.*, **36** (8), 705–711.

Degidi, M., Artese, L., Piattelli, A. *et al.* (2012) Histological and immunohistochemical evaluation of the peri-implant soft tissues around machined and acid-etched titanium healing abutments: A prospective randomised study. *Clin. Oral Invest.*, **16**, 857–866.

Glauser, R., Schupbach, P., Gottlow, J. and Hammerle, C.H. (2005) Periimplant soft tissue barrier at experimental one-piece mini-implants with different surface topography in humans: A light-microscopic overview and histometric analysis. *Clin. Implant Dent. Relat. Res.*, **7** (Suppl. 1), S44–S51.

Glauser, R., Zembic, A. and Hammerle, C.H. (2006) A systematic review of marginal soft tissue at implants subjected to immediate loading or immediate restoration. *Clin. Oral Implants Res.*, **17** (Suppl. 2), 82–92.

Hermann, J.S., Buser, D., Schenk, R.K. *et al.* (2001) Biologic width around one- and two-piece titanium implants. *Clin. Oral Implants Res.*, **12** (6), 559–571.

Linkevicius, T. and Vaitelis, J. (2015) The effect of zirconia or titanium as abutment material on soft peri-implant tissues: A systematic review and meta-analysis. *Clin. Oral Implants Res.*, **26** (Suppl. 11), 139–147.

Nevins, M., Kim, D.M., Jun, S.H. *et al.* (2010) Histologic evidence of a connective tissue attachment to laser microgrooved abutments: A canine study. *Int. J. Periodontics Restorative Dent.*, **30** (3), 245–255.

Pontes, A.E., Ribeiro, F.S., Iezzi, G. *et al.* (2008) Biologic width changes around loaded implants inserted in different levels in relation to crestal bone: Histometric evaluation in canine mandible. *Clin. Oral Implants Res.*, **19**, 483–490.

Sculean, A., Gruber, R. and Bosshardt, D.D. (2014) Soft tissue wound healing around teeth and dental implants. *J. Clin. Periodontol.*, **41** (Suppl. 15), S6–S22.

Tallarico, M., Canullo, L., Caneva, M. and Ozcan, M. (2017) Microbial colonization at the implant-abutment interface and its possible influence on periimplantitis: A systematic review and meta-analysis. *J. Prosthodont. Res.*, **61** (3), 233–241.

Vignoletti, F., de Sanctis, M., Berglundh, T. *et al.* (2009) Early healing of implants placed into fresh extraction sockets: An experimental study in the beagle dog. III: Soft tissue findings. *J. Clin. Periodontol.*, **36** (12), 1059–1066.

Weber, H.P., Buser, D., Donath, K. *et al.* (1996) Comparison of healed tissues adjacent to submerged and non-submerged unloaded titanium dental implants: A histometric study in beagle dogs. *Clin. Oral Implants Res.*, **7** (1), 11–19.

You, T.M., Choi, B.H., Li, J. *et al.* (2009) Morphogenesis of the peri-implant mucosa: A comparison between flap and flapless procedures in the canine mandible. *Oral Surg. Oral Med. Oral Pathol. Oral Radiol. Endod.*, **107**, 66–70.

Zhao, B., van der Mei, H.C., Subbiahdoss, G. *et al.* (2014) Soft tissue integration versus early biofilm formation on different dental implant materials. *Dent. Mater.*, **30** (7), 716–727.

Chapter 55

Bouchard, P., Malet, J. and Borghetti, A. (2001) Decision-making in aesthetics: Root coverage revisited. *Periodontol. 2000*, **27** (1), 97–120.

Esposito, M., Maghaireh, H., Grusovin, M.G. *et al.* (2012) Interventions for replacing missing teeth: Management of soft tissues for dental implants. *Cochrane Database Syst. Rev.*, **2**, CD006697.

Jung, J.E., Siegenthaler, D.W. and Hammerle, C.H. (2004) Postextraction tissue management: A soft tissue punch technique. *Int. J. Periodont. Restorat. Dent.*, **24** (6), 545–553.

Klinge, B. and Flemmig, T.F. (2009) Tissue augmentation and esthetics (Working Group 3). *Clin. Oral Implants Res.*, **20** (Suppl. 4), 166–170.

Rotundo, R., Pagliaro, U., Bendinelli, E. *et al.* (2015) Long-term outcomes of soft tissue augmentation around dental implants on soft and hard tissue stability: A systematic review. *Clin. Oral Implants Res.*, **26** (Suppl. 11), 123–138.

Scharf, D.R. and Tarnow, D.P. (1992) Modified roll technique for localized alveolar ridge augmentation. *Int. J. Periodont. Restorat. Dent.*, **12** (5), 415–425.

Sculean, A., Chappuis, V. and Cosgarea, R. (2017) Coverage of mucosal recessions at dental implants. *Periodontol. 2000*, **73** (1), 134–140.

Seibert, J.S. and Salama, H. (1996) Alveolar ridge preservation and reconstruction. *Periodontol. 2000*, 11, 69–84.

Thoma, D.S., Benic, G.I., Zwahlen, M. *et al.* (2009) A systematic review assessing soft tissue augmentation techniques. *Clin. Oral Implants Res.*, **20** (Suppl. 4), 146–165.

Wennstrom, J.L., Bengazi, F. and Lekholm, U. (1994) The influence of the masticatory mucosa on the peri-implant soft tissue condition. *Clin. Oral Implants Res.*, **5** (1), 1–8.

Chapter 56

Esposito, M., Grusovin, M.G. and Worthington, H.V. (2013) Interventions for replacing missing teeth: Antibiotics at dental implant placement to prevent complications. *Cochrane Database Syst. Rev.*, 7, CD004152.

Chapter 57
Further reading

Hofschneider, U., Tepper, G., Gahleitner, A. and Ulm, C. (1999) Assessment of the blood supply to the mental region for reduction of bleeding complications during implant surgery in the interforaminal region. *Int. J. Oral Maxillofac. Implants*, **14** (3), 379–383.

Manning, J.E. (2004) Fluid and blood resuscitation, in *Emergency Medicine: A Comprehensive Study Guide* (ed. J. Tintinalli), McGraw-Hill, New York, p. 227.

Chapter 58

Branemark, P.I., Adell, R., Albrektsson, T. *et al.* (1984) An experimental and clinical study of osseointegrated implants penetrating the nasal cavity and maxillary sinus. *J. Oral Maxillofac. Surg.*, **42** (8), 497–505.

Chen, S.T., Beagle, J., Jensen, S.S. *et al.* (2009) Consensus statements and recommended clinical procedures regarding surgical techniques. *Int. J. Oral Maxillofac. Implants*, **24** (Suppl.), 272–278.

Giglio, J. and Laskin, D. (1998) Perioperative errors contributing to implant failure. *Oral Maxillofac. Surg. Clin. North Am.*, **2**, 197–202.

Chapter 59

Devine, M., Taylor, S. and Renton, T. (2016) Chronic post-surgical pain following the placement of dental implants in the maxilla: A case series. *Eur. J. Oral Implantol.*, **9** (Suppl. 1), 179–186.

Goodacre, C.J., Bernal, G., Rungcharassaeng, K. *et al.* (2003) Clinical complications with implants and implant prostheses. *J. Prosthet. Dent.*, **90** (2), 121–132.

Lin, C.S., Wu, S.Y., Huang, H.Y. *et al.* (2016) Systematic review and meta-analysis on incidence of altered sensation of mandibular implant surgery. *PLoS One*, **11** (4), e0154082.

Park, S.H. and Wang, H.L. (2005) Implant reversible complications: Classification and treatments. *Implant Dent.*, **14** (3), 211–220.

Vetromilla, B.M., Moura, L.B., Sonego, C.L. *et al.* (2014) Complications associated with inferior alveolar nerve repositioning for dental implant placement: A systematic review. *Int. J. Oral Maxillofac. Surg.*, **43** (11), 1360–1366.

Chapter 60

Hofschneider, U., Tepper, G., Gahleitner, A. and Ulm, C. (1999) Assessment of the blood supply to the mental region for reduction of bleeding complications during implant surgery in the interforaminal region. *Int. J. Oral Maxillofac. Implants*, **14** (3), 379–383.

Manning, J.E. (2004) Fluid and blood resuscitation, in *Emergency Medicine: A Comprehensive Study Guide* (ed. J. Tintinalli), McGraw-Hill, New York, p. 227.

ten Bruggenkate, C.M., Krekeler, G., Kraaijenhagen, H.A. *et al.* (1993) Hemorrhage of the floor of the mouth resulting from lingual perforation during implant placement: A clinical report. *Int. J. Oral Maxillofac. Implants*, **8** (3), 329–334.

Chapter 61

Academy Report (2013) Peri-implant mucositis and peri-implantitis: A current understanding of their diagnoses and clinical implications. *J. Periodontol.*, **84** (4), 436–443.

Albrektsson, T. and Isidor, F. (1994) Consensus report of session IV, in *Proceedings of the 1st European Workshop on Periodontology* (ed. N.P. Lang NP), Quintessence, London, pp. 365–369.

Berglundh, T., Lindhe, J. and Lang, K. (2008) Peri-implant pathology, in *Clinical Periodontology and Implant Dentistry*, 5th edn (eds J. Lindhe, N.P. Lang and T. Karring), Blackwell, New York, pp. 529–538.

Coli, P., Christiaens, V., Sennerby, L. and Bruyn, H. (2017) Reliability of periodontal diagnostic tools for monitoring peri-implant health and disease. *Periodontol. 2000*, **73** (1), 203-217.

Derks, J., Schaller, D., Håkansson, J. *et al.* (2016) Effectiveness of implant therapy analyzed in a Swedish population: Prevalence of peri-implantitis. *J. Dent. Res.*, **95** (1), 43–49.

Ellegaard, B., Baelum, V. and Karring, T. (1997) Implant therapy in periodontally compromised patients. *Clin. Oral Implants Res.*, **8** (3), 180–188.

Heitz-Mayfield, L.J., Schmid, B., Weigel, C. *et al.* (2004) Does excessive occlusal load affect osseointegration? An experimental study in the dog. *Clin. Oral Implants Res.*, **15** (3), 259–268.

Isidor, F. (1996) Loss of osseointegration caused by occlusal load of oral implants: A clinical and radiographic study in monkeys. *Clin. Oral Implants Res.*, **7** (2), 143–152.

Isidor, F. (1997) Histological evaluation of peri-implant bone at implants subjected to occlusal overload or plaque accumulation. *Clin. Oral Implants Res.*, **8** (1), 1–9.

Jepsen, S., Berglundh, T., Genco, R. *et al.* (2015) Primary prevention of periimplantitis: Managing peri-implant mucositis. *J. Clin. Periodontol.*, **42** (Suppl. 16), S152–S157.

Lang, N.P. and Berglundh, T. (2011) Periimplant diseases: Where are we now? Consensus of the Seventh European Workshop on Periodontology. *J. Clin. Periodontol.*, **38** (Suppl. 11), 178–181.

Lang, N.P., Berglundh, T., Heitz-Mayfield, L.J. *et al.* (2004) Consensus statements and recommended clinical procedures regarding implant survival and complications. *Int. J. Oral Maxillofac. Implants*, **19** (Suppl.), 150–154.

Lang, N.P., Bragger, U., Walther, D. *et al.* (1993) Ligature-induced peri-implant infection in cynomolgus monkeys. I. Clinical and radiographic findings. *Clin. Oral Implants Res.*, **4** (1), 2–11.

Meyle, J. (2008) Peri-implant diseases: Consensus report of the Sixth European Workshop on Periodontology. *J. Clin. Periodontol.*, **35** (8 Suppl.), 282–285.

Mombelli, A. (1999) Prevention and therapy of peri-implant infections, in *Proceedings of the 3rd European Workshop on Periodontology* (eds N.P. Lang, T. Karring and J. Lindhe), Quintessence, Berlin, pp. 281–303.

Roos-Jansåker, A.M., Lindahl, C., Renvert, H. and Renvert, S. (2006) Nine- to fourteen-year follow-up of implant treatment. Part II: Presence of peri-implant lesions. *J. Clin. Periodontol.*, **33** (4), 290–295.

Schou, S., Holmstrup, P., Reibel, J. *et al.* (1993a) Ligature-induced marginal inflammation around osseointegrated implants and ankylosed teeth: Stereologic and histologic observations in cynomolgus monkeys (Macaca fascicularis). *J. Periodontol.*, **64**, 529–537.

Schou, S., Holmstrup, P., Stoltze, K. *et al.* (1993b) Ligature-induced marginal inflammation around osseointegrated implants and ankylosed teeth. *Clin. Oral Implants Res.*, **4**, 12–22.

Weyant, R.J. and Burt, B.A. (1993) An assessment of survival rates and within-patient clustering of failures for endosseous oral implants. *J. Dent. Res.*, **72** (1), 2–8.

Chapter 62

Carcuac, O., Derks, J., Charalampakis, G. *et al.* (2016) Adjunctive systemic and local antimicrobial therapy in the surgical treatment of peri-implantitis: A randomized controlled clinical trial. *J. Dent. Res.*, **95** (1), 50–57.

Esposito, M., Grusovin, M.G., Tzanetea, E. *et al.* (2010) Interventions for replacing missing teeth: Treatment of perimplantitis. *Cochrane Database Syst. Rev.*, **6**, CD004970.

Heitz-Mayfield, L.J. and Mombelli, A. (2014) The therapy of peri-implantitis: A systematic review. *Int. J. Oral Maxillofac. Implants*, **29** (Suppl.), 325–345.

Kotsakis, G.A., Konstantinidis, I., Karoussis, I.K. *et al.* (2014) Systematic review and meta-analysis of the effect of various laser wavelengths in the treatment of peri-implantitis. *J. Periodontol.*, **85** (9), 1203–1213.

Listl, S., Fruhauf, N., Dannewitz, B. *et al.* (2015) Cost-effectiveness of non-surgical peri-implantitis treatments. *J. Clin. Periodontol.*, **42** (5), 470–477.

Louropoulou, A., Slot, D.E. and Van der Weijden, F. (2014) The effects of mechanical instruments on contaminated titanium dental implant surfaces: A systematic review. *Clin. Oral Implants Res.*, **25** (10), 1149–1160.

Renvert, S., Polyzois, I. and Maguire, R. (2009) Re-osseointegration on previously contaminated surfaces: A systematic review. *Clin. Oral Implants Res.*, **20** (Suppl. 4), 216–227.

Salvi, G.E. and Ramseier, C.A. (2015) Efficacy of patient-administered mechanical and/or chemical plaque control protocols in the management of peri-implant mucositis: A systematic review. *J. Clin. Periodontol.*, **42** (Suppl. 16), S187–S201.

Further reading

Ellegaard, B., Baelum, V. and Karring, T. (1997) Implant therapy in periodontally compromised patients. *Clin. Oral Implants Res.*, **8** (3), 180–188.

Heitz-Mayfield, L.J., Schmid, B., Weigel, C. *et al.* (2004) Does excessive occlusal load affect osseointegration? An experimental study in the dog. *Clin. Oral Implants Res.*, **15** (3), 259–268.

Isidor, F. (1996) Loss of osseointegration caused by occlusal load of oral implants: A clinical and radiographic study in monkeys. *Clin. Oral Implants Res.*, **7** (2), 143–152.

Isidor, F. (1997) Histological evaluation of peri-implant bone at implants subjected to occlusal overload or plaque accumulation. *Clin. Oral Implants Res.*, **8** (1), 1–9.

Mombelli, A. (1999) Prevention and therapy of peri-implant infections, in *Proceedings of the 3rd European Workshop on Periodontology* (eds N.P. Lang, T. Karring and J. Lindhe), Quintessence, Berlin, pp. 281–303.

Roos-Jansåker, A.M., Lindahl, C., Renvert, H. and Renvert, S. (2006) Nine- to fourteen-year follow-up of implant treatment. Part II: Presence of peri-implant lesions. *J. Clin. Periodontol.*, **33** (4), 290–295.

Weyant, R.J. and Burt, B.A. (1993) An assessment of survival rates and within-patient clustering of failures for endosseous oral implants. *J. Dent. Res.*, **72** (1), 2–8.

Chapter 63

Albertini, M., López-Cerero, L., O'Sullivan, M.G. *et al.* (2015) Assessment of periodontal and opportunistic flora in patients with peri-implantitis. *Clin. Oral Implants Res.*, **26** (8), 937–941.

Esposito, M., Grusovin, M.G., Tzanetea, E. *et al.* (2010) Interventions for replacing missing teeth: Treatment of perimplantitis. *Cochrane Database Syst. Rev.*, **6**, CD004970.

Heitz-Mayfield, L.J. and Lang, N.P. (2010) Comparative biology of chronic and aggressive periodontitis vs. peri-implantitis. *Periodontol. 2000*, **53**, 167–181.

Jepsen, S., Berglundh, T., Genco, R. *et al.* (2015) Primary prevention of periimplantitis: Managing peri-implant mucositis. *J. Clin. Periodontol.*, **42** (Suppl. 16), S152–S157.

Monje, A., Aranda, L., Diaz, K.T. *et al.* (2016) Impact of maintenance therapy for the prevention of peri-implant diseases: A systematic review and meta-analysis, *J. Dent. Res.*, **95** (4), 372–379.

Pontoriero, R., Tonelli, M.P., Carnevale, G. *et al.* (1994) Experimentally induced peri-implant mucositis: A clinical study in humans. *Clin. Oral Implants Res.*, **5** (4), 254–259.

Salvi, G.E. and Ramseier, C.A. (2015) Efficacy of patient-administered mechanical and/or chemical plaque control protocols in the management of peri-implant mucositis: A systematic review. *J. Clin. Periodontol.*, **42** (Suppl. 16), S187–S201.

Salvi, G.E. and Zitzmann, N.U. (2014) The effects of anti-infective preventive measures on the occurrence of biologic implant complications and implant loss: A systematic review. *Int. J. Oral Maxillofac. Implants*, **29** (Suppl.), 292–307.

Schou, S., Holmstrup, P., Reibel, J. *et al.* (1993) Ligature-induced marginal inflammation around osseointegrated implants and ankylosed teeth: Stereologic and histologic observations in cynomolgus monkeys (Macaca fascicularis). *J. Periodontol.*, **64** (6), 529–537.

Serino, G., Turri, A. and Lang, N.P. (2015) Maintenance therapy in patients following the surgical treatment of peri-implantitis: A 5-year follow-up study. *Clin. Oral Implants Res.*, **26** (8), 950–956.

Further reading

Grusovin, M.G., Coulthard, P., Worthington, H.V. *et al.* (2010) Interventions for replacing missing teeth: Maintaining and recovering soft tissue health around dental implants. *Cochrane Database Syst. Rev.*, **8**, CD003069.

Index

Note: page numbers in *italics* refer to figures; those in **bold** to tables or boxes

Implant Dentistry at a Glance, Second Edition. Jacques Malet, Francis Mora and Philippe Bouchard.
© 2018 John Wiley & Sons Ltd. Published 2018 by John Wiley & Sons Ltd.
Companion website: www.wiley.com/go/malet/implant